Psychosocial Stress and Cancer

Psychosocial Stress and Cancer

Edited by

Cary L. Cooper

University of Manchester
Institute of Science and Technology

JOHN WILEY & SONS

Chichester · New York · Brisbane · Toronto · Singapore

Library of Congress Cataloging in Publication Data:
Main entry under title:

Psychosocial stress and cancer.

Includes index.
1. Cancer—Psychosomatic aspects. 2. Stress (Psychology)
3. Cancer—Psychological aspects. 4. Cancer—Social aspects.
I. Cooper, Cary L. [DNLM: 1. Stress, Psychological—Complications.
2. Neoplasms—Etiology. QZ 202 P974]
RC262.P79 1984 616.99′408 84–5264

ISBN 0–471–90477–5

British Library Cataloguing in Publication Data:

Cooper, Cary L.
Psychosocial stress and cancer.
1. Cancer 2. Stress (Physiology)
3. Stress (Psychology)
I. Title
616.99′4071 RC262

ISBN 0–471–90477–5

Phototypeset by Input Typesetting Ltd, London.
Printed in Great Britain by
St Edmundsbury Press, Bury St Edmunds, Suffolk

Acknowledgements

To my wife and colleague Rachel, for all the help, support and encouragement.

To my baby daughter, Laura for her social support!

To my secretary, Lesley, who laboured long on the manuscript.

To the Leverhulme Trust for their support for our research in this field.

Contributors

Professor Hymie Anisman
Professor of Psychology, CarletonUniversity, Ottawa, Canada.

Dr Linas A. Bieliauskas
Associate Professor, Department of Psychology and Social Sciences, Rush-Presbyterian-St Luke's Medical Center, Chicago, USA.

Professor Cary L. Cooper
(*Editor*)
Professor of Organisational Psychology, University of Manchester Institute of Science and Technology, Manchester, UK.

Dr T. Cox
Senior Lecturer, Department of Psychology, University of Nottingham, Nottingham, UK.

Professor H. J. Eysenck
Department of Psychology, Institute of Psychiatry, Maudsley Hospital, London, UK.

Professor Frances Lomas Feldman
School of Social Work, University of Southern California, Los Angeles, USA.

Professor C. Allen Haney
Department of Sociology, University of Houston, Texas, USA.

Dr Bruce W. Heller
Associate Professor of Psychiatry, Langley Porter Institute, University of California, San Francisco, USA.

Dr Jill Irwin
Associate Professor, Carelton University, Ottawa, Canada.

Professor E. S. Paykel
Professor of Psychiatry, St George's Hospital Medical School, London, UK.

Mrs B. Rao
Research Assistant, Department of Psychiatry, St George's Hospital Medical School, London, UK.

Dr Paul J. Rosch
President, The American Institute of Stress, New York, USA.

Dr Lydia Temoshok
Associate Professor of Psychiatry, Langley Porter Institute, University of California, San Francisco, USA.

Contents

SECTION FOUR MANAGING PSYCHOSOCIAL FACTORS IN CANCER PATIENTS

SECTION FIVE METHODOLOGICAL OVERVIEW OF STUDIES IN PSYCHOSOCIAL STRESS AND CANCER

Introduction

While a great deal of research has been undertaken linking stress with heart disease (Cooper, 1983), particularly emphasising the importance of psychosocial factors, similar research work in the field of cancer is only just beginning. As in various fields in the medical sciences, the first research work linking stress and cancer took place in the laboratory, in animal research (Bammer and Newberry, 1981). Sophisticated controlled research in animals has indicated some link between stress and the formation and development of carcinoma.

More recent research on humans indicates that various life events, personality predispositions, immunological and central nervous system interactions etc, may trigger the cancer process, or at the very least, accelerate its development.

It is the purpose of this volume to highlight some of the important issues, concepts, research and, in some cases, methodological approaches in the fields linking psychosocial stress and cancer. The volume will be broken down into a number of different sections. In the first section we will start with a historical piece, emphasising the theoretical and empirical background of research in this field. This will provide us with the foundation stones for extending the development of theory and research linking psychosocial stress and cancer. In addition, another chapter in this section will briefly review some of the recent research orientations in terms of the psychosocial precursors to cancer. This piece will not attempt to raise any detailed methodological or conceptual issues, but will merely clarify two fields of interest for researchers.

In the second section, more in-depth analyses are carried out on several potential social-psychological precursors to cancer. Professor Eysenck, for example, attempts to explore the relationship between stress-prone personality types and lung cancer. One of the most important fertile areas of cancer research must lie in the area of personality predispositions and psychometrics. By focusing in on one specific form of cancer (i.e. lung cancer), Professor Eysenck attempts to look at the mediation of the personality – cancer relationship. Another chapter in this section will explore the relationship between psychological depression and cancer. An effort will be made to solidify the available research in this area into an integrated conceptual framework. This will help to highlight some of the suggestive evidence of the triadic link between depression, stress and cancer.

In addition, one of the most lucrative areas of research focus over the last 20 years has been on the stress of life events and cancer. This has been such an important area of attention, but the research methodologies have been too broad and varied. Professor Paykel attempts to assess the various ways in which life events can be systematically measured, raising issues which are fundamental to future research in what appears to be one of the most fruitful arenas for investigation.

In the third section we are concerned about the way in which the psychosocial factors may influence the aetiology and development of cancer. It is important to establish the link between social-psychological stimuli and the possible bodily mechanisms (e.g. the immune system), which may causally influence the formation and/or development of the carcinoma. In this section we provide a review of this process by one European research worker and by an North American team. They both provide illuminating information on the psycho-physiological process involved in cancer pathology. If future research into the link between psychosocial stress and cancer is to develop adequately, our understanding of the mechanisms underlying the causal chain of events is central if there is to be credibility in preventative work in the future.

The fourth section of the volume looks at the way in which the psychosocial factors may be managed in terms of patients with cancer. If there is a link between the social-psychological environmental factors and some forms of cancer, then it follows that if someone is suffering from a carcinoma, that the development of such a disease process could be positively altered by the management of psychosocial factors. It is certainly the case that many treatment methods for cancer patients are working on the premise that the right social-psychological environment may inhibit the disease process and/or provide the best opportunity for effective therapy. The chapters in this section will highlight some of these issues.

And finally, we conclude the volume by a comparative summary of the various methodological approaches utilized in studies exploring the field of psychosocial oncology. This highlights not only the medical outcomes, but the way in which the research design, instruments and methodology were approached. This should provide us with the 'methodological crevasses' that other researchers failed to avoid in their efforts to climb this newly discovered and difficult mountain of research.

REFERENCES

Bammer, K. and Newberry, B. H. (1981). *Stress and Cancer*. Toronto: C. J. Hogrefe Inc.

Cooper, C. L. (1983). *Stress Research: Issues for the Eighties*. New York and Chichester: John Wiley & Sons.

Section One
Overview: A Review of Historical and Research Orientations

Psychosocial Stress and Cancer
Edited by C. L. Cooper

Chapter 1
Stress and Cancer

Paul J. Rosch
President, American Institute of Stress, New York, USA

The notion that cancer might in some way be related to stress or emotional factors is as old as the history of recorded medicine. Galen's treatise on tumors, *De Tumoribus*, noted that melancholy women (who presumably had too much black bile (Gr. melas chole) were much more susceptible to cancer than other females. It is interesting that the earliest English definition of cancer appearing in 1601 was: 'Cancer is a swelling or sore coming of *melancholy* bloud, about which the veins appeare of a blacke or swert colour spread in the manner of a creifish [crayfish] claws.'

It is difficult to find much written about cancer in the medical literature until 1701, at which time the English physician, Gendron, emphasized the effect of 'disasters of life as occasion much trouble and grief' in the causation of cancer. Eighty years later, Burrows attributed the disease to 'the uneasy passions of the mind with which the patient is strongly affected for a long time.' Other authors such as Nunn in 1822, emphasized that emotional factors influenced the growth of tumors of the breast, and Stern noted that cancer of the cervix in women was more common in sensitive and frustrated individuals.

In the mid 1800s, Walshe's *The Nature and Treatment of Cancer* called attention to the 'influence of mental misery, sudden reverses of fortune and habitual gloomings of the temper on the disposition of carcinomatous matter. If systematic writers can credited, these constitute the most powerful cause of the disease.' Toward the end of the century, another English physician, Snow, reviewed more than 250 patients at the London Cancer Hospital and concluded that 'the loss of a near relative was an important factor in the development of cancer of the breast and uterus.'

Such concepts were replaced, however, in the 20th century with emphasis being directed to external agencies. Currently, a host of carcinogens in the air we breathe or the foods we ingest have been incriminated. Others search for a viral cause, but there is always the implication of attack from without. This is consistent with our view of illness in general and the germ theory of disease.

The discovery of the microscope and micro-organisms by Leeuwenhoek, Pasteur's subsequent identification of microbes and the convincing conclusions of Koch's Postulates confirmed direct causal relationships between bacteria and disease. The subsequent success of vaccines and the dramatic life-saving response to antibiotics seemed to settle any doubts. People became sick because something attacked them from outside. Little attention was directed to determinants of resistance or susceptibility to disease. Few questioned why certain individuals exposed to the same tubercle bacillus, hepatitis virus, or carcinogen, remained healthy.

The discovery of vitamins, other essential nutrients and enzymes and their relationship to a host of deficiency diseases again seemed to demonstrate the validity of the concept that illness was most likely due to either the presence or absence of some *external* factor.

Our contemporary approach has also been shaped largely by the important influence of the 17th century French philosopher, René Descartes, whose concepts dominated medical thought well into the present century. Descartes viewed the human body as a machine. Illness occurred when some part of this machine broke down. In order to repair the malfunction, it would be necessary to learn more and more about the function of even the smallest working parts, and this was the province of medicine. In this reductionist mechanistic hypothesis, the *mind* (or *spirit*) was viewed as a distinctly separate and unrelated entity. Problems in such areas were considered to be far beyond man's comprehension and relegated solely to the province of the Church. Thus for Descartes, there could be no mind/body relationship or interaction. Galileo had proven that scientific methods were capable of providing mechanical interpretations of the physical universe, and Descartes extended this type of logic to living things.

This Cartesian dissociation of mind and body actually represented a radical departure from the classical roots of medicine which preached the totality of the human condition and the inseparability of mind and body. Plato in one of his dialogues noted: 'Hippocrates, the Asclepiad, says that "The nature of the body can only be understood as a *whole*, for this is the great error of our day in the treatment of the human body, that physicians separate the soul from the body".' Subsequently, Virgil defined good health as: *mens sana in corpore sano* (a sound mind in a sound body).

Such insightful observations of classical philosophers, as well as the comments of 18th and 19th century physicians previously noted, should be evaluated in terms of the abilities and opportunities of such individuals to view the patient as a person. Practitioners had the time to take and evaluate a detailed history, which perhaps emphasized the emotional setting and life style of the patient, as well as a host of other personal factors often unavailable or overlooked by today's preoccupied physicians whose diagnoses more often depend on sophisticated laboratory studies. Furthermore, the background and training for medicine was much more heavily weighted in the humanities, literature, and philosophy. Such physicians quite likely *knew* the patient *better* and *longer*, knew the *family*, the nature and significance of environmental and personal background events, and more importantly, had more time to spend with the patient. Thus by virtue of education, orientation and a more personalized approach, earlier physicians might well have had a greater sensitivity and awareness to possible subtle relationships between stress and malignancy than is now possible in the frenetic pace of today's super-specialized oncology practice.

Lest this be misinterpreted as a denigration of the modern physician, it should be noted that not all members of the profession were insensititve to possible relationships between stress and cancer. Evans, a Jungian psychoanalyst in the 1920s, pointed out that many cancer patients had lost a close personal emotional relation before the onset of illness (Evans, 1926), and over the last three decades there has been a steady increase in interest in this subject. David Kissen, the distinguished British chest surgeon at Brompton Hospital, utilizing psychological tests, called attention to the fact that there were certain predominant personality profiles in patients with cancer of the lung. He characterized such traits as being associated with an inability to express true emotions or to get things off their chests (Kissen, 1966). Schmale and Iker at the University of Rochester were able to predict the diagnosis of cancer of the cervix with considerable accuracy in women who were entirely asymptomatic but who had suspicious Pap smears, merely by evaluating a simple personality questionnaire. They concluded that this disorder occurred most often in individuals with a 'helpless-prone personality' or with a sense of hopeless frustration due to some irresolvable conflict during the preceding 6 months (Schmale and Iker, 1971).

In studies of life histories of sets of twins, Greene, a hematologist also at the University of Rochester, found that the twin out of each set, who contracted and died of leukemia, had experienced a psychological upheaval in contradistinction to the healthy twin who had not undergone any emotional trauma (Greene and Swisher, 1969). In another 15 year study of patients with lymphoma or leukemia, Greene found that those diseases were most apt to occur in a setting of emotional loss or separation which engendered deep feelings of anxiety, anger, sadness, or hopelessness (Greene, 1962).

Lawrence LeShan, a New York psychoanalyst, has been preoccupied with this subject for the past 25 years. Utilizing Rorschach techniques, a variety of questionnaires, and detailed personal interviews with patients as well as close relatives, he concluded that the most important factors in the development of malignancy were: a loss of *raison d'être* (hopelessness/helplessness), an inability on the part of the individual to express anger or resentment, a marked amount of self-dislike and distrust, and most *significantly*, *loss* of an important emotional relationship (LeShan, 1977).

About 35 years ago, Caroline Thomas at Johns Hopkins Hospital began a psychosocial study of medical students (Thomas, 1977; Thomas and Duszynski, 1974), since they could be closely observed during their 4 years of medical training, and as physicians, could be relied upon to cooperate in subsequent follow-up studies. She was initially concerned with determining possible factors that might have predictive value for hypertension and coronary heart disease, and she accumulated detailed data dealing with demographic, familial and genetic factors, as well as physiologic, psychologic and metabolic characteristics. As the study progressed, the statistics suggested that in addition to hypertension there were also possible predictable precursors for mental illness, emotional disturbance, suicide and cancer. Thomas' data suggest that cancer tends to occur in individuals who are low-key, *non-aggressive*, and unable to adequately express their emotions. Many of the individuals tended to be rather lonely persons without any close parental affiliation, or who had figuratively 'lost their parent.'

One might suspect that writers or poets might be expected, by virtue of keen powers of observation, to appreciate such relationships, and indeed, Tolstoy's *The Death of Ivan Iliyich* bears such a theme. It was reitcrated by the American poet W. H. Auden in 'Miss Gee':*

Doctor Thomas sat over his dinner
  Though his wife was waiting to ring,
Rolling his bread into pellets,
  Said, 'Cancer's a funny thing.

Nobody knows what the cause is,
  Though some pretend they do;
It's like some hidden assassin
  Waiting to strike at you.

Childless women get it,
  And men when they retire;
It's as if there had to be some outlet
  For their foiled creative fire.'

Emotional loss and frustration of ambitions due to political defeat were viewed by several commentators as playing an important role in the cancers of Napoleon, Ulysses S. Grant, Robert Taft and Hubert Humphrey.

Apart from its possible causative role in the development of cancer, stress has also been implicated in determining the rate of spread and the ultimate course of an established malignancy. All physicians have had the experience of seeing a malignant tumor spread like wildfire despite all therapeutic efforts, whereas in another patient of the same age and sex, an apparently identical malignancy behaves in a rather indolent fashion, with or without treatment. Some authors have alleged that the rate of tumor growth can be predicted based upon certain personality traits similar to those described above. One frequently quoted study, done about 30 years ago by Blumberg *et al.* (1954) examined two groups of cancer patients, all of whom knew their diagnosis and were matched for age, intelligence, and the state of their cancers. The patients were studied following their initial treatment when they were, relatively speaking, 'feeling well.' Those patients dying in less than 2 years were compared with those living for more than 6 years and were found to have significantly poorer outlets for emotional discharge.

Almost 20 years ago, Stavraky conducted a similar study on 204 cancer patients (Stavraky *et al.*, 1969) and concluded that the group with the most favorable outlook were those who were able to show strong feelings under severe stress without loss of emotional control. Again, we encounter the feeling that 'giving up' or loss of '*raison d'être*' may be an important factor in whether the patient survives and in determing the course of the disease.

Nicholas Rogentine, an immunologist at the National Cancer Institute, reported on a group of patients who had apparently been operated on successfully for malignant melanoma, a particularly lethal form of skin cancer (Rogentine *et al.*, 1977). He found that relapse did not occur among patients who maximized the significance of their illness, again supporting the theory that repression and denial are related to a more discouraging prognosis. A Johns Hopkins study of terminal breast cancer patients showed that feisty, combative females survived longer than trusting, complacent individuals (Derogatis *et al.*, 1979). Similar findings were reported by a study at King's College (London) of 160 asymptomatic women, admitted for breast tumor biopsy, who underwent a series of interviews, psychological tests, medical and psychiatric histories. A significant correlation was established between cancer diagnosis and extreme anger suppression, especially in females under 50 years of age (Greer and Morris, 1975). Interestingly enough, this anger suppression also correlated with altered immunoglobulin IgA levels and degree of metastasis 1 year after surgery (Pettingale *et al.*, 1977).

Such findings reinforce the efforts of Le Shan (1977), Simonton *et al.*, 1978), Achterberg and Lawlis (1978) and others in encouraging patients to take an active participatory role and positive, aggressive stance in the management of their malignancy.

Considerable research on the effects of stress on cancer growth in laboratory animals also provide corroborative data. Workers in the school of the great Russian psychologist and physiologist, Pavlov, reported that dogs subjected to severe and chronic stress had a marked increase in malignancy of internal organs. Vernon Riley at the Pacific Northwest Research Foundation in Seattle selected a strain of mice that was highly cancer-prone. Under usual laboratory conditions, 60% of the animals developed tumors within 8–18 months after birth. When the research team placed the mice behind a protective barrier insulating them from the stress of normal laboratory commotion and noise, only 7% of the mice developed cancer during a 14-month period (Riley and Spackman, 1976). Conversely, another experiment showed that by merely slowly rotating the animals on a turntable one could significantly increase the incidence of cancer rates (Riley, 1981). Research at Stanford University School of Medicine explored the effects of stress on viral-induced mammary tumors in mice. Tumor growth was significantly increased by stressing the animals with electric shock immediately following the virus inoculation. They also noted that female mice which spontaneously displayed a fighting or antagonistic behavior tended to have smaller tumors (Solomon, 1969). This same phenomenon has been observed in human breast cancer patients, where females who were 'bitchy' or antagonistic seemed to enjoy a better prognosis (Greer *et al.*, 1979)

Thus both by anecdotal report, as well as clinical and laboratory research, there is considerable evidence that stress can significantly influence susceptibility and resistance to cancer, as well as the course of the disease. How could such effects be mediated?

A wide range of external substances and factors have been implicated as the cause of various cancers due to carcinogenic activities of a physical or chemical nature (solar or x-irradiation, asbestos, coal tar, excessive local heat, etc.). The two most important internal mechanisms which have been demonstrated to influence malignant growth are hormonal factors and the immunologic competency of the individual. It is most important to recognize that the central nervous system plays a dominant role in the control of these important determinants of malignant activity. The role of stress is emphasized by noting that both endocrine and immune function are so sensitive to its influence that they are used to measure or characterize its effects in humans.

It has been suggested that malignant cells intermittently develop in various tissues and organs. In susceptible individuals, such cells are able to gain a foothold and multiply into clinically detectable malignant lesions, while in others, an efficient immune system is able to recognize and destroy such abnormal cells. When exposed to some foreign agent such as a pathogenic bacteria or virus, we respond by producing very specific antibodies, as well as more non-specific substances such as interferons or properdin to combat or increase resistance to the offending agent. This property is exploited in a variety of immunization techniques in which a susceptible patient is exposed to an attenuated form of the virus which stimulates a variety of immune defenses to thwart subsequent infection by the same or similar agents.

Conversely, decreased immune defenses are associated with increased susceptibility to, and rapid spread of, infections. The herpes simplex virus appears to be constantly present in the cell but is usually quiescent. When resistance is lowered, its clinical expression is manifested by sores and lesions in various mucous membranes and oral and genital regions of the body. In the mouth, such lesions are commonly referred to as 'cold sores' or 'fever blisters,' acknowledging that they occur during periods of increased stress and lowered resistance. It is also of interest to note that the clinical appearance of two closely related viruses are linked with cancer. Patients with herpes zoster infection (commonly known as shingles) are thought to exhibit diminished immunologic defenses and reportedly have a higher incidence of cancer. Herpes simplex II virus, which is responsible for recurrent genital lesions, is said to predispose to cervical cancer. The virus or agency that presumably causes AIDS has not been identified as yet but theoretically might represent another dramatic example. Primary immunodeficiency diseases confer a risk of malignancy 100 times greater than that seen in the general population (Filipovich, 1983).

Similarly, adrenal-cortical hormones interfere with the body's immune system or ability to make antibodies. This property is used clinically to prevent rejection of organ transplants or grafts that the body perceives as foreign. When cortisone was first made available, it was noted that many patients, being treated for chronic disorders such as rheumatoid arthritis, suffered a reactivation of previously quiescent tuberculosis, presumably due to inhibition of a previously effective defense mechanism. The effect of cortisone and other similar adrenal-cortical-type hormones are now clinically recognized as causing a rapid spread of other bacterial or viral infections and consequently are contraindicated in infection. In kidney transplant patients, where cortisone, and other immunosuppressive agents are routinely used to prevent rejection and there may be an eventual 20–30% incidence of malignancy in the recipient.

We know very little about the composition and range of activity of the immune system. What is more confusing is that all the agencies utilized to treat cancer, including radiation, immunosuppressors and certain steroid hormones, have also been demonstrated to cause cancer. Selye's research clearly demonstrated that stimulation of the adrenal cortex was the hallmark of the organism's response to acute stress. As part of this 'alarm reaction' there was also a marked involution of lymphatic tissue and of the thymus, major producers of immune system components. Thus, because of strong effects on both endocrine and immune factor, stress would appear to have profound potential properties on susceptibility to malignancy as well as its clinical course.

Recent research on leukocyte production of ACTH and interferon production following experimental viral infection suggests that immune and endocrine responses to stress are controlled by separate mechanisms (Smith *et al.*, 1983). Psychologists Klaus and Marjorie Bahnson of the Eastern Pennsylvania Psychological Institute found a strong correlation between depression and decreased immunologic capacity but not adrenal function (Bahnson and Bahnson, 1966). Bartrop in Australia showed that loss of a spouse was followed by a marked reduction in immune system function 2 to 6 weeks after the event (Bartrop *et al*, 1977). This response also occurred without evidence of any significant change in adrenal hormonal activity, further suggesting a direct communication between the brain and the immune system. These findings have now been confirmed and expanded at Mount Sinai Hospital in New York by Schleifer and Stein who also measured T-cell mitogenic activity in the husbands of patients with terminal breast cancer (Schleifer *et al.*, 1983).

Research findings on University of Ohio medical students (Kiecolt-Glaser *et al.*, 1983a) reveal that social stress as measured by the Holmes-Rahe and UCLA Loneliness Scales had strong effects on other parameters of immune system function such as natural 'killer cell' activity. The high-stress high-loneliness group had the lowest natural killer cell activity with the reverse being true for the low stress, low-loneliness cohort. Similarly, hospitalized psychiatric patients, who scored highest on such scales, had lowest levels of natural killer cell activity as well as poor lymphocyte responses to mitogenic stimuli (Kiecolt-Glaser *et al.*, 1983b). Killer cells are known to play a vital role in preventing the development and spread of malignant tumors. Other studies by Borysenko's group at Beth Israel in Boston of dental students showed a high correlation between academic stress and poorer motivation and a decreased rate of salivary secretion of immunoglobulin A (Jemmott *et al.*, 1983). Interferons, one of the basic defenses against viral infections, are now also being intensively investigated in the treatment of cancer, and are suppressed under conditions of emotional stress.

T-cell lymphocytes have receptor sites for ACTH, metenkephalin, endorphins, and other small brain peptides, again strongly suggesting direct central nervous system communication with these mediators of immune activity. Recent advances in the rapidly expanding new discipline of psychoneuroimmunology appear to confirm this hypothesis. One recent report studied the effect of adding endorphins to the blood of healthy volunteers *in vitro*. Mixing the treated blood with tumor cells resulted in a 14%–32% increase in natural killer lymphocyte activity when compared with a mixture of normal untreated blood and malignant cells. The investigators postulate that beta-endorphin receptors on lymphocytes may be the mechanism whereby anger and aggressiveness combat cancer and compensate for steroid-induced suppression of the immune system (Kay and Morley, 1983).

Thus it seems clear that stress can cause disturbances in many areas of immune system competency, and that impaired immune system function predisposes to malignant growth. But this is merely *evidence*, and evidence is not *proof*. It is difficult to *prove* that stress causes cancer, simply because it is impossible to satisfactorily define or quantify stress, and equally difficult to identify the precise time of origin of malignancy. Nevertheless, the implications are intriguing and are of more than theoretical interest. All the great integrative and adaptive resources that the body has at its disposal operate on a system of opposing checks and balances (Selye and Rosch, 1954a,b). The autonomic nervous system has antagonistic sympathetic and parasympathetic activity. Endocrine function, to a large extent, is governed by self-regulating feedback systems between target glands and peripheral metabolites or pituitary activity. Therefore, one might suspect that if noxious influences depress immune system function, there are likely to be opposing forces which produce opposite effects. This hypothesis is a basic precept that has been emphasized throughout the development of the stress concept.

During the latter half of the 19th century, the great French physiologist Claude Bernard first promulgated the theory that one of the most characteristic features of living organisms is their ability to maintain the constancy of what he termed the internal environment (*milieu interieur*). Thus, despite dramatic changes in the environment, such as sub-zero arctic temperatures or the excessive heat of the tropics, body temperature remains constant. This is achieved by a series of adaptive responses, such as vasoconstriction and shivering to generate heat, or vasodilatation and sweating to provide cooling. Similarly, the blood level of glucose or sodium tends to remain constant despite variations in intake because of appropriate changes in hormonal responses or excretory patterns. The health of the organism therefore depends upon effective communication between its internal components as well as communications with the external environment. Good health or resistance to stress depends upon the integration, coordination, and communication between complex sophisticated mechanisms designed to maintain the integrity and constancy of this internal environment.

In the early part of this century, these theories were expanded by the Harvard physiologist, Walter Cannon, who coined the term 'homeostasis' or the steady state to describe this phenomenon essential to life and good health. Cannon studied the changes which occurred when this status quo was severely threatened by the stress of acute fear. His research suggested that under such circumstances, there was a powerful stimulation of the sympathetic nervous system and release of adrenalin which called into play a host of physiological and biochemical reactions which would have survival value. There was a release of glycogen stores in the liver to provide an elevation of blood sugar for increased energy, the pupils dilated to permit better visual acuity, the blood clotted more quickly to minimize loss from internal hemorrhage or wounds, the blood pressure rose and there was increased circulation to the brain to improve decision making. Blood was shunted away from the gut, where it was not immediately needed for digestive processes, to the large muscles of the arms and legs to prepare primitive man for life-saving 'fight or flight' (Cannon, 1914).

Bernard and Cannon provided the theoretical and experimental substructure for the brilliant and revolutionary research of Hans Selye whose studies of the effects of stress in laboratory animals were elucidated in his general adaptation syndrome (Selye, 1946). Improved laboratory techniques allowed Selye to study the premier role of the pituitary – adrenal cortical axis in the response to acute stress. After thousands of experiments, he concluded that despite variable or even opposite stressors, such as extreme heat or cold, psychological frustration, loud noise or blinding light, or exhausting physical exercise, the organism's response was identical. The changes observed appeared to be a consequence of marked stimulation of the pituitary – adrenal cortex axis resulting in the production of large amounts of glucocorticoids. These cortisone-like hormones similarly offered immediate protective benefits by reducing inflammation and edema, and sustained elevation of blood sugar by gluconeogenesis due to the catabolic effects on protein stores, but the effect could not be sustained.

Following this acute response, which Selye termed 'the alarm reaction,' certain stereotyped changes could be observed macroscopically and microscopically. They included enlargement and hypertrophy of the adrenal cortex (particularly the zona glomerulosa), involution or dissolution of the thymus and lymphatic tissues, and gastric ulcerations. If the stressor persisted, the animal entered a second 'stage of resistance', during which adaptive responses were maximized, and finally, persistent stress led to a 'stage of exhaustion' and death. Selye termed this tripartite response, 'the general adaptation syndrome,' and viewed it as a 'non-specific' response to any stressor. Autopsy studies during various phases of the 'general adaptation syndrome' revealed pathologic changes indistinguishable from findings in patients with rheumatoid arthritis, peptic ulcer, hypertension, and myocardial necrosis, and he reasoned that such disorders in humans might also be likely to be due to stress, labelling them 'diseases of adaptation.'

Implicit in the theories of Cannon and Selye, and most important for this presentation, is the teleological premise that biological responses to stress must have had some purposeful design in primitive times or in lower forms of life. However, in higher stages of evolution and as responses to chronic psychological rather than acute physical stressors, they were now inappropriate and quite probably harmful if not fatal. It is equally apparent that nature often hyperreacts to a stimulus or need with responses that are exaggerated. We see this in the occasional development of disfiguring keloids in scar formation, or the local response to excessive heat in clay pipe smokers where malignancy occurs at the site of injured tissue attempting to repair itself.

A similar phenomenon occurs in evolution. In discussing this subject over

25 years ago, I described the theory of 'opportunism' in the adaptational process, in which the organism responds or fulfills a need with whatever means are available, even if such a response may ultimately prove harmful (Rosch, 1958). The example I utilized in that earlier work was the tremendous variation in the development of horns by some 23 species of African antelope. The marked differences in anatomical configuration and functional effect did not seem to serve any rational purpose, and in some instances were disadvantageous and prohibitively unwieldy. In rewriting that article today, I should choose the development of malignancy in man as a better example.

As one descends the phylogenetic scale and examines lower forms of life, it becomes apparent that the incidence of cancer decreases progressively. Conversely, the ability of the organism to regenerate tissues, organs, or even parts of the body increases proportionately. Among simpler organisms, certain types of invertebrates have the ability to sever parts of their anatomy when irritated. Obviously, this capacity has survival value only if the animal possesses an equally remarkable ability to regenerate the cast-off portion from the available cell remnants. The starfish can grow a new appendage; the salamander can regenerate its tail. Humans, however, do not have such regenerative powers.

I would suggest that the human cancer chromosome – or whatever typology one might care to apply (genome, DNA molecule) – is the modern vestige or replica of this regenerative trait, once so essential to the organism's survival and adaptation, but which now may become life-threatening. Thus, although the primitive cellular response to loss, injury, or irritation is purposeful new growth or regeneration, this capability is not preserved in the higher animals, and in man, surfaces as new growth or neoplasia with far more sinister consequences. Experiments involving the injections of chemicals, known to cause cancer in laboratory animals and humans, into the limb or eye of the newt support such a hypothesis. When a carcinogen is injected into its limb, the newt promptly grows an accessory limb; in response to injection into the lens of the eye, the newt regenerates a new lens. In brief, the same carcinogenic stimulus can produce either purposeful regeneration or fatal malignancy – depending upon the evolutionary development of the organism (Rosch, 1979).

The leap from physical to emotional loss should not be troublesome. Even the ability to regenerate lost or injured tissue must involve something more than a simple local response and include central nervous system responses to activate endocrine, immune and autonomic attempts at repair. With man's highly developed cerebral cortex, emotional loss may very well evoke similar reparative processes so essential to primitive survival.

Man is unique in that he responds not only to actual danger but also its anticipation due to complex cognitive processes or symbolic signals. Such threats, or the anticipation of noxious stimuli, may elicit responses of far greater magnitude and duration than the actual injury itself. One can think of many examples of this, such as the anxiety and apprehension of individuals waiting in the dentist's office prior to a tooth extraction, or a child anticipating a spanking. Such physiological responses when sustained may be far more damaging that the actual trauma *per se*. A sharp rise in blood pressure may serve some useful purpose in an endangered animal. However, that same response in an irritated executive, boiling over from some minor vexation, is a grossly inappropriate reaction that could result in a stroke far more dangerous than the provocative irritant itself. Emotional stress in humans may have much more profound effects than physical stress, as demonstrated by studies of racing car drivers, or comparing stress-related hormonal changes in the coxswain and crew members during competition. Such stress, especially if severe, repetitive, or prolonged, may result in primitive responses once useful to our progenitors but which now quite likely contribute to hypertension, stroke, coronary heart disease, peptic ulcer, arthritis, cancer and a host of other disorders involving immune competency (Rosch, 1980a).

It is clear that the great adaptive and integrative mechanisms at the body's disposal operate on a system of opposing checks and balances. As we have seen, the autonomic nervous system achieves homeostasis through the equilibrium provided by antagonistic sympathetic and parasympathetic influences. The endocrine system similarly is stabilized by a self-regulating cybernetic feedback mechanism in which target gland hormone levels control further pituitary stimulation. Therefore, if distress (noxious influences) can cause depression of immune competency that predisposes to cancer, is it not likely that there are opposing forces which counteract such influences or enhance immune function? Can 'good' stress (eustress) in the form of a sense of positive control, produce endocrine, immune or other responses that resist or prevent cancer growth?

Nearly a decade ago, J. I. Rodale, in a book entitled, *Happy People Rarely Get Cancer*, noted that certain types or groups of people appeared to be relatively resistant to malignancy. Various studies also indicate that nuns, Mormons, Christian Scientists and Seventh Day Adventists also have low incidences of cancer. There is other evidence that stress reducing life styles and positive emotions, all of which provide a sense of control, offer protection. In studying cases of spontaneous remission in cancer, Ikemi (1978) concluded that a powerful faith or strong positive belief system was the common denominator. Anecdotal but irrefutable reports of cancer cures from shrines, faith healing, various non-traditional approaches such as laetrile, krebiozen, acupuncture, macrobiotic diets, etc., also suggest that the benefits derived may be due to resultant emotional or psychological attitudes rather than therapies judged to be medically worthless.

For years, medicine has observed the results of the 'placebo' effect, but has yet to satisfactorily explain the cause or the means by which it is mediated. While generally acknowledged to exist, this phenomenon is poorly understood but appears to exert many of its beneficial effects by allaying anxiety. It may well be that pursuing *any* strategy in which one has faith provides an important sense of control which in some way activates potential self-healing mechanisms. While it is not possible to scientifically define stress, it is quite clear that its hallmark is being out of control. It is becoming increasingly apparent that progressive loss of control is a characteristic of civilization and cancer rates may correlate with such stressful and disruptive effects on the 'internal environment' and homeostasis.

This concept is far from novel and was actually suggested by Tanchou in his 'Memoir on the Frequency of Cancer' presented to the French Academy of Sciences in 1843 (as quoted in Le Conte, 1846):

> M. Tanchou is of the opinion that cancer, like insanity, increases in a direct ratio to the civilization of the country, and of the people. And it is certainly a remarkable circumstance, doubtless in no small degree flattering to the vanity of the French *savant*, that the average mortality rate from Cancer in Paris during 11 years is about 0.80 per 1,000 living annually, while it is only 0.20 per 1,000 in London! Estimating the intensity of civilization by these data, it clearly follows that Paris is four times more civilized than London!

The renowned medical missionary, Dr. Albert Schweitzer, echoed a similar theme when he wrote:

> On my arrival in Gabon in 1913, I was astonished to encounter no cases of cancer. . . . I cannot, of course, say positively that there was no cancer at all, but like other frontier doctors, I can only say that if any cases existed, they must have been quite rare. In the course of the years, we have seen cases of cancer in growing numbers in our region. My observations incline me to attribute this to the fact that the natives are living more and more after the manner of the whites . . . .(quoted in Stefansson, 1960).

The celebrated anthropologist and Arctic explorer, Vilhjalmur Stefansson, in his book actually entitled, *Cancer: Disease of Civilization?* (Stefansson, 1960) noted the absence of cancer in the Eskimos upon his initial arrival in the Arctic, but a subsequent increase in the incidence of the disease as closer contact with white civilization was established. He quotes Sir Robert McCarrison, a physician who surveyed 11,000 Hunza natives in Kashmir from 1904–1911, and concluded that cancer was unknown among them. In addition to their diet, the Hunzas were 'far removed from the refinements of civilization. Certain of these races are of magnificent physique, preserving until late in life the character of youth; they are unusually fertile and long-lived and endowed with nervous systems of notable stability . . . .'

Dr. Morley Roberts' *Malignancy and Evolution* (1926) contained the observation: 'I take the view commonly held that, whatever its origin, cancer is very largely a disease of civilization.' He was referring to a wide body of literature, such as Dr. Charles Powell's *The Pathology of Cancer* (1908) which stated: 'There can be little doubt that the various influences grouped under the title of civilization play a part in producing a tendency to Cancer.'

In an article in the journal *Cancer*, in July 1927, Dr. William Howard Hay wrote:

> A study of the distribution of cancer, among the races of the entire earth, shows a cancer ratio in about proportion to which civilized living predominates; so evidently something inherent in the habits of civilization is responsible for the difference of cancer incidence as compared with the uncivilized races and tribes. Climate has nothing to do with this difference, as witness the fact that tribes living naturally will show a complete absence until mixture with more civilized man corrupts the naturalness of habit, and just as these habits conform to those of civilization, even so does cancer begin to show its head . . . .

One of the most persuasive arguments is to be found in Dr. Alexander Berglas' work, *Cancer: Its Nature, Cause and Cure*, published in Paris in 1957. Throughout this book runs the theme that cancer is a disease from which primitive peoples are relatively or wholly free. Berglas declared: 'there is as yet no remedy for cancer; it is not infectious, and it is the most frequent cause of death in highly developed countries (exclusive of death due to wear and old age); . . . everyone is threatened with death from cancer because of our *inability to adapt to present day living conditions*.' It is in his Preface that one finds the most significant, prophetic and useful commentary:

> Over the years, cancer research has become the domain of specialists in various fields. Despite the outstanding contributions of the scientists, we have been getting farther away from our goal, the curing of cancer. This specialized work, and the knowledge gained through the study of individual processes, had the peculiar result of becoming an obstacle to the whole.
>
> More than thirty years in the field of cancer research have convinced me that it is not to our advantage to continue along this road of detailed analysis. I have come to the conclusion that cancer may perhaps be just another intelligible natural process whose cause is to be found in our environment and mode of life.

Cancer research has focused almost entirely on its *epidemiology*, which by definition studies the demographics of illness – where, when, and among what populations it occurs. Thus we have become preoccupied with a variety of environmental carcinogens or suspicious viruses. A more sophisticated approach was provided by the Russian scientist, Danishevsky (quoted by Paul, 1950) who divided epidemiologic climates into two categories: a 'macroclimate' which deals with quantifiable factors such as temperature, humidity, atmospheric pressure, or pollution, and a 'microclimate' which represents the sum of the intimate sociologic, spiritual, and habitational conditions that exist in any given individual. It is this 'microclimate' which now requires intensive investigation and what is required is an *endemiological* approach (Rosch, 1980b).

Such information is surfacing, as in the recent study by Jenkins (1983). The report revealed a startling increase in mortality in those areas where poverty, crowded housing, divorce and fragmented families were prevalent. We are just beginning to appreciate the important effect of such chronic, insidious, poorly quantified but lethal psychosocial stress. As in acutely stressful situations due to external factors, or the self-induced stress in the adrenalin addicted individual with Type A coronary prone behavior (Rosch, in press), *lack of control* is the characteristic common to all. That also happens to be the best definition of the cancer cell – a cell out of control.

Bernard had equated good health with good communication. But the cancer cell does not communicate, doesn't respond. Could it be that in developing a strong faith or sense of control or by utilizing visual imagery to treat cancer, we are reasserting our ability to do something about our condition, to say to our bodies, 'I'm in control of things.' Can that message somehow filter down through the body's communication network to various organs and even tissues? We have seen that the brain has direct communication links to white cells involved in the body's immune defenses to cancer. Can we not tune into that conversation or influence the vocabulary and dialogue?

Louis Pasteur, the great microbiologist and proponent of the germ theory of disease, engaged in many debates with his famous contemporary Claude Bernard. On his deathbed, he allegedly stated: '*Bernard avait raison. Le germe n'est rien, c'est le terrain qui est tout.*' ('Bernard was right. The microbe is nothing, the soil is everything.') We are all exposed daily to a host of potential carcinogens in the air we breathe or the foods we ingest. What determines resistance to malignant change is not clear, but we are becoming increasingly aware that behavioral attitudes and exaggerated or inappropriate stress-related responses must be considered in any approach to the problem of who develops cancer and what the consequences will be. In the final analysis, we are left with what every good physician knows intuitively. 'Many times it is much more more important to know what kind of patient has the disease than what kind of disease the patient has.'

REFERENCES

Achterberg, J. and Lawlis G. F. (1978) *Imagery of Cancer*, Institute for Personality and Ability Testing, Champaign, Ill.

Bahnson, C. B., and Bahnson, M. J.: (1966). Role of the ego defenses: Denial and repression in the etiology of malignant neoplasm, *Ann, N. Y. Acad. Sci.* **125**, 827–845.

Bartrop, R. W., Lazarus, L., Luckhurst, E., Kiloh, L. G., and Penny, R (1977). Depressed lymphocyte function after bereavement, *Lancet*, **i**, 834–836.

Blumberg, E. M., West, P. M., and Ellis, F. W. (1954). A possible relationship between psychological factors and human cancer, *Psychosom. Med.*, **16**, 277–286.

Cannon, W. J. (1914). The emergency function of the adrenal medulla in pain and the major emotions, *Am. J. Physiol.*, **33**,356–372.

Derogatis, L. R., Abeloff, M. D. and Melisaratos, N (1979). Psychological coping mechanisms and survival time in metastatic breast cancer, *J. A. M. A.*, **242**, 1504–1508.

Evans, E. (1926). *A Psychological Study of Cancer*, Dodd, Mead, New York.

Filipovich, A. H. (1983). Lymphoma in persons with naturally occurring immunodeficiency disorders. Paper presented at International Society for Experimental Hematology Meeting, London, 1983.

Greene, W. A. (1962). The psychosocial setting of the development of leukemia and lymphoma, *Ann. N. Y. Acad. Sci.*, **125**, 794–802.

Greene, W. A., and Swisher, S. N.: (1969). Psychological and somatic variables associated with the development and course of monozygotic twins discordant for leukemia, *Ann. N. Y. Acad. Sci.*, **164**, 394–408.

Greer, S., and Morris, T. (1975). Psychological attributes of women who develop breast cancer: A controlled study, *J. Psychosom. Res.*, **19**, 147–153.

Greer, S. Morris, T., and Pettingale, K. W. (1979). Psychological response to breast cancer: Effect on outcome, *Lancet*, **ii**, 785–787.

Ikemi, Y. (1978). Premorbid psychological factors as related to cancer incidence, *J. Behavior. Med.*, **1**, 45.

Jemmott, J. B., Borysenko, J. Z., Borysenko, M., *et al.* (1983). Academic stress, power motivation, and decrease in secretion rate of salivary secretory immunoglobulin A., *Lancet*, **ii**, 1400–1402.

Jenkins, C. D. (1983). Social environment and cancer mortality in men, *N. Engl. J. Med.* **308**, 395–398.

Kay, N. E., and Morley, J. E. (1983). Paper presented at American Federation for Clinical Research Meeting, Washington, D.C., 1983.

Kiecolt-Glaser J. N., Garner, W., Speicher, C., Penn, G. M., Holliday, B. S., and Glaser, R. (1984a). Psychosocial modifiers of immunocompetence in medical students, *Psychosom. Med.* **46**, 7–14.

Kiecolt-Glaser, J. N., Ricker, D., George, J., Messick, G., Speicher, C., Garner, W., and Glaser, R. (1984b). Urinary cortisol levels, cellular incompetence and loneliness in psychiatric patients., *Psychosom. Med.* **46**, 15–24.

Kissen, D. M. (1966). The significance of personality in lung cancer in men, *Ann. N. Y. Acad. Sci.*, **125**, 820–826.

LeConte, J. (1846) Statistical researches on cancer, *Southern Medical and Surgical Journal*, (Augusta, GA), May 1846, pp. 273–274.

Le Shan, L. L. (1977). *You Can Fight for Your Life*, M. Evans, New York.

Paul, J. R. (1950). Epidemiology, in *Research in Medical Science*, (Eds. D. E. Greer and W. E. Knox) Macmillan, New York.

Pettingale, K. W., Greer, S., and Dudley, E. H. T. (1977). Serum IgA and emotional expression in breast cancer patients, *J. Psychosom. Res.* **21**, 395–399.

Riley, V. (1981). Psychoneuroendocrine influences on immunocompetence and neoplasia, *Science*, **212**, 1100–1109.

Riley, V., and Spackman, S. (1976). Modifying effects of a benign virus on the malignant process and the role of physiological stress on tumor incidence, in *Fogarty*

International Center Proceedings, vol. 28, pp. 319–336, US Government Printing Office, Washington, D.C.
Rogentine, G. N., Docherty, J. P., van Kammen, D. P., Fox, B. H., and Bunney, W. E. (1977). Psychosocial and biological factors in the prognosis of clinical stage II melanoma. Paper presented with partial, preliminary results at the Annual Meeting, American Psychosomatic Society, Atlanta, 1977.
Rosch, P. J. (1958). Growth and development of the stress concept and its significance in clinical medicine, in *Modern Trends in Endocrinology*, pp. 278–297. Paul B. Hoeber, New York, Butterworths, London.
Rosch, P. J. (1979). Stress and cancer: A disease of adaptation? in *Stress and Cancer*, (Eds. J. Tache, H. Selye and S. B. Day), pp. 187–212, Plenum Press, New York.
Rosch, P. J. (1980a). Lifestyle and cancer, *N. Y. State Med. J.*, **80**, 2034, 2038.
Rosch, P. J. (1980b). Some thoughts on the endemiology of cancer, in *Readings in Oncology*, (Eds, S. B. Day, E. V. Sugarbaker and P. J. Rosch) pp. 1–6, The International Foundation for Biosocial Development and Human Health, New York.
Rosch, P. J. (1983). Stress addiction: Causes, consequences, and cures, *Directions in Psychiatry*, **3**, 2–7.
Schleifer, S. J., Keller, S. E., Camerino, M., Thornton, J. C., and Stein, M. (1983). Suppression of lymphocyte stimulation following bereavement, *J.A.M.A.*, **250**, 374–377.
Schmale, A. H., and Iker, H. D. (1971). Hopelessness as a predictor of cervical cancer, *Soc. Sci. Med.*, **5**, 95–100.
Selye, H. (1946). The general adaptation syndrome and the diseases of adaptation, *J. Clin. Endocrinol.*, **6**, 117–120.
Selye, H., and Rosch, P. J. (1954a). The renaissance in endocrinology, in *Medicine and Science*, pp. 30–49, International University Press, New York.
Selye, H., and Rosch, P. J. (1946). Integration of endocrinology, in *Glandular Physiology and Therapy*, pp. 1–100, J. B. Lippincott Co., Philadelphia.
Simonton, B. C., Mathews-Simonton, S. and Creighton, J (1978). *Getting Well Again*, J. P. Tacher, Los Angeles.
Solomon, G. F. (1969). Emotions, stress and central nervous system and immunity, *Ann. N. Y. Acad. Sci.*, **164**, 335–343.
Smith, E. M., *et al* (1983). Virus-induced corticosterone and hyphosectomized mice: A possible lymphoid adrenal axis, *Science*, **218**, 1311–1312.
Stavraky, K. M., Buck, O. W., Lott, S. S., and Wanklin, J. M. (1969). Psychological factors in the outcome of human cancer, *J. Psychosom Res.* **12**, 251–259.
Stefansson, V. (1960). *Cancer: Disease of Civilization*?, Hill and Wang, New York.
Thomas, C. B. (1977). *Habits of Nervous Tension: Clues to the Human Condition*, The Precursors Study, 725 N. Wolfe Street, Baltimore, MD.
Thomas, C. B., and Duszynski, K. R. (1974). Closeness to parents and the family constellation in a prospective study of five disease states: Suicide, mental illness, malignant tumor, hypertension and coronary heart disease, *Johns Hopkins Med. J.*, **134**, 251–270

Psychosocial Stress and Cancer
Edited by C. L. Cooper

Chapter 2
The Social Psychological Precursors to Cancer

Cary L. Cooper
Department of Management Sciences, University of Manchester, Institute of Science and Technology, Manchester M60 1QD, UK

Over the last couple of decades, there has been an enormous amount of attention devoted to the field of occupational/life stress and coronary heart disease (CHD) (Cooper and Marshall, 1976; Glass, 1977; Greenberg, 1980; Cooper, 1981). There have been large scale prospective national studies, such as the Western Collaborative (Rosenman *et al.*, 1967) and the Framingham Studies (Haynes *et al.*, 1980), which have enhanced our understanding of the stressors and processes of coronary heart disease. A prominent feature of this research effort is the concentration on what has been termed in the medical profession as the 'psychosocial' factors, that is, the personality and social psychological precursors to CHD. While research into coronary heart disease and stress has been growing, developing and bearing valuable information, the same cannot be said of other potentially stress-related illnesses, particularly cancer. Although psychological research work has been conducted in the field of cancer, it has not been as systematic or as concrete as in the field of cardiovascular disease. Much of this research has been published in disparate journals and tends to be retrospective in design. Nevertheless, there is a wide body of seminal knowledge available, and in order for us to make progress, it is essential to bring it together to see 'where we are' and 'where we should be going.' The purpose of this chapter is to review the existing research work on the effect of personality and other social psychological factors in the aetiology of cancer. This will also help us to highlight some of the methodological weaknesses of the current research and suggest future developments.

THE RELATIONSHIP OF PSYCHOLOGICAL FACTORS TO CANCER

It was in the late 19th century that attention was first drawn to the possible link of stress and cancer by Paget (1870) who observed that 'the cases are so frequent in which deep anxiety, defended hope and disappointment are quickly followed by the growth and increase of cancer, that we can hardly doubt that mental depression is a weighty addition to the other influences favouring the development of the cancerous constitution.' Herbert Snow (1893) in his acclaimed book *Cancer and the Cancer Process* noted that 'We are logically impelled to inquire if the great majority of cases of cancer may not own a neurotic origin?. . . . We find that a number of instances in which malignant disease of the breast and uterus follows immediately antecedent emotion of a depressing character is too large to be set down to chance, or to that general liability to the buffets of ill fortune which the cancer patients, in their passage through life, share with most other people not so afflicted.' Throughout the early part of the 20th century, further suggestions have been made about the relationship between psychosocial factors and cancer, culminating in a book by Evans (1926) on *A Psychological Study of Cancer*, in which she suggested that one of the leading causes of cancer was the loss of a love object or an important emotional relationship. Her analysis of cancer patients led her to believe that some people experiencing grief directed their psychic energy inward, against their own natural body defences.

There have been a number of explanations of just how stress may cause disease. Foque (1931), for example, believed that there was a multiplicity of secondary causes for cancer, such as x-rays, chemicals and viruses. However, in his view, the cells had to be in a receptive state before the cancerous process could start. He believed in 'the role of sad emotions as activators and secondary causes in the activation of human cancers.' These, he added, 'through the instrumentality of the nervous system's effect on metabolism, act on the endocrine balances of the body in such a way that the cell is pu into a state where it is sensitive and receptive to the carcinogen'.

Fox (1978), however, suggested that there are two primary cancer-causing mechanisms: (1) 'carcinogenesis, the production of cancer by an agent o mechanism overcoming existing resistance of the body', and (2) 'lowere resistance to cancer, which permits a potential carcinogen normally insuffi cient to produce cancer to do so' (e.g. weakened emotional state). This latte mechanism involves the immunosuppresion system of the body, with a 'immune deficient' individual at risk of one form of cancer or anothe depending on the vulnerability of particular organs.

Selye (1979), on the other hand, suggested that all organisms go throug a 'general adaptation syndrome,' which passes through three stages:

1. *Alarm Reaction*, which is comprised of a *shock phase* ('the initial and immediat

reaction to a noxious agent') and a *countershock phase* ('a mobilisation of defences phase in which the adrenal cortex becomes further enlarged and secretes more corticicoid hormones').

2. *Stage of Resistance*, which involves adapting to the stressor stimulus, but decreasing one's ability to cope with subsequent stimuli.

3. *Stage of Exhaustion*, which follows a period of prolonged and severe adaptation.

He goes on to say that the hormonal attack (particularly adrenocorticotrophic hormone or ACTH) on the body, is the ultimate cancer producing weapon if it is activated at a frequent, continuous and high level.

Selye (1979) believes that stress plays some role in the development of all diseases, and 'these effects may be curative (as illustrated by various forms of externally-induced stress such as shock therapy, physical therapy, and occupational therapy) or damaging, depending on whether the biochemical reactions characteristic of stress (e.g. stress hormones or nervous reactions to stress) combat or accentuate the trouble'.

Although the exact bodily and psychological mechanisms are still not entirely clear, the evidence is mounting that there is some link between psychosocial/personality factors and certain forms of cancer, even though the methodological weaknesses in the existing research leave something to be desired.

Most of the research in this field can be sub-divided into two categories: those studies which focus on the relationship between various psychometric predispositions and cancer, those which examine the emotional history or adverse life events and the pathogenesis of cancer.

Whereas Fox (1978) and Selye (1979) emphasise the physiological or bodily reactions and processes of stress, Haney (1977), Kissen (1969) and others have concentrated on the psychological processes that may lead to cancer. Kissen has argued that adverse life events and loss of a love object can lead to cancer by the psychological mechanisms of 'despair, depression and hopelessness'. He suggests 'adverse life situations in an individual with poor emotional outlets, and therefore, with diminished ability to effectively sublimate or dissipate an emotional situation, are likely to result in such effects as depression, despair and hopelessness. It is also possible that adverse life situations may directly precipitate such effects whatever the personality, but it must be conceded that their manifestation is more likely in those with poor emotional outlets.' Haney (1977) argues that personality predispositions may not be directly linked to cancer, but will help to determine 'which psychic and somatic insults to which the individual will be exposed and the meaning of these exposures will have for the individual'. There is likely to be a psychocarcinogenic process in operation, which works in such a way that the stressor and bodily predispositions interact and co-vary in the direction of an ultimate carcinoma, one feeding the other.

PERSONALITY PREDISPOSITIONS AND CANCER

Bacon *et al.* (1952) provided one of the earliest suggestions of a cancer personality. They investigated 40 women with cancer of the breast, and detailed psycho-analytic case histories of patients. They concluded that these patients have six important behavioural characteristics;

(1) a masochistic character structure;
(2) inhibited sexuality;
(3) inhibited motherhood;
(4) inability to discharge or deal appropriately with anger, aggressiveness or hostility, covered over by a facade of pleasantness;
(5) an unresolved hostile conflict with the mother, handled through denial and unrealistic sacrifice; and
(6) delay in securing treatment.

Bacon and her colleagues were inclined to believe that there might be a connection between the psyche and cancer, and that 'it is possible for emotional forces at times to provide a catalyst for the cancer reaction.' Le Shan (1959) was one of the first to suggest that cancer may result from the loss of a loved one or some significant other, particularly in persons who are prone to feelings of hopelessness, depression, low self-esteem and introjection. Many of the early researchers in this field have observed that malignancies seem to be associated with what Kissen (1963) and others (Dattore *et al.* 1980) have termed 'general emotional inhibition, denial and repression'.

Le Shan and Worthington (1955) did some of the early work in this field by comparing 152 cancer patients and 125 patients with other or no illness using a projective test developed by Worthington. The cancer group differed from the control in the following ways: (1) they had difficulty expressing hostile feelings; (2) they had suffered the loss of a dear one prior to diagnosis; and (3) they showed greater potential anxiety about the death of a parent.

Kissen (1963) carried out a study among 335 patients, of whom 161 had been diagnosed as having lung cancer, while the others had some other less severe illness. He instrumented a childhood behaviour disorder questionnaire and the Maudsley Personality Inventory, and found that the cancer patients suffered from 'a diminished outlet for emotional discharge', both in their childhood experiences and in their present adult lives. Booth's (196 Rorschach work on 93 lung cancer patients and 82 tubercular patients revealed similar patterns among the cancer patients. He found that cancer patients responded very differently to the inkblots than tubercular patients, emphasising emotional repression, the inward direction of anger and the vulnerability to emotional loss.

Studies in the late 1960's and early 1970's used more sophisticated psychometric measures, but still suffered from inadequate or non-representative sampling and inappropriate comparison groups. They, nevertheless, came up with similar findings to the early work. Pauli and Schmid (1972) carried out an investigation among 57 patients with histologically verified breast cancer and compared them to a group of 34 women with benign disorders of the reproductive organs, using the MMPI. They found that the patients with mastocarcinoma were significantly different on depression, hypochondriasis, and paranoia. Grissom *et al.* (1975) compared healthy subjects and patients with bronchial carcinoma and found that their cancer patients had significantly lower 'personal integration' scores on the Tennessee Self Concept scales. Individuals with this pattern of behaviour frequently direct their frustration, anger and failure inward, and are vulnerable to the loss of an important relationship.

There have been a great number of studies which have explored the psychometric differences between cancer patients and other patients or normals, but they all suffer from being retrospective. The major problem with these investigations stems from the nature of the primary sample, who are usually diagnosed cancer patients. It is extremely difficult in these circumstances to disentangle the interrelationship between cancer and personality. There is enough evidence available to suggest that the awareness of having cancer can alter various personality measures. (Craig and Abeloff, 1974), which could make methodological nonsense of existing findings. Prospective work in this field is now under way in the U.S.A. Paffenbarger (1977), for example, is engaged in a long-term cohort study of over 35,000 former Harvard students and 16,500 University of Pennsylvania students (of both sexes), on whom physiological and psychological data have been accumulating over a large number of years.

In the meantime, there are a number of premorbid personality studies already available to test some of Kissen's (1963) theories that repression is the fundamental personality mechanism in cancer pathogenesis, particularly in people who have suffered the loss of a love object. To this end, Dattore *et al.* (1980) carried out a very well-designed study of 200 patients on whom premorbid MMPI personality data were available through Veterans Administration Hospital records, 75 cancer and 125 non-cancer patients. Extensive screening of records was involved to ensure comparable samples. They found that the two groups were significantly different on three scales; Repression, Depression and Denial of Hysteria. Their findings on repression were in the direction of earlier studies, that cancer patients showed significantly higher scores. Their results on depression were unexpected but understandable. They found cancer patient had significantly lower depression scores than controls. They argued 'since depression represents such a threatening emotion to the cancer patient, one would expect to see relatively little acknowledgement of depression by subjects in the cancer group'. Similar results were found by Thomas and Greenstreet (1973) in their study of 1,076 graduates of Johns Hopkins Medical School. These former students were followed for a number of years, and the small group who developed cancer differed from those who developed other illnesses (e. g. mental illness, hypertension, etc.) and from disease-free controls in being significantly lower on depression and anxiety scales. And finally, Dattore *et al.* (1980) found cancer patients scored lower on the Denial of Hysteria measure, which they interpreted to indicate that they were more *insightful* and *introceptive* than non-cancer patients, which is also consistent with earlier theoretical speculations.

Other research has shown the opposite, that extraverts are more prone to cancer. Hagnell (1966) carried out an epidemiological survey of 2,550 Swedish women over a 10 year period. It was found that a significantly higher proportion of women who had developed cancer had been originally rated as having a 'substable' personality. This classification of personality types was developed by a Swede, Sjobring (1963) in which he describes four dimensions: (1) capacity factor; (2) stability factor; (3) solidity factor; and (4) validity factor. The 'substable' personality is described as 'warm, hearty, concrete, heavy, industrious, interested in people, social, tending to personal interrelations and inhibition.' Hagnell's finding did not support earlier or subsequent research observations, as his results show that cancer patients were 'substable' more often than one might expect. 'Substability' in Sjobring's system has traits in common with Eysenck's classification of 'extraversion', which refers to the outgoing, uninhibited social proclivities of a person. Thus, Cooper and Metcalfe (1973) prompted by Hagnell's findings, carried out a survey on 47 women with cancer, using the Maudsley Personal Inventory, which assesses extraversion. They concluded that women who develop breast cancer do have significantly higher extraversion scores and that this is a 'constitutionally determined' characteristic of these patients rather than a 'temporary reaction' to their illness. This finding confirms Hagnell's result, but does not agree with Kissen's hypothesis that cancer is associated with individuals who have 'poor emotional outlets' and repress their feelings.

In addition, a great deal of recent work has been carried out on the link between clinical depression and cancer. Bieliauskas and Garron (1982) provide an excellent review of most of this research. Many early studies have indicated, mostly retrospectively, that cancer patients tend to suffer from some form of psychological depression (Levine *et al.*, 1978). Probably the best designed prospective study in the field is by Shekelle and his colleagues (Shekelle *et al.*, 1981), in an epidemiological investigation of 2020 men from whom clinically assessed depression had been measured by the MMPI some 17 years before the mortality records had been examined. For those males who had scored at the top end of the depression scale, there were twice the incidence of deaths due to cancer than for those who did not score at the high end of the depression continua. The data indicates that the risk was prevalent during the whole 17 year period but was most prominent between 12 and 17 years. Bieliauskas and Garron (1982) indicate that

> 'because of the prospective nature, the long period, the use of quantitative measures, attention to their risk factors, and the large number of subjects, this study provides significant evidence of prospective increases in risk of cancer death with increased depression.'

Nevertheless, there were a number of methodological weaknesses. First, the MMPI absolute depression scores for the cancer deaths were not in the pathological range, only linearly more depressive than for the non-cancer deaths. Second, we only have a 'one point in time' measurement of depression (i.e. 17 years ago) and don't have information about the changes that may have taken place in the psychological state of the individuals assessed. While all the results point in a similar direction, with the exception of the few mentioned above, the methodological weaknesses here are very great indeed. Most of these studies suffer from inappropriate samples, uncoordinated and unreliable measuring instruments, inadequate comparison groups, retrospective as opposed to prospective data gathering, and a disregard for fitting the research work into any kind of conceptual or theoretical framework. The issue of an appropriate control group is particularly important, and the difficulties of interpretation in this respect were highlighted in a recent study by Watson and Schuld (1977). They took a sample of cancer patients and matched control groups and found no significant differences on any of the MMPI scales between the two. Although the data were collected on a premorbid basis (i.e. well before any clinical diagnosis of cancer), the sample was comprised of individuals for whom psychopathology had been diagnosed (i.e. they were psychiatric patients). In addition, the malignancy group contained a large proportion of people with alcohol-related problems, six times as many as in the control group (Kellerman, 1978). These kinds of studies create a great deal of confusion in the cancer field and could be controlled by more careful research designs. As Perrin and Pierce (1959) suggest, each study of cancer and personality should contain ideally two control groups, one of subjects who have some chronic, non-cancerous disease sufficient to cause him/her anxiety about his/her health, and the other a comparison group of 'healthy' subjects.

LIFE EVENTS AND CANCER

A second category of studies in this field has been to focus in on recent stressful life events and the onset of cancer. In this respect, the Holmes and Rahe (1967) Social Readjustment Rating Scale (SRRS) has been used extensively as a measuring tool. There are several problems with this instrument, which may make the research in this area less fruitful than it could otherwise be. First, the SRRS lists a number of events which may be symptoms or consequences of illness rather than critical incidences (e.g. change in number of marital arguments, fired from work, sex difficulties, etc.). Second, each event on the SRRS has differential meaning for each subject, yet they are rigidly enumerated in scoring. And finally, the illness itself may impede or prevent the patient from accurately recalling past events, as Napier *et al.* (1972) have found.

Nevertheless, a great deal of attention has been directed to life events research. Indeed, in Le Shan's (1959) early review of 75 studies on psychological factors in the development of malignant disease, he concluded 'the most consistently reported, relevant psychological factor has been the loss of a major emotional relationship prior to the first-noted symptoms of neoplasm'. He later carried out a large-scale epidemiological study (LeShan, 1966) into mortality rates among different groups of people likely to be affected by loss of a close emotional relationship. He predicted that cancer mortality rates should be highest for widowed, next highest for divorced, and lowest for married and then single persons, if the theory of loss of emotional relationships was valid. He analysed epidemiological data from a number of studies, age-adjusting the mortality rates, and found that the data were consistent with this hypothesis.

Muslin *et al.* (1966) carried out an investigation of 165 women who were about to have a breast biopsy. They were interviewed and given a life events questionnaire prior to diagnosis, and in the end they were able to produce 37 matched pairs of malignant and benign subjects. They found that twice as many diagnosed cancer patients had 'a permanent loss of a first degree relative or other person whom the subject specifically stated was emotionally important to her', than did the benign group.

Schmale and Iker (1966) explored the same phenomena among a group of women who were reporting for a cone biposy as a result of a positive Pap test. They were given psychological tests and interviewed prior to diagnosis and none of the subjects had any gross abnormality that would lead the physician to suspect cervical cancer. On the basis of high life events scores 6 months prior to the first positive Pap smear, the authors then predicted who would ultimately be diagnosed as having cervical cancer. It was found that there was a significantly high level of accuracy in their judgements, based almost solely on life events immediately preceding the first tests.

On the other hand, Schonfield (1975), who interviewed 112 Israeli women on the day before biopsy of a breast lump, found no evidence that stressful life events, particularly losses, precede the onset of cancer. Data from this study show that patients who were subsequently found to have benign tumours of the breast had higher scores (more stress) on Holmes and Rahe's Social Readjustment Rating Scale than those who had malignancies. However, he found that patients who were subsequently found to have malignant tumours, had a higher covert anxiety and MMPI Lie scale scores. This could possibly be the result of the physician unconsciously transmitting to them his own anxiety about their breast lump.

In addition, Snell and Graham (1971) in their study of 352 breast cancer patients and 670 patients with other types of cancer and non-neoplasmic diseases, could find no difference between these two groups in the experiencing of a single event or a cumulative number of events by themselves or by members of their families. They pointed out the shortcomings of their methodology and also suggested that there may be events of a different type, not studied by them, which may be related to the development of cancer of the breast.

In recent years a great deal of sustained work has been carried out by Greer and his colleagues (Greer and Morris, 1975; Greer, 1979). In a recent study on premorbid breast cancer, Greer (1979) studied 160 women admitted to hospital for a breast tumor biopsy . . . a breast tumor was defined as being 'a tumor with or without palpable axillary nodes, with no deep attachment and no distant metastases', that is, women with either very early breast cancer which is operable or women with some breast disease which is benign. These patients were interviewed on the day prior to the biopsy and detailed information was collected on stressful life events (e.g. events which caused them severe and prolonged emotional distress). These events were verified by husbands or close relatives. Additional psychometric data were also collected on depression, hostility, extraversion/neuroticism and other social and psychiatric states. After the operation, 69 were found to have breast cancer and 91 a benign breast disease. The cancer and controls (i.e. benign group) were matched in most respects (e.g. social class, marital state, etc.), except that the cancer patients were significantly older.

No significant differences were found in respect of the occurrence of stressful life events, including loss of a loved person, or depression, or denial as the characteristic response to life stresses. Although an effort was made to design the research in a way that would minimise the effects of diagnosed cancer on personality and the recall of life events, the author admits himself that 'we had no control over what surgeons told patients before admission'. In addition, he was unable to control for the fear of having an operation which could result in the removal of a breast and the diagnosis of breast cancer. As well, the cancer group were significantly older, which could have biased the results. But most important of all, since breast cancer may take several years to develop and the stressful life events responsible may take place years before that, there is a strong potential 'memory falsification' problem. What is really needed, as Greer himself suggests, are large scale prospective studies with more sophisticated control groups.

There have been other studies which have explored traumatic life events and cancer, without using the SRRS. For example, Smith and Sebastian (1976) examined the emotional history of 44 cancer patients and 44 patients with physical abnormalities which were non-cancerous. Structured interviews were carried out to try and identify the frequency, intensity, and duration of emotional states in each person's life, which involved questions about family life, childhood, social and sexual life, career, religion, etc. Their aproach was far more open-ended then the traditional life events research just reviewed, in that they relied on interview responses to the following question:

> 'I am going to ask you to remember events that have occurred in your life which have made you feel very concerned, emotional, stressed and so forth. I will ask you to relate the kind of events that provoked emotional feelings in you, the date of the event and the intensity and duration of the events and emotional conditions. We will begin with early childhood and end up with questions about your present life situation.'

Critical incidents were then recorded and rated as either high, medium or low, and the intensity and duration of the emotional events for each person were rated on a 15 point scale. It was found that there were significantly more frequent and intense emotional events prior to diagnosis among cancer patients than the comparison group.

Another interesting study among these lines was undertaken by Witzel (1970) among 150 cancer patients and 150 patients with other serious diseases. He took personal histories of past illnesses and found that non-cancer patients had a significantly larger number of reported incidents of medical problems throughout their lives than cancer patients. They reported being out-patients three times more often than cancer patients, being in a hospital bed three times more often, having temperatures in excess of 38.5°C seven times more often, and experiencing twice as many minor illnesses and operations. The authors contend that this does not necessarily contradict the other research on adverse life events, because these critical medical incidents may signal the disease process itself. As Fox (1978) has suggested 'developing cancer had mobilised the immune response, which is capable of fighting many diseases, and which, because of its aroused status, could do so more successfully than that of non-cancer patients'.

Some other research in this area is being undertaken which attempts to predict cancer from the psychosocial factors. One such study was carried out by Horne and Picard (1980) among lung cancer patients. The sample included 110 male patients, who were selected on the basis of the 'presence of an undiagnosed, subacute or chronic lung lesion visible on previous roentgenographic examination'. They were then interviewed extensively on a variety of psychosocial factors: childhood stability, job stability, marriage stability, lack of plans for the future and recent significant loss. A composite score was devised for each patient on the basis of these five life areas. The patient clinical pathology from 15 to 38 months after the psychosocial interview was determined, to see if predictions could be made from the life events to the diagnosis. The composite score was predictive in 80% of the patients with benign lung disease and in 61% of lung cancer patients. In fact, the predictive power of the psychosocial factors was as good as information on smoking history.

The majority of the studies relating to psycho-social factors in cancer have been done on a retrospective basis. Criticisms which have been made regarding the methodology of these studies are:

(*a*) lack of, inadequate or inappropriate control groups;
(*b*) vagueness in description of method of measurement of psychological factors;
(*c*) use of psychological measures which are often inadequately validated;
(*d*) most of the techniques depend on the recall responses of patients and there are inherent problems in this approach to research. The subject's response depends on: (1) the personality of the interviewer and the degree and speed of establishing rapport; (2) the status of the interviewer (a doctor as opposed to nurse or social worker or lay interviewer); (3) the physical environment in which the investigation is conducted; and (4) the health status of the subjects (those seeking medical help may be more positively motivated than healthy subjects).

Nevertheless, the area of stressful life events and the pathogenesis of cancer is a potentially fruitful field of future research and must be seriously considered. At the very least, adverse life events must act as an intervening if not primary source, of illness behaviour. As Haney (1977) has recently suggested 'adverse life events may produce situations and circumstances which heighten the individual's belief in his susceptability or increase the perceived threat. Adverse life events may exacerbate existing and often otherwise well tolerated symptoms and reduce the individual's tendency to deny them or delay help-seeking.'

Currie (1974) aptly sums up the present state of research by saying, in the context of tumor immunology, but which applied equally well to the field of cancer and the psychological processes, 'our knowledge . . . is primitive because the methodology is primitive. With the development of refined . . . methods, will come a refinement in our knowledge of the subject.'

NOTE: Material in this chapter has been published by the author in the Journal of Human Stress; the author would like to thank the publishers Heldref Publications for permission to use it here.

REFERENCES

Bacon, C. L., Rennecker, R., and Cutler, M. (1952). Psychosomatic survey of cancer of the breast, *Psychosomatic Medicine*, **4**, 453–460.

Bieliauskas, L. A., and Garron, D. C. (1982). Psychological depression and cancer, *General Hospital Psychiatry*, **4**, 56.

Booth, G. (1964). *Cancer and Culture: Psychological Disposition and Environment* (A Rorschach Study), Unpublished.

Cooper, C. L. (1981). *The Stress Check*. Prentice-Hall Inc., Englewood Cliffs, New Jersey.

Cooper, C. L. and Marshall, J. (1976). Occupational sources of stress, *Journal of Occupational Psychology*, **49**, 11–28.

Cooper, A. J., and Metcalf, M. (1963). Cancer and extraversion, *British Medical Journal*, 6 July, 18–19.

Craig, T. J., and Abeloff, M. D. (1974). Psychiatric symptomatology among hospitalised cancer patients, *American Journal of Psychiatry*, **131**, 1323–1327.

Currie, G. A. (1974). *Cancer and the Immune Response*, Edward Arnold, London.

Dattore, P., Shontz, F., and Coyne, L. (1980). Premorbid personality differentiation of cancer and non-cancer groups, *Journal of Consulting and Clinical Psychology*, **48** (3), 388–394.

Evans, E. (1926). *A Psychological Study of Cancer*. Dodd-Mead, New York.

Foque, E. (1931). Le problem au cancer dans sel aspects psychiques, *Hospital Gazette* (Paris), **104**, 827.

Fox, B. H. (1978). Premorbid psychological factors as related to cancer incidence, *Journal of Behavioural Medicine*, **1** (1), 45–133.

Glass, D. (1977). *Behaviour Patterns, Stress and Coronary Disease*, LEA, New Jersey.

Greenberg, H. (1980). *Coping with Job Stress*. Prentice-Hall Inc., Englewood Cliffs, New Jersey.

Greer, S. (1979). Psychological enquiry: a contribution to cancer research. *Journal of Psychological Medicine*, **9**, 81–89.

Greer, S., and Morris, T. (1975). Psychological attributes of women who develop breast cancer: a controlled study, *Journal of Psychosomatic Research*, **19**, 147–153.

Grissom, J., Weiner, B., and Weiner, E. (1975). Psychological correlates of cancer, *Journal of Consulting and Clinical Psychology*, **43**, 113.

Hagnell, O. (1966). The Premorbid personality of persons who develop cancer in a total population investigated in 1947 and 1957, in *Psycho-physiological Aspects of Cancer, Annals of New York Academy of Science*, 846.

Haney, C. A. (1977). Illness behaviour and psychosocial correlates of cancer, *Journal of Social Science and Medicine*, **11** (4), 223–228.

Haynes, S., Feinleib, M., and Kannel, W. (1980). The relationship of psychological factors to coronary heart disease in the Framingham Study, *American Journal of Epidemiology*, **111** (1), 37–58.

Holmes, T. H., and Rahe, R. H. (1967). The social readjustment rating scale. *The Journal of Psychosomatic Medicine*, **11**, 213–218.

Horne, R. L., and Picard, R. S. (1980). Psychosocial risk factors for lung cancer, *Psychosomatic Medicine*, **41**, 503–514.

Kellerman, J. (1978). A note on psychosomatic factors, *Journal of Consulting and Clinical Psychology*, **46**, 1422–1523.

Kissen, D. (1963). Personality characteristics in males conducive to lung cancer, *British Journal of Medical Psychology*, **36**, 27–36.

Kissen, D. (1969). The present status of psychosomatic cancer research, *Geriatrics*, **24**, 129.
LeShan, L., and Worthington, R. E. (1955). Some psychological correlates of neoplastic disease: preliminary report, *Journal of Clinical and Experimental Psychopathology*, **16**, 281.
LeShan, L. (1959). Psychological states as factors in the development of malignant disease: a critical review, *Journal of the National Cancer Institute*, **22**, 1–18.
LeShan, L. (1966). An emotional life-history pattern associated with neoplastic disease, *Annual New York Academy of Science Journal*, **125**, 780–793.
Levine, P. M., Silberfarb, P. M., and Lipowski, A. J. (1978). Mental disorders in cancer patients: a study of 100 psychiatric referrals, *Cancer*, **42**, 1385–1391.
Muslin, H. L., Gyarfas, K., and Pieper, W. J. (1966). Separation experience and cancer of the breast, *Annual New York Academy of Science Journal*, **125**, 802–806.
Napier, J. A., Metzner, H., and Johnson, B. C. (1972). Limitations of morbidity and mortality data obtained from family histories. A report from the Tecumseh studies, *American Journal of Public Health*, **62**, 30–35.
Paffenbarger, R. S. (1977). Psychosocial Factors in Students Predictive of Cancer, *Grant No. 1R01 CA 225 74–01, National Cancer Institute*, Bethesda, Md.
Paget, J. (1870). *Surgical Pathology*, Longman Green, London.
Pauli, H., and Schmid, V. (1972). Psychosomatic aspects in the clinical manifestation of mastocarcinoma, *Journal of Psychotherapy and Medical Psychology*, **22** (2).
Perrin, G. M., and Pierce, I. R. (1959). Psychosomatic aspects of cancer: A review, *Psychosomatic Medicine*, **5**, 397–421.
Rosenman, R., Friedman, M., and Jenkins, C. D. (1967). Clinically unrecognised myocardial infarction in the Western Collaborative Group Study, *American Journal of Cardiology*, **19**, 776–782.
Schmale, A. H., and Iker, H. P. (1966). The affect of hopelessness and the development of cancer, *Journal of Psychosomatic Medicine*, **28**, 714–721.
Schonfield, J. (1975). Psychological and life-experience differences between Israeli women with benign and cancerous breast lesions, *Journal of Psychosomatic Research*, **19**, 229.
Selye, H. (1979). Correlating stress and cancer, *American Journal of Proctology, Gastroenterology, Colon and Rectal Surgery*, **30** (40), 18–28.
Shekelle, R. B., Raynor, W. J., Ostefeld, A. M., *et al.* (1981). Psychological depression and 17 year risk and death from cancer, *Psychosomatic Medicine*, **43**, 117–125.
Sjobring, H. (1963). *La personality, structure et developpment*, Doin, Paris.
Smith, W. R., and Sebastian, H. (1976). Emotional history and pathogenesis of cancer, *Journal of Clinical Psychology*, **32** (4), 63–66.
Snell, L., and Graham, S. (1971). Social trauma as related to cancer of the breast, *British Journal of Cancer*, **25** (4), 721.
Snow, H. (1893). *Cancer and the Cancer Process*, Churchill, London.
Thomas, C. B., and Greenstreet, R. L. (1973). Psychobiological characteristics in youth as predictors of five disease states: Suicide, mental illness, hypertension, coronary heart disease and tumor, *Johns Hopkins Medical Journal*, **132**, 16–43.
Watson, C., and Schuld, D. (1977). Psychosomatic factors in the etiology of neoplasmas, *Journal of Consulting and Clinical Psychology*, **45** (3), 455–461.
Witzel, L. (1970). Anamnese and zweiterkrankungen bei patienten mit bosartigen neubildungen. (Anamnesis and second diseases in patients with malignant tumors.) *Med. Klin.*, **65**, 876–879.

Section Two
Psychosocial Precursors to Cancer

Psychosocial Stress and Cancer
Edited by C. L. Cooper

Chapter 3
Depression, Stress, and Cancer

Linas A. Bieliauskas
Associate Professor, Rush-Presbyterian-St. Luke's Medical Center, Chicago, Illinois, USA

Relationships between psychological depression and cancer and between stress and cancer have been widely promulgated. While there has been no solid evidence proving that such relationships exist either in a concommitant or aetiological sense, a number of investigations have provided at least suggestive support that depression and/or stress may somehow increase the risk of cancer morbidity or mortality. Studies in this area are diverse, including a variety of designs, perspectives of different disciplines, use of different independent and dependent variables, and focus on both animal and human models. It is the purpose of this chapter to attempt to integrate this wide variety of research within a more cohesive conceptual framework, one which may serve to bring together some of the suggestive evidence of relationships between depression, stress, and cancer.

DEPRESSION AND CANCER

It is commonly believed that psychological depression is a frequently occurring phenomenon in patients with cancer. Writers at least as far back as Galen believed that a melancholic state increased the proneness to cancer (Hueper, 1942). Clinical studies, using psychiatric descriptions of depression, have reported its presence in a majority of cancer patients (Fras *et al.*, 1967; Levine *et al.* 1978; Peck, 1972). In such studies, however, the structure of interviews conducted with patients was not well specified, control samples were often lacking or inadequate, and statistical analyses were suspect. When an objective, controlled assessment of depression has been made in patients with cancer, a significant increase in depression has not been found (Leiber *et al.*, 1976; Plumb and Holland, 1977). On the basis of a critical review of such studies, Bieliauskas and Garron (1982) concluded that there was no evidence that patients with cancer are more depressed, in a psychiatric sense, than anyone else.

One of the more common errors of earlier studies of depression in cancer patients was to document depression in those cancer patients for whom psychiatric referral had been made. Such patients constitute a necessarily biased sample and should not be considered as representative of cancer patients as a whole. A very recent study (Derogatis *et al.*, 1983) assessed 215 randomly accessed, newly admitted cancer patients with a common protocol. Psychiatric diagnoses were made according to *DSM-III* criteria. The prevalence of significant depression was at six per cent, a rate not disparate from that seen in any random sample of patients with medical disorders. This finding supports the argument that while some cancer patients are significantly depressed, the widespread notion that cancer patients are generally depressed is not supported by the evidence.

However, there have been studies which link *pre-morbid* depression with an increase of risk for mortality from cancer. Shekelle *et al.* (1981) reported a doubling in the risk of death from cancer in a group of men who had scored highest on the depression (D) scale of the MMPI (Hathaway and McKinley, 1951) measured 17 years earlier. This risk remained intact when controlled for well-known risk factors for cancer of smoking, alcohol use and age. Nevertheless, on further exploration of the data, we found that these high scores were not in what is considered the pathological range for depression (Bieliauskas and Garron, 1982). This suggested that, at least in patients with cancer, it might be better to view depression as a continuous variable rather than a present/absent pathological condition, a perspective endorsed by Hoch (1972).

In a related study, Bieliauskas and Shekelle (1983) reported that two behavioral characteristics which could be identified in the sample of patients with high D MMPI profiles were a decreased percentage of time in bed spent sleeping, and an increased report of being frequently nervous or upset. While such behaviors are consistent with the presence of depression, they are also found with almost any psychiatric disturbance. Therefore, it seems quite possible that a depressive-like, probably chronic state of mild 'distress' is the active risk factor which was being measured rather than clinical depression itself. The Derogatis *et al.* (1983) study of the prevalence of psychiatric disorders among patients with cancer seems to buttress this interpretation. They found that while only six per cent of their patients could be classified as clinically depressed, 47% of their patients received some sort of psychiatric diagnoses; of these, 85% could be accounted for by features of depression and anxiety. On the basis of these findings as well, it appears that a depressive-like state of chronic mild distress may be both a risk factor for mortality from cancer and a presenting feature in a significant proportion of patients with cancer (up to 40%).

The distinction between clinical psychological depression and a depressive-like state of distress is an important one. It emphasizes the need to use broad based instruments in assessing depression and/or distress in conducting research or clinical assesssment in patients with cancer. If only depression of clinical proportions is documented or instruments restricted to pure symptoms of depression are used, it is likely that important psychological contributions to risk of cancer or important psychological concommitants of cancer will be missed or misinterpreted.

STRESS AND CANCER

Studies of the effects of stress on cancer in humans received impetus from early explorations of the influence of psychosocial loss on cancer (LeShan and Worthington, 1956). Le Shan (1959) concluded that the loss of a major emotional relationship prior to the first symptoms of neoplasm is one of the most consistently reported psychological contributors to risk of cancer. However, many of the early studies reviewed had major methodological and design difficulties such as poor definitions of loss and inadequate or lacking controls. For example, it is not adequate to simply describe a variety of events as representing 'loss' in cancer patients; many studies did so *ex post facto*. In an attempt to improve on this kind of methodology, Muslin *et al.* (1966) used a standard questionnaire which documented permanent separations from all first-degree relatives and close friends of female patients admitted for breast biopsy. They found no differences in such separations between those patients with malignant versus benign biopsy results.

It is also not enough to look at cancer patients, note an incidence of loss at some point in their lives, and conclude that this is a progenitor of cancer. This, again, was a flaw in earlier studies. To support a hypothesis of increased cancer risk following loss, it is necessary to look at the incidence of such loss and then examine whether that loss is related to an increased incidence of cancer. Helsing and Szklo (1981) and Helsing *et al.* (1982) conducted a prospective study of a major psychosocial loss which is known to lead to increased rates of mortality – bereavement. They found increased rates of mortality only among male individuals, not females, following bereavement; this increase in mortality among males was causally non-specific. On the basis of major weaknesses in studies supporting a relationship between loss and cancer and negative findings in well-designed studies, Bieliauskas and Garron (1982) concluded that there is no evidence to support significant emotional loss as a stressor which is a significant precursor of cancer. In fact, there does not appear to be any evidence that an increase in the experience of stressors *per se* is linked to the risk of cancer.

Animal studies, on the other hand, have demonstrated that subjection to various stressors can increase tumor growth, though the timing and nature of the stressors are critical in the kind of effects which will be observed (Riley, 1981). For example, if rats are stressed following tumor implant, tumor enhancement occurs provided the stressor is acute; if animals are placed in a chronic 'social stress' producing situation (such as housing exposed to noise, crowding, etc.) tumor enhancement also generally occurs. Sklar and Anisman (1981a) summarize the research findings as follows (p. 98): 'Enhancement of tumor development has usually been reported in studies using acute, uncontrollable physical stress, chronic social stress, or stimulating housing conditions. Chronic, uncontrollable physical stress has tended to be associated with tumor inhibition.'

Beyond experiments with the timing and nature of stressors, Sklar and Anisman (1979) have strongly suggested that the crucial factor affecting tumor growth is not the presence of a stressor itself, but rather the ability to cope with the stressor. They demonstrated that inescapable shock will cause earlier appearance of an induced tumor in rats while escapable shock will produce no such effect. Acute social stress, such as changing housing conditions for rats, will also promote tumor development; however, if coping methods are available and used, such as fighting, tumor growth is not increased (Sklar and Anisman, 1980).

However, one must keep in mind that the type of tumor which is studied also will affect the kinds of results one sees when the organism is exposed to stressors. Tumors which occur spontaneously respond differently from tumors which are chemically induced or result from transplantation; the former tend to be facilitated by stressors while the latter tend to be inhibited (Newberry, 1981). In humans, one would suspect that we would be most concerned with chronic social stress and its influence on tumors that tend to occur spontaneously. An exact translation of the animal literature to humans is thus premature at this time.

The emphasis on the coping process rather than exposure to stressors *per se* as the risk factor for cancer has begun to be appreciated in human research. Notice was taken of the importance of patterns of human reactions by LeShan and Worthington (1956) who described patients with cancer as having difficulty expressing hostile feelings. Kissen (1966) and Kissen *et al.* (1969) compared patients who were eventually shown to have cancer of the lung with patients who were shown to have other lung disease after biopsy. They reported a general inhibition of emotion in the patients with cancer. Schmale and Iker (1966a, b) demonstrated an increased sense of hopelessness in females who were later shown to have malignant versus benign tissue changes following biopsy of the cervix. Greer *et al.* (1979) found that more favorable outcome following mastectomy for breast cancer in women was associated with a 'fighting spirit' while poorer outcome was associated with either hopeless/helpless feelings or a 'stoic acceptance' of their disease.

The data from these investigators suggests that hopelessness and/or an inability to effectively express emotions are characteristic of patients who may have cancer and may possibly be a precursor of cancer. Both of these emotional states can be interpreted as either giving up or reacting ineffectively to life stressors. They can thus be seen as reflecting a poor coping style and could buttress the proposal of Sklar and Anisman (1979) that it is the pattern of coping with stress and not exposure to stressors alone which affects tumor growth. The advantage of this viewpoint is evident in a recent report by Levy (1983). In studying metastatic disease in women with cancer of the breast, she found that increased survival time is associated with increased distress and psychiatric symptomatology. While at first glance these reactions may appear to be at odds with earlier findings of a potentiation of cancer with increased distress, hopelessness, and emotional inhibition, one must keep in mind that the patients studied by Levy already had cancer, and had been treated for it. The studies of Kissen and his colleagues and Schmale and Iker mentioned above concerned themselves with patients who were admitted for biopsy but as yet did not have knowledge of their disease. In a sample such as Levy's, it is quite conceivable that an ability to express emotions, even if they are 'negative,' is an effective coping mechanism; that is, the ability to effectively express an appropriate reaction of distress in the face of a life threatening illness will likely be more adaptive than denial or suppression of such emotions. Such an interpretation would be in line with the earlier cited findings of Greer *et al.* (1979).

PSYCHONEUROIMMUNOLOGY

A commonly proposed route for the effect of psychological stress on cancer has been via the immune system. Selye (1979) suggests that hormonal release commonly associated with 'stress', particularly ACTH, is the likely cancer-producing agent, especially if it is activated frequently and continuously. The effects of ACTH-related and other hormonal release on immune system changes have been documented. Catecholamines and corticosteroids are associated with the stress response and are seen as likely mediators of immunologic changes (Borysenko, 1982a). Corticosteroids and epinephrine both have significant inhibitory influences on the immune system response (Borysenko and Borysenko, 1982). Such immune system changes at the time of stress, if sustained, may well be relevant to development of cancer.

Of particular interest to those interested in possible behavioral effects on risk of cancer is the finding that at least certain immune system responses may be subject to conditioning procedures. Ader and Cohen (1975) and Rogers *et al.* (1979) report that immunosuppression can be conditioned in rats by pairing of saccharin with injection of an immunosuppressing compound; eventually, simple presentation of the saccharin leads to measured immunosuppression. This finding is the basic paradigm of 'psychoneuroimmunology.'

Implications of psychoneuroimmunology for cancer are found in the work of Sklar and Anisman (1981a) who point out that stress increases both the utilization and synthesis of catecholamines. If coping responses are available, the utilization rates decline and there are minimal changes in amine availability. Furthermore, if physical stress is chronic and coping is not available, a physiological adaptation takes place nevertheless and catecholamine depletion is reduced. Finally, previous stressor exposure will sensitize the organism such that a re-exposure to a previously experienced stressor, even at a mild (ordinarily non-stressing) level, will induce norepinephrine depletion. Without the previous exposure, such depletion would not occur. Sklar and Anisman (1981b, p. 391) conclude: 'Thus stress may produce its effects on the immune system via the mediation of neurochemical and hormonal mechanisms. In addition, the hormonal changes themselves may directly influence tumor development.'

Therefore, physiological adaptation to stress over time, modification of physiological response when coping occurs in response to a stressor, and physiological indicators of the effect of a learned association with a previously stressing stimulus all argue towards the strong possibility of behavioral (including learned behavioral) influence on immune system response. In conjunction with their earlier work demonstrating the effects of stress and coping on tumor development, Sklar and Anisman (1981a, p. 116) feel that 'consistent with the effects on tumor development and neurochemical activity, it appears that coping factors may influence stress-induced hormonal activation.'

Unfortunately, at this time there is no *direct* evidence of a link between stress, immunologic reactivity, and development of cancer. However, in addition to the work described above, additional *suggestive* evidence has developed several other possible links between immune activity and tumor growth. Recently, a subgroup of lymphocytes, natural killer (NK) cells have been implicated as serving an anti-carcinogenic immune surveillance function in terms of being able to acquire spontaneous cytotoxic properties (Pross and Baines, 1976). Macrophages, as well, have been shown to have spontaneous anti-tumor capability (Chow *et al.*, 1979). Both macrophages and NK cells may decrease tumor activity and both are inhibited by stress (Riley, 1981; Borysenko, 1982a).

The functioning of these possible aspects of immune-related tumor inhibition has begun to be studied in humans. Locke (1982) reports decreased NK activity in college students experiencing high degrees of life stress who concomittantly exhibit poor adaptive ability, as evidenced by increased psychiatric symptomatology. In these students, the experience of life stressors alone did not cause changes in NK activity. Such change was evident only when psychiatric symptomatology accompanied the presence of life stressors, a relationship which Locke interprets as reflecting a deficient coping style.

Levy (1983), in her study, also found increased NK activity in her patients who had undergone mastectomy for breast cancer who exhibited the previously described increase in psychological disturbance and who were in the better outcome group. As noted previously, however, this apparent increase in psychiatric symptomatology may well be interpreted as 'improved' coping in that these patients were aware of their disease and the risk of their status. As such, increased symptomatology may reflect a more efficient means of expressing and dealing with distress than a silent resignation. This is an important difference between the group she studied and the one examined by Locke (1982), a group of healthy college students. This difference provides a plausible explanation which may make the seemingly disparate results of the two studies compatible.

Once again, it is emphasized that an exact linear relationship between stress, NK or macrophage activity, and effect on tumor has not been clearly demonstrated. However, the evidence suggests there is a complex association. Furthermore, current investigations of such an association go well beyond the cited studies on NK and macrophage activity, including changes in mast cells, intracellular cyclic AMP levels, etc. Current thinking regarding these issues is nicely reviewed by Locke and Kraus (1982), and Borysenko (192b) who concludes (p.33) that 'while the inability to cope with relatively recent stressful situations is not biologically compatible with a role as an aetiologic variable, it is possible that chronic endocrine changes consistent with life-history of deficient coping may have an aetiologic role.'

However, as a caveat, it should be kept in mind that Riley (1981) reminds us that the relationship between stressors and changes in the immune system will have relevance only for tumors which are under partial or complete immunological control. Not all cancers are such and we must remain cautious about knowledge of effects of stress on tumors studied in animal models which are induced and/or implanted and on potential roles for inferring relationships between changes in the human immune system and expression of neoplasia.

DEPRESSION AND STRESS

The relationship between studies of depression and cancer and between stress and cancer may be inferred from the foregoing discussion. To return to my initial point, it appears that those studies which do demonstrate either a premorbid or concommitant association between psychological depression and cancer identify a chronic depressive-like state of distress either as a risk factor (Bieliauskas and Garron, 1982) or prevalent symptom (Derogatis *et al.*, 1983). A clinical depression *per se* does not seem to be associated with either. It does not require a major leap in logic to infer that this depressive-like state of distress is probably a manifestation of an inefficient coping style when dealing with stressors.

Similarly, the animal and human studies of stress, psychoneuroimmunology, and cancer find that effective coping has a striking impact on both tumor development and on immune system-related hormonal changes which can be expected to influence tumor growth. The fundamental finding in these studies is that it is not exposure to a stressor *per se* but the ability to cope with it effectively which is most likely to influence neoplasia.

Herein is the potential link between depression and stress in relationship to cancer; studies in both areas are likely to be measuring an inefficient coping style when they report a significant relationship to cancer.

Apart from the inferences I have drawn from the relationships between studies which have been reviewed, there has been other suggestive evidence that depression and stress research, as it relates to cancer, often addresses chronic deficiencies in coping ability. To begin with, the indicator of depression used in the Shekelle *et al.* (1981) study was the MMPI *D* scale. As we have discussed, however, the significant elevations on this scale in the group of patients dying from cancer were of non-pathological proportions and unlikely to be indicating the presence of a clinical depression. A description of the MMPI *D* scale as a behavioral measure provides further support for my interpretation of the findings (Webb *et al.*, 1981, p. 16):

> 'In general, it is the best single, and a remarkably effective, index of psychic distress, immediate satisfaction, comfort, and security; it tells something of how individuals evaluate themselves and their role in the world and of their optimism – pessimism.'

As can be seen, this description is quite compatible with a self-perception of successful or unsuccessful coping with life stressors.

Further support for the relationship between depression and stress studies is found in a recent article by Kaplan, *et al.* (1983). These investigators conducted a prospective evaluation of the relationship between indicators of self-rejection and deprivation of social support in 1633 seventh grade children, and the occurrence of life stress events during the subsequent 10 years, and a measure of psychological distress 10 years later. One measure of self-rejection was a 'self-derogation' scale, scores on which were expected to interact significantly with stressing life events 'on the assumption that a self-rejecting person has a deficit in coping/adaptive/defensive resources that permits the occurrence and fails to mitigate the effects of self-devaluing circumstances' (Kaplan *et al.*, 1983, p. 231). The authors found a significant relationship between self-derogation and psychological distress 10 years later. A similar relationship was found between perceived rejection by peers and by family. As predicted, a significant interaction effect was found between measures of self-rejection and subsequent stressing life events, with the implication that such individuals are particularly vulnerable to such events.

The similarity between measures of self-derogation and perceived rejection and depressive-like symptomatology is obvious. In addition there is clear application of the measure of self-derogation to coping style. The dependent measure of psychological distress, used by the investigators, appears to reflect the presence of a chronic pattern of poor coping which seems to reflect a special vulnerability to life stressors with such a pattern.

Finally, some authors have pointed more directly to links between depression and stress. Borysenko (1982b) points out that hypersecretion of cortisol, one of the best documented physiological responses to stress, frequently accompanies endogenous depression. Biochemical changes in other amines, most notably norepinephrine and dopamine, have also been reported by a number of investigators in depression, but the results are often contradictory (Green and Costain, 1979). Miller (1982) makes a more direct argument, suggesting that stressing factors often produce symptoms of depression which, in turn, can lead to behaviors which can either increase the risk of cancer (i.e. smoking, obesity, etc.) or decrease the chance of its detection (i.e. failure to report symptoms, non-compliance with medical regimens, etc.).

The arguments put forward by the latter studies, however, are less relevant to the main thesis of this chapter, that deficiency in coping style is often the cogent measure in studies of depression and stress and cancer. Those studies address changes with depression of clinical proportions rather than changes associated with a depression-like chronic state of distress. Biochemical and behavioral changes would not necessarily be expected to be the same in both circumstances. Nevertheless, to the extent that some similarities between the range of symptoms of psychological depression and stress response are noted, there is the suggestion that there may be some common ground.

CONCLUSIONS

Based on the studies reviewed, the following points appear to be justified: (*a*) there is no clear evidence of increased clinical depression either as a risk factor for cancer or as a prevalent feature of patients with cancer; (*b*) there is evidence for a chronic depressive-like state of distress as both a risk factor for cancer mortality and as a concommitant symptom of many patients with cancer; (*c*) the most significant relationship between stress and cancer appears to be the inability to cope with stressors effectively, not exposure to stressors *per se*; this is true both for effects on tumor growth and on immune system-related hormonal changes which can affect neoplasia; (*d*) both measures of depression and measures of stress, as they relate to cancer, are likely to be measures of poor coping style in the presence of stressors.

The deficient ability to cope with stressors in both promoting risk for cancer and as a prominent feature in at least some patients with cancer serves as a link between studies of animal models of neoplastic development and studies of vulnerability to cancer and adaptation to cancer in humans. It is re-emphasized that at this point, no direct functional link between measures of depression and stress and cancer is proven. The speculation about such relationships currently rests at the stage of inference.

However, the apparent importance of coping style in studies of behavioral relationships to cancer carries several implications for research designed to elucidate such relationships. First, investigations of depression should not concentrate on measurement of depression of clinical proportions alone; a range of depressive-like symptoms of distress should be examined. Second, investigations of the effect of stressors on either tumor development itself or on possible physiological mediating mechanisms must address coping ability in a direct fashion; relationships between exposure to stressors alone and such dependent variables are unlikely to be found. Finally, investigations of psychological change in patients with cancer, whether they are designed to clarify relationships to survival issues or to psychological adaptation issues, should include assessments of coping style.

Some apparent disparities between various research approaches may be resolvable if the issue of coping ability is addressed as it relates to cancer. It is hoped that the highlighting of reasons for such a view point may be of value in the further exploration of the potentially exciting establishment of firm relationships between behavioral factors and cancer.

REFERENCES

Ader, R., and Cohen, N. (1975). 'Behaviorally conditioned immunosuppression', *Psychosom. Med.*, **37**, 333–340.

Bieliauskas, L. A., and Garron, D. C. (1982). 'Psychological depression and cancer', *Gen. Hosp. Psychiat.*, **4**, 187–195.

Bieliauskas, L. A., and Shekelle, R. B. (1983). 'Stable behaviors associated with high-point D MMPI profiles in a non-psychiatric population', *J. Clin. Psychol.*, **39**, 422–426.

Borysenko, J. Z. (1982a). 'Behavioral – physiological factors in the development and management of cancer', *Gen. Hosp. Psychiat.*, **4**, 69–74.

Borysenko, J. A. (1982b). 'Higher cortical function and neoplasia: psycho-neuroimmunology', in *Biological Mediators of Behavior and Disease: Neoplasia* (Ed. S. M. Levy), pp. 29–54, Elsevier, New York.

Borysenko, M., and Borysenko, J. (1982). 'Stress, behavior, and immunity: animal models and mediating mechanisms', *Gen. Hosp. Psychiat.*, **4**, 59–67.

Chow, D. A., Greene, M. I., and Greenburg, A. H. (1979). 'Macrophage-dependent, NK-cell-dependent "natural" surveillance of tumors in syngenic mice', *Int. J. Cancer*, **23**, 788–797.

Derogatis, L. R., Morrow, G. R., Fetting, J., Penman, D., Piasetsky, S., Schmale, A. M., Henrichs, M., and Carnicke, C. L. M. (1983). 'The prevalence of psychiatric disorders among cancer patients', *J. Am. Med. Assoc.*, **249**, 751–757.

Fras, I., Litin, E. M., and Pearson, J. S. (1967). 'Comparison of psychiatric symptoms in carcinoma of the pancreas with those in some other intra-abdominal neoplasms', *Am. J. Psychiat.*, **123**, 1553–1562.

Green, A. R., and Costain, D. W. (1979). 'The biochemistry of depression', in *Psychopharmacology of Affective Disorders* (Eds. E. S. Paykel and A. Codden), pp. 14–40, Oxford, New York.

Greer, S., Morris, T., and Pettingale, K. W. (1979). 'Psychological response to breast cancer: effect on outcome', *Lancet*, **2**, 785–787.

Hathaway, S. T., and McKinley, J. C. (1951). *The Minnesota Multiphasic Personality Inventory Manual*, Psychological Corporation, New York.

Helsing, K. J., Comstock, G. W., and Szklo, M. (1982). 'Causes of death in a widowed population', *Am. J. Epid.*, **116**, 524–532.

Helsing, K. J., and Szklo, M. (1981). 'Mortality after bereavement', *Am. J. Epid.*, **114**, 41–52.

Hoch, P. A. (1972). *Differential Diagnosis in Clinical Psychiatry*, Aronson, New York.

Hueper, W. C. (1942). *Occupational Tumors and Allied Diseases*, Charles C. Thomas, Baltimore.

Kaplan, H. B., Robbins, C., and Martin, S. S. (1983). 'Antecedents of psychological distress in young adults: self-rejection, deprivation of social support, and life events', *J. Health Soc. Behav.*, **24**, 230–244.

Kissen, D. M. (1966). 'The significance of personality in lung cancer in men', *Ann. N. Y. Acad. Sci.*, **125**, 820–826.

Kissen, D. M., Brown, R. I. F., and Kissen, M. (1969). 'A further report on personality and psychosocial factors in lung cancer', *Ann. N. Y. Acad. Sci.*, **164**, 535–544.

Leiber, L., Plumb, M. M., Gerstenzang, M.L., and Holland, J. (1976). 'The communication of affection between cancer patients and their spouses', *Psychosom. Med.*, **38**, 379–389.

LeShan, L. (1959). 'Psychological states as factors in the development of malignant disease: a critical review', *J. Nat. Cancer Inst.*, **22**, 1–18.

LeShan, L., and Worthington, R. E. (1956). 'Some recurrent life history patterns observed in patients with malignant disease', *J. of Nerv. Ment. Dis.*, **124**, 460–465.

Levine, P. M., Silberfarb, P. M., and Lipowski, Z. J. (1978). 'Mental disorders in cancer patients. A study of 100 psychiatric referrals', *Cancer*, **42**, 1385–1391.

Levy, S. (1983). 'Emotional response and disease outcome in breast cancer: immunological correlates', *The Society of Behavioral Medicine 4th Annual Scientific Sessions*, p. 45.

Locke, S. E. (1982). 'Stress, adaptation, and immunity', *Gen. Hosp. Psychiat.*, **4**, 49–58.

Locke, S., and Kraus, L. (1982). 'Modulation of natural killer cell activity by life stress and coping ability', in *Biological Mediators of Behavior and Disease: Neoplasia* (Ed. S. M. Levy), pp. 3–28, Elsevier, New York.

Miller, N. E. (1982). 'Some behavioral factors relevant to cancer', in *Biological Mediators of Behavior and Disease: Neoplasia* (Ed. S. M. Levy), 113–122, Elsevier, New York.

Muslin, H. L.; Gyarfas, K., and Pieper, W. J. (1966). 'Separation experience and cancer of the breast', *Ann N. Y. Acad. Sci.*, **125**, 802–806.

Newberry, B. H. (1981). 'Stress and mammary cancer', in *Stress and Cancer* (Eds. K. Bammer and B. H. Newberry), pp. 233–244, Hogrefe, Toronto.

Peck, A. (1972). 'Emotional reactions to having cancer', *Am. J. Roentgen. Nuc. Med.*, **114**, 541–599.

Plumb, M. M., and Holland, J. (1977) 'Comparative studies of psychological functioning in patients with advanced cancer: I. Self-reported depressive symptoms', *Psychosom. Med.*, **39**, 264–276.

Pross, H. F., and Baines, M. G. (1976). 'Spontaneous human lymphocyte-mediated cytotoxicity against tumor target cells. I. The effect of malignant disease', *Int. J. Cancer*, **18**, 593–604.

Riley, V. (1981). 'Psychoendocrine influences on immunoreeption and neoplasia', *Science*, **212**, 110–1109.

Rogers, M. P., Dubey, D., and Reich, P. (1979). 'The influence of the psyche and the brain on immunity and disease susceptibility', *Psychosom. Med.*, **41**, 147–174.

Schmale, A. H., and Iker, H. P. (1966a). 'The affect of hopelessnes and the development of cancer. I. Identification of uterine cervical cancer in women with atypical cytology', *Psychosom. Med.*, **28**, 714–721.

Schmale, A. H., and Iker, H. P. (1966b). 'The psychological setting of uterine cervical cancer', *Ann. N. Y. Acad. Sci.*, **125**, 807–813.

Selye, H. (1979). 'Correlating stress and cancer', *Am. J. Proct. Gastro. Col. Rect. Surg.*, **30**, 18–28.

Shekelle, R. B., Raynor, W. J., Ostfeld, A. M., Garron, D. C., Bieliauskas, L. A., Liu, S. C., Maliza, C., and Paul, O. (1981). 'Psychological depression and 17 year risk of death from cancer', *Psychosom. Med.* **43**, 117–125.

Sklar, L. S., and Anisman, H. (1980). 'Social stress influences tumor growth', *Psychosom. Med.*, **42**, 347–365.

Sklar, L. S., and Anisman, H. (1981a). 'Contributions of stress and coping to cancer development and growth', in *Stress and Cancer* (Eds. K. Bammer and B. H. Newberry), pp. 98–136, Hogrefe, Toronto.

Sklar, L. S., and Anisman, H. (1981b). 'Stress and cancer', *Psychol. Bull.*, **89**, 369–406.

Sklar, L. S., and Anisman, H. (1979). 'Stress and coping factors influence tumor growth', *Science*, **205**, 347–365.

Webb, J. T., McNamara, K. M., and Rodgers, D. A. (1981). *Configural Interpretation of the MMPI and CPI*, Ohio Psychology Publishing, Columbus.

Psychosocial Stress and Cancer
Edited by C. L. Cooper

Chapter 4
Lung Cancer and the Stress-Personality Inventory

H. J. Eysenck
Professor of Psychology, Institute of Psychiatry, Maudsley Hospital, London, UK

1. PSYCHOSOMATIC DISEASE AS A SCIENTIFIC CONCEPT

The concept of psychosomatic diseases has become very popular in recent times, but has also encountered a good deal of criticism. Some of this criticism is directly related to the terms used in describing the relationship; an inevitable implication of the term 'psychosomatic' is the postulation of a Cartesian duality between psyche and soma, which is being bridged in some magical fashion in the production of disease. Philosophers and scientists are very chary of accepting this duality, and although it cannot be said that any of the alternative theories has achieved a dominant position, both the dual aspect and the epiphenomenon view are fairly widely accepted by scientists. Monistic theories have difficulties commensurable with those of Cartesian dualism, and are probably not very widely held nowadays.

Another and possibly much more cogent reason for criticising the concept of psychosomatic disease, and the research done on it, is the close association that has become apparent between psychosomatic disease and Freudian theory. The obvious inability of psychoanalytic treatment to deal even with the neurotic disorders for which it was originally created (Rachman and Wilson, 1980), and the failure of empirical research to support the psychoanalytic theories of Freud and his followers (Eysenck and Wilson, 1973) have made such psychoanalytic theories and interpretations of psychosomatic disorders unpalatable, and the failure of psychoanalysts to provide evidence of cures has been equally substantial in reducing interest in these theories. In addition, research on psychosomatic disorders has often made use of projective techniques of low reliability and little validity, leading to conclusions which are essentially projections of previously held opinions, rather than having objective validity.

A quite different approach to the problem is mediated by the conception of man as a biosocial animal (Eysenck, 1980a, b, c). Such an approach rejects the frequently observed division of psychologists into biotropes and sociotropes, with the attending overemphasis on biological or social determinants of behaviour, and adopts the view that biological and social factors are inevitably both important and relevant in human behaviour. Such an approach leads to attempts to quantify the relative importance of these different factors in any given situation, for any particular group of individuals (Binnie-Dawson, 1982).

Such an approach may be illustrated by looking at recent models of neurosis and criminality. It is suggested that neuroses are produced by the conditioning of autonomic (emotional) responses, and can be cured by their extinction (Eysenck, 1983a). On the other hand, antisocial conduct is believed to be due to the failure of a conditioning process along Pavlovian lines to produce a 'conscience', capable of deterring the individual from such conduct (Eysenck, 1977). Pavlovian conditioning, of course, is a biological phenomenon, and individual differences in conditionability are largely determined by genetic factors, and associated with personality (Eysenck, 1967, 1981). Social factors determine the content of the conditioning; i.e., while it is usually social behaviour that is being conditioned, it is also possible for antisocial behaviour to be so conditioned! (Raine and Venables, 1981). It is particularly important in this connection to note that personality is not conceived, as it is in much psychoanalytic speculation, as being socially determined (e.g. by interactions with parents during early childhood, etc.), but is conceived of rather as having a strong genetic determination, and as being closely dependent upon anatomical and neurophysiological structures and processes (Eysenck, 1967, 1981). The evidence for these assertions is strong, and if we conceive of personality in this fashion, then the possibility of psychosomatic disease assumes a much more realistic aspect. We do not now have a confrontation between mental and physical events, or between biological and social determinants, but rather an interaction between one set of biochemical and physiological events and another. Social influences, such as stress, are conceived of as producing hormonal, physiological and other biological effects, and may thus interact with personality and other psychological variables in a manner which does not present the contradictions involved in Cartesian dualism. As T. H. Huxley pointed out: 'No psychosis without a neurosis', i.e. no psychic events without an underlying neural event. It is on such a dual-aspect or epiphenomenal view of the relationship between body and mind that the theories discussed in this paper are based.

2. PERSONALITY AND LUNG CANCER

It should be noted that just as much of the literature on psychosomatic diseases is based on very poor evidence, the same must be said about the link between stressful life experiences and disease (Kasl, 1983). This author reviews the evidence available at the moment, and points out the difficulties of applying the notion of 'cause' and 'effect' to the complex interactions apparent in human behaviour. 'For example, the many sides of poverty are seen in the co-existence or co-occurrence of a large number of interrelated problems: physical illness, mental illness, low income, unemployment, social disorganisation, racial discrimination, broken families, poor housing, slum location, crime and delinquency, alcoholism and drug abuse, and so on. A scientist who boldly steps in and imposes causal arrows on these variables had better have a strong research design to back him up.' (p. 97). As Kasl points out, no such strong designs seem to bolster up the many conclusions drawn by research workers in the field. In this connection, it is interesting to compare the two edited volumes on stressful life events by Dohrenwend and Dohrenwend (1974, 1981). In the earlier volume there was a large section dealing with content, i.e. empirical findings, and a small section on methodology, whereas the later volume is overwhelmingly methodological, with novel empirical findings almost entirely absent. Kasl (1983) raises the question whether at the moment methodological research should replace substantive research until our methodology is properly organised. We must note, therefore, that there is little reason for confidence in existing stress research, insofar as it is related to disease, and that in this the development has been very similar to that of the psychosomatic disease concept.

The notion of psychosomatic disease is intimately related to the concept of individual differences in susceptibility; were all people similarly liable to develop a given disease, the notion of psychosomatic causes would seem to be unnecessary. Given that people of different personality show differential incidence of disease, it becomes reasonable to ask what it is in the personality of these people that causes them to develop, or not to develop the disease in question. It was with this notion in mind that Kissen and Eysenck (1962) began to investigate with the use of objective tests various theories about the relationship between cancer and personality which has been voiced over the past millenia. There is a long history of theories linking emotion with cancer, going back to the Greek physician Galen (A.D. 131–201); more recent theories have been reviewed in a number of papers quoted by Kissen and Eysenck. Using a short form of the M.P.I., a questionnaire which measures neuroticism and extraversion, these authors tested 116 male lung cancer patients and 123 lung cancer controls, both groups being patients at surgical and medical chest units tested *before* diagnosis. Patients and controls were subdivided into age groups before a comparison of their scores was made. Patients were also subdivided into those with and without psychosomatic disorders of the types at that time recognised.

It was found that the control group had much higher N scores than the cancer group, regardless of psychosomatic involvement. The highly significant finding there gave some support to the hypothesis that lung cancer patients differ from other patients with respect to personality, the major differences being with respect to lack of, or suppression of, emotionality in cancer patients.

As regards extraversion, differences were only found in comparing the groups with psychosomatic disorder, where the cancer group was considerably more extraverted than the control group. This differentiation was found in all the age groups; in patients without psychosomatic disorders, a similar trend was found only for the younger age groups. Kissen (1964a, b) took up the relationship between lung cancer and lack of neuroticism, and again found that the lung cancer patients had very significantly lower N scores than did the other patients. From the obtained figures he calculated lung cancer mortality rates per 100,000 men aged 25 and over by levels of neuroticism scores, and found that people with very low scores had a mortality rate of 296, those with intermediate scores of 108, and those with very high scores of only 56! Thus very low scorers on N have about a six-fold possibility of developing lung cancer as compared with very high scorers.

More recently, Berndt *et al.* (1980), using Eysenck's E.P.I. questionnaire, compared control groups of patients with patients who *after* completion of the questionnaire were found to suffer from breast cancer or bronchial carcinoma. Large numbers of patients and controls were used, and very significant differences were obtained with cancer patients having neuroticism scores lower than controls (Eysenck, 1981). In this study no significant differences were found for extraversion.

In 1962, Hagnell reported on the results of an epidemiological survey of the 2,505 inhabitants of two adjacent rural parishes in the South of Sweden. This survey was started in 1947 and included an interview during which a personality assessment was made on each subject. Ten years later the procedure was repeated and the subsequent history of each subject examined. During this follow-up it was observed that a significantly higher proportion of women who had developed cancer had been originally rated as extraverted. This finding would seem to support the theory put forward by Walshe (1846), who had claimed that 'women of high colour and sanguinous temperament were more subject to mammary cancers than those of different constitutions'.

A study by Coppen and Metcalfe (1963) was in good agreement with Hagnell's findings. They contrasted 47 patients who had a malignant tumour (32 had cancer of the breast, 4 had cancer of the uterus, and 11 had cancer of other parts of the body), with two control groups. They found that the cancer group had significantly higher extraversion scores than both control groups, with the subgroups of cancer patients all having very similar means. They concluded: 'Although the nature of this association is by no means clear one may perhaps speculate that certain constitutional factors predispose individuals to develop malignant tumours. Extraversion may be one manifestation of this constitutional difference which may also be related to physique and to hormonal activity.'

Later studies by Kissen, summarised in his 1968 paper, report an extension of the works so far discussed, using different methods of personality assessment; the general findings tend to support the original relationship between lung cancer and low neuroticism. Trends were also found for high extraversion and lung cancer patients, but the trend is rather weaker.

More recently Greer and Morris (1975), using breast cancer patients, studied a consecutive series of 160 women at hospital for breast tumour biopsy. They used detailed structured interviews and standard tests, including the M.P.I., conducting the interviews and tests on the day before operation without knowledge of the provisional diagnosis. Information obtained from patients was verified in almost all cases by separate interviews with husbands or close relatives. The principal finding was the significant association between the diagnosis of breast cancer and the behaviour pattern, persisting throughout adult life, of abnormal release of emotions. 'This abnormality was, in most cases, extreme suppression of other feelings. Extreme expression of emotions, though much less common, also occurred in a higher proportion of cancer patients than controls.' No relation was found with extraversion. A study by Abse *et al.* (1974) concerned with lung cancer patients, tended to bear out the hypothesis on the relationship between lung cancer and low emotionality, although the methods used for ascertaining personality differences seem to have been rather subjective.

Various other studies give indirect support to relationships between personality and cancer discussed in this section (e.g. Ure, 1969; Pettingale *et al.*, 1977; Achterberg *et al.*, 1976, 1977; Krasnoff, 1959; Evans *et al.*, 1965; Kissen and Rowe, 1969; Stavraky, 1968).

A rather different type of study suggests a similar kind of conclusion, i.e. that strong anxiety and other emotions may be *negatively* correlated with lung cancer. Eysenck (1980d) has reviewed a long list of studies, beginning with the work of Bahnson and Bahnson (1964a) suggesting that: 'Cancer is an alternative to psychosis'. Psychosis is certainly prominently associated with strong emotional reactions (except in burnt out schizophrenics), and it is widely observed that psychotics appear to be relatively immune to lung cancer, in spite of the fact that smoking is very prevalent among them. Levi and Waxman (1975) have put forward the suggestion that the low incidence of cancer in schizophrenics may be the result of a metabolic defect, related to a lack of labile methyl groups, but this hypothesis is no better supported than other biochemical theories. The fact remains that the incidence of cancer in psychotics is less than one-third of that occurring among normal people, and this fact certainly calls for an explanation.

In concluding this section, it may be useful to draw attention to a study by Rae and McCall (1973) which relates extraversion and neuroticism, on the one hand, to both smoking and lung cancer, on the other. The authors attempted to demonstrate that an association between cancer and personality holds internationally. National extraversion and anxiety levels in eight advanced countries, and statistics of the number of cigarettes smoked per adult per annum in these countries, were compared with mortality rates per 100,000 of the population due to lung cancer (males and females separately) and cancer of the cervix (females only).

Rank order correlations were calculated between national personality levels and cancer mortality rate. There was a highly significant correlation between extraversion and male lung cancer (0.66) and between extraversion and female lung cancer (0.72). Corresponding correlations for cigarette smoking and lung cancer, for males and females combined, were quite insignificant (0.07). For cancer of the cervix a correlation with extraversion was again significant (0.64), whereas for cigarette consumption it was insignificant (0.45). Correlations between anxiety and lung cancer were negative in both sexes (-0.52 and -0.71). Thus the investigation of individual correlations within one country, indicating a positive correlation between lung cancer and extraversion, and a negative one between lung cancer and neuroticism, are confirmed in these comparisons between countries. It would appear that lung cancer is positively correlated with extraversion, negatively with neuroticism, although of course it would be most desirable to have these relationships confirmed on larger samples.

3. STRESS AND CANCER

It has often been found in retrospective studies that life stress events frequently precede the appearance of different forms of neoplasia (e.g. Bahnson and Bahnson, 1964; Greene, 1966; Horne and Picard, 1979; Jacobs and Charles, 1980). Greene and Swisher (1969) investigated the effect of genetic factors by looking at leukemia in monozygotic twins discordant for the illness, and found that psychological stress was an important feature in the origins of the disease. Reviews by Bloom *et al.* (1978) and Fox (1978) give a good account of the literature.

It seems that loss of spouse has been one of the stressors most frequently studied, and a number of investigations (Bloom *et al.*, 1978; Greene, 1966; LeShan., 1966; Lombard and Potter, 1950; Murphy, 1952, Peller, 1952; Ernster *et al.*, 1979) are in agreement in showing that cancer appeared in higher than expected frequency among such individuals. Retrospective studies are of course subject to many difficulties (Fox, 1978; Sklar and Anisman, 1981), but agreement seems to be fairly close (but see Kasl, 1983). Some theories furnish an explanation for the influence of emotional, psychosocial and anxiety-stimulated stress influencing the growth of neoplasia. Such stress produces increased plasma concentration of adrenal corticoids, and other hormones, through well known neuroendocrine pathways (Riley, 1981). These corticoid concentrations are known to enter elements of the immunological apparatus, and this may leave the subject vulnerable to the action of latent oncogenic viruses, newly transferred cancer cells, or other incipient pathological processes that are normally held in check by an intact immunological apparatus. Riley describes studies supporting the view that increased plasma concentrations of adrenal corticoids have adverse effects on the thymus and thymus-dependent T-cells, i.e. elements which constitute the major defence system against various neoplastic processes and other pathologies. He cites studies which show that anxiety-stress can be quantitatively induced, and the consequences measured through specific biochemical and cellular effects, always provided that proper baselines of these conditions are obtained in the experimental animals by the use of low-stress protective housing and handling techniques.

The facts, linking stress with cancer both in humans and animals, pose a paradox for the investigator because there is an apparent contradiction between this work and that on personality. If stress can produce or facilitate the growth and metastasis of cancers, then one would expect cancer to be associated with *high* levels of neuroticism, and with psychosis. There is no doubt that a psychotic condition is highly stressful to the individual concerned, and similarly the evidence is overwhelming that a higher degree of emotional instability, such as is found in high N scorers, is both productive of stress-inducing situations, and increases the level of stress experienced by the individual. Thus we have an apparent contradiction, in the sense that those personality traits which generate stress in the individual also apparently seem to protect him against cancer, in spite of the fact that stress has frequently been shown to induce cancer. Does this apparent contradiction have an explanation?

Eysenck (1983b) has suggested an explanation in terms of what he calls the 'inoculation effect'. It is clear from animal studies that we need to distinguish carefully between acute and chronic stress. It appears from studies surveyed by Eysenck (1983b) that while acute stress increases the incidence of spontaneous tumours, chronic stress has the opposite effect. It seems that this generalization also holds for the development of metastases. Zimel *et al.* (1977) have shown that acute stress may exacerbate metastases, but that under conditions of chronic shock administration, the formation and growth of metastases was inhibited, very much in the way that chronic stress inhibited the induction and growth of primary tumours.

There seems to be a remarkable parallel among the stress effects on neurochemical, hormonal and immunological functioning. As Sklar and Anisman (1981) point out: 'Acute stress results in depletion of catecholamines and increases of ACh, increased synthesis and secretion of hormones and immuno-suppression. Adaptation in these biological mechanisms is observed with chronic stress, such that normal levels of functioning or alteration opposite to those induced by acute stress are apparent. '(p. 391). We may thus conclude that there is some evidence that acute stress produces tumour *growth*, chronic stress tumour *reduction*, and also that acute stress exacerbates metastases, while chronic stress inhibits metastases. As Eysenck (1983b) has pointed out, 'We may perhaps call this effect "an inoculation effect"; it is as if the previous experience of stress inoculates the animal against subsequent stress, making it less effective, or reversing the biological changes produced.' (p. 128).

Gray *et al*. (1981) have reviewed psychological experimentation relevant to the inoculation efect. Brown and Wagner (1964) may be quoted as reporting a typical defining experiment in this context. Two groups of rats were studied in a situation where they were trained to run an alley for food reward, one group being given continuous reinforcement, the other also receiving electric shocks, initially of low intensity, but gradually increasing in intensity on successive trials. In the second phase of the experiment, both groups were given reward together with a high-intensity shock on every trial. Comparing the two groups, it was found that the group which previously received shock shows much less reluctance to go to food-plus-shock than did the group that did not receive shock.

A similar paradigm is that of 'learned helplessness' (Seligman *et al*. 1971). In this type of experiment, one group of rats is given a single session in which it is exposed to inescapable electric shock. It is then trained in a task in which it is again shocked, but in which it is possible to escape from the shock, or avoid it, by jumping from side to side of the shuttle-box in which they are being trained. The control group without exposure to the initial inescapable shocks is also tested in the shuttle-box. It is usually found that the group with the 'learned helplessness' experience is worse at escaping from shock in the shuttle-box than the control group. However, when the experiment is now repeated with the 'learned helplessness' group given 15 daily sessions of inescapable shock before the shuttle-box test, such animals are just as good at learning to escape shock as the controls. Miller (1976) has termed this effect 'toughening up', and Weiss *et al*. (1975) have reported a similar experiment, identical to the one mentioned above, except that, in place of the inescapable shock sessions, the rats were made to swim in cold water for 3 to 4 minutes before the shuttle-box test session. Like inescapable shock, this treatment impaired shuttle-box performance, and also like inescapable shock, 15 consecutive day sessions of 'cold swim' can overcome the initial deficit, so that shuttle-box performance tested after the final swim is normal.

'Frustrative non-reward' can be used in a similar way to shock or 'cold swim' (Gray, 1975). Like these other stressors, frustrative non-reward elicits a rise in plasma corticosterone (Goldman *et al.*, 1973). This technique has been used in experiments similar to those quoted above, where again two groups of rats are trained to run in an alley for food reward. One is the control or continuous reinforcement group; the second is trained with a partial reinforcement schedule. In the test phase of the experiment, the simple extinction paradigm is used, and it is found that the experimental group continues to run to the now empty goal box much more persistently than the control group (Lewis, 1960). As Gray *et al.* (1981) summarise these findings: 'In each of these four experiments the animal is exposed repeatedly to a stressor (shock, non-reward, cold-swim) and comes in consequence to show reduced behavioural responses to the stressor. In these cases, then, the animal develops tolerance for the stressor to which it is exposed.' (p. 154).

Not only do we find direct tolerance effects, outlined above, but also evidence of cross-tolerance. Thus exposure to the punishment schedule gives rise to increased resistance to extinction, and conversely, exposure to partial reinforcement schedule gives rise to increased resistance to punishment (Brown and Wagner, 1964). Exposure to repeated inescapable shock can also be shown to lead to increased resistance to extinction (Chen and Amsel, 1977). In addition, Weiss *et al.* (1975) have shown that repeated exposure to shock prevents cold swim from impairing shuttle-box performance, and repeated exposure to cold swim prevents inescapable shock from having this effect. Gray *et al.* (1981) conclude that: 'Cross-tolerance has been demonstrated in both directions for the pairs, shock and non-reward, shock and cold swim; the pair, non-reward and cold swim does not appear to have been investigated as yet.' (P. 154). Gray *et al.* (1981) report research into possible neuromechanisms for stress tolerance of this kind, but a discussion of this theory would take us too far. Let us merely end this section by drawing attention to the close similarities of these experiments and the 'inoculation effect' postulated to account for the beneficial effects of chronic stress, as opposed to the deleterious effects of acute stress.

4. EXTRAVERSION – INTROVERSION: THE CONDITIONING OF THE IMMUNE REACTION

The possible mediation of the personality – cancer relation in respect to neuroticism via the inoculation effect does not of course explain the correlation between extraversion and cancer, and an alternative and quite different theory has to be elaborated. Again this must inevitably be quite speculative, because to date no one has given any constructive thought to this relationship. Eysenck (1984) has suggested a possibility which derives from the well-established fact that introverts have higher resting levels of cortical arousal than extraverts (Eysenck, 1967, 1981), and that Pavlovian conditioning is facilitated by high levels of arousal. The resulting prediction that introverts would tend to condition better than extraverts has found considerable support (Levey and Martin, 1981), and while there are many qualifications relating to the strength of the unconditioned stimulus, the appetitive or aversive nature of the stimulus, etc., on the whole it may be said that for many purposes this generalization holds.

These findings are very relevant to a consideration of the relationship between personality and lung cancer because there is good evidence that immune reactions can be conditioned, using Pavlovian paradigms (Ader, 1981; Ader and Cohen, 1975; Rogers *et al.*, 1976; Wayner *et al.* 1978; Cohen *et al.*, 1979). The evidence suggests that carcinogenic cells continue to be produced in the body on a more or less random basis, and that the influence of the immune reaction is paramount in deciding whether or not these will develop into metastising carcinomas. Hence anything that can influence the development of immune reactions is of vital importance in the study of the development of cancer. If it is indeed true, as it seems to be, that the immune reaction can be conditioned, then obviously individual differences in conditionability would have far-reaching effects on the development of cancers. If introverts succeed in developing the immune reaction more rapidly, more strongly and more lastingly than do extraverts, then we would have here an explanation of the correlation between cancer and extraversion.

Conditioning the immune reaction has utilised in the main the taste aversion paradigm (Garcia *et al.*, 1974; Riley and Clark, 1977). In this passive avoidance situation, injection of a drug immediately followed the ingestion of a novel, distinctly flavoured drinking solution. A single such pairing of the flavoured solution with the aversive effects of the drug leads to a drastic reduction of the further consumption of the solution, even though tests may be conducted months later. Ader and Cohen (1975) applied this conditioning procedure in order to suppress an immune response. They injected cyclophosphamide (CY) into rats that had just drunk a saccharine solution. Later on, when the animals were exposed to the saccharine solution at the same time that sheep erythrocytes were injected, the investigators found a reduced serum antibody response. Their conclusion was that pairing of the injection of CY, which is of course a potent immunosuppressive drug, with consumption of the saccarine solution produced not only conditioned taste aversion, but also conditioned suppression of the humoral immune response. This conditioned immunosuppression in rats challenged with the thymus-dependent antigen sheep erythrocytes, has since been replicated by Rogers *et al.* (1976) and Wayner *et al.* (1978). Cohen *et al.* (1979) have found the same effects, using mice challenged with the thymus-independent antigen 2,4,6-trinitrophenyl-lipopolysaccharide. These experiments do seem to give powerful support to the idea that immune suppression (and presumably therefore also immune facilitation) can be conditioned along Pavlovian lines.

More recently, Bovbjerg *et al*. (1982) have reported experiments undertaken to extend the conditioning phenomenon to include the other major class of immune reactions, the cellular response. They conditioned suppression of a regional graft-versus-host reaction, using injection of parental strain lymphoid cells into the footpads of F_1 hybrid offspring. Injecting the recipients with CY dramatically reduces the cullular response. In the conditioning trial, three injections of CY at 10 mg/kg were used and compared with a condition in which two of the three injections of CY administered after grafting were replaced by re-exposure to conditioned stimuli (i.e. a saccarine solution and an injection of saline). The results suggested that conditioned immunosuppression did indeed affect the popliteal GvHR, a cellular immune response.

As already noted, all these studies have dealt with the suppression of the immune reaction, but if the mechanism works as outlined, then it would seem to follow that the strengthening of the immune reaction should also be possible through Pavlovian conditioning. In fact, it would seem that in everyday life immunosuppression is much less likely to occur than immuno-enhancement, possibly through chronic stress reactions as pointed out in previous sections of this chapter. The whole field clearly needs urgent replication of such studies that have been carried out with the variable of individual differences included in the experimental paradigm. As Eysenck and Eysenck (in press) have pointed out, there is now evidence that personality dimensions corresponding to extraversion – introversion and neuroticism – stability can be found and measured in animals, and hence there should be no particular difficulty in carrying out such studies of individual differences, or possibly strain differences.

It should be noted that the postulated effects of conditioning might also affect the negative correlation between neuroticism and lung cancer. As Eysenck (1981) has pointed out, under certain specified conditions strong anxiety reactions may facilitate the conditioning process, as postulated by Spence and Spence (1966); this would lead to a positive correlation between anxiety/neuroticism and conditioning. Thus a conditioning mechanism may also mediate a better conditioning of the immune reaction in high N scorers, particularly as a strong degree of emotion necessary for producing the effects is more likely to be found under conditions of environmental stress. Here too direct examination of the hypothesis by means of suitably planned experiments is obviously a sine qua non for the acceptance of the speculations contained in this section. Enough is known about the relationship between conditioning and personality to make fairly confident predictions, but confident prediction is no substitute for experimental verification.

5. THEORIES OF LUNG CANCER

There are many theories of cancer causation, most of which can be subsumed under two headings. First we have the very popular set of theories implicating external factors, such as cigarette smoking, air pollution, asbestos, etc. in the causation of cancer. External theories of this kind are usually based on epidemiological evidence, and this evidence often suffers greatly from poor statistical treatment, bad experimental design, and other avoidable causes (Eysenck, 1980). Smoking, in particular, has often been implicated in these theories, but the evidence does not suggest that confident assertions can at the moment be made. This is not to doubt the possibility, or even the probability, that external factors do facilitate the development of cancers. It is merely pointed out that with respect to specific relationships the evidence may not be as satisfactory as one might wish, and that the theories which have been developed are not normally specific enough to be tested by research paradigms which are anything other than circumstantial.

A second important group of theorists denies the importance of external factors, and instead advocates a concept of *spontaneous malignancy*, resulting from the intrinsic instability of complex biological structures such as genes (Burch, 1976; Oeser, 1979). These theories are rather complex, but rely mostly on mathematical models plotting age developments of the disease in detail. There certainly is considerable evidence for such spontaneous malignancy, but this theory is not necessarily opposed to one which postulates the importance of external factors. Such external factors might facilitate the *growth* and *spreading* of spontaneous malignancies, e.g. by impairing the immune system, or in other ways. The picture is a complex and involved one, and nothing is to be gained by exaggerating the influence of any particular causal factor. Indeed, few of the researchers and writers involved in these controversies seem to take to heart Hume's criticism of the very concept of causality, criticisms which have peculiar force in relation to this field in view of the likely multiplicity of causal factors, none of which can with any certainty be labelled 'the' cause.

Certainly, when we look at any specific agent, such as cigarette smoke, as a causal element in the development of lung cancer, the evidence makes it clear that this is neither *necessary* nor a *sufficient* cause. Out of ten heavy smokers, only one will die of lung cancer; hence smoking clearly is not a sufficient cause. Out of ten people who die of lung cancer, one will be a non-smoker, hence smoking is clearly not a necessary cause. The search for single causes is probably more motivated by social than by scientific demands, and this has led to a very serious deterioration in the quality of research devoted to these problems (Eysenck, 1980d).

There is some agreement on the fact that both within and across nations correlations can be found between the incidence of lung cancer and the smoking of cigarettes. Here again, of course, one should really be more specific. Kreyberg (1962) found a relationship between smoking and his Group 1 lung tumours (squamous carcinomas), but none between smoking and his Group 2 lung tumours (adenocarcinomas). This provides difficulties for those who argue that the recent increase in lung cancer in females is due to their having taken up smoking; the increase has been in adenocarcinomas, which were thought not to be related to smoking! Another difficulty with the data is that there are good reasons for doubting the reliability of diagnosis as far as lung cancer is concerned (Eysenck, 1980d); such cancers used to be greatly under-diagnosed as the cause of death, and are now probably greatly over-diagnosed. In spite of these and other difficulties it will probably be wise to accept the existence of a correlation between these two variables, but the interpretation of this corrrelation as having a causal basis, i.e. that cigarette smoking *causes* lung cancer (or is instrumental in its growth and spreading) is far from mandatory, and may be mistaken. Eysenck (1980d) and Burch (1976) have looked carefully at the evidence presented, and have arrived at the conclusion that the evidence was far from conclusive. What might be called the 'causal' hypothesis is certainly a possible interpretation, but alternative hypotheses are also tenable, such as those of Burch and Oeser.

Eysenck (1984) has presented a theory which is radically different from, and may be supplementary to, those discussed so far. This hypothesis is shown in diagrammatic form in Figure 4. 1, and attempts to relate lung cancer, stress, personality and smoking in terms of certain underlying genetic factors. Put briefly, the hypothesis suggests that genetic factors are in part responsible for both the smoking of cigarettes and the occurrence of lung cancer, either directly or through the intermediary of personality. The correlation between smoking and lung cancer would, on this hypothesis, be indirect (non-causal), and due to the similarity of the genetic factors responsible for *both* smoking and lung cancer.

To substantiate the general scheme outlined in Figure 4.1, we must provide evidence: (1) that genetic factors are involved in the causation of lung cancer; (2) that genetic factors are involved in the maintenance of the smoking habit; (3) that genetic factors are implicated in the development of personality; (4) that personality is related to smoking; (5) that personality is related to lung cancer; (6) that stress is related to smoking; and (7) that stress is related to lung cancer. Furthermore, we should be able to point to experimentally established causal factors mediating some of these relationships. We have already discussed items (5) and (7); we will here take up some of the remaining points.

There seems to be little doubt about the importance of genetic factors in the causation of lung cancer. Lynch (1976) has provided a general overview of the field of cancer genetics, and as regards lung cancer in particular, we

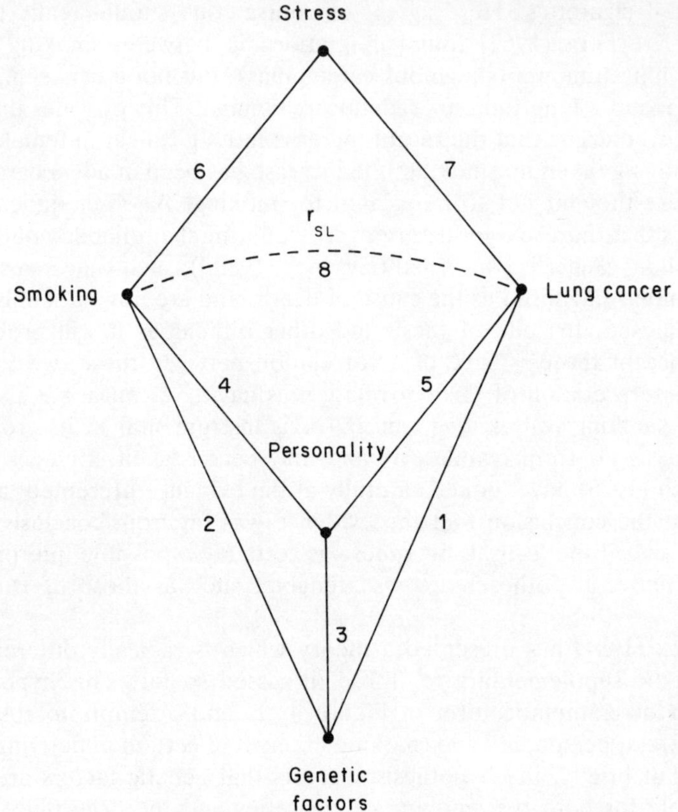

Figure 4.1: Path analysis of factor linking stress, personality, smoking and lung cancer.

have the work of Tokuhata (1964, 1976) and Tokuhata and Lilienfeld (1963a, b) which would seem to establish a firm genetic basis for lung cancer. These investigators studied first-degree relatives of 270 lung cancer probands and first-degree relatives of 270 controls, matched for race, sex, age and residence. Deaths from lung cancer among non-smoking first-degree relatives of probands were found to be 3.8 times greater than expected on the basis of those observed in non-smoking first-degree relatives of controls. The corresponding ratio among smokers was 2.3. Combining both sexes, as well as smokers and non-smokers, the probability that these differences between probands and controls could have arisen by chance was calculated at $p < 0.0006$. This seems good evidence for the existence of a strong genetic predisposing factor in the development of cancer. For all causes of death, and for all cancers, similar ratio differences were found, with that for all cancers being very much higher than that for all causes of death. It is interesting that among the relatives of probands a significantly higher proportion were smokers than among the relatives of controls; this suggests the influence of genetic factors in smoking.

Many other studies are cited in Eysenck (1984) to demonstrate the genetic determination of cancer. Burch (1976) concluded from these studies that: '(*a*) smoking and lung cancer are positively associated; (*b*) certain genes predispose to lung cancer; (*c*) certain genes predispose to smoking; (*d*) the net positive familial association between lung cancer and all causes of death is genetically based; (*e*) the net positive familial association between lung cancer and all cancers has a genetic basis; (*f*) the net positive familial association between lung cancer and fatal non-malignant respiratory diseases has a genetic basis; and (*g*) the net negative familial association between lung cancer and fatal disease other than under (*e*) has a genetic basis . . . although these data support genetic hypotheses of positive and negative association between smoking and disease, they do not exclude additional causal factors.'

The literature on the influence of genetic factors on smoking behaviour is large (e.g. Fisher, 1958a, b, c; Shields, 1962; Todd and Mason, 1959; Friberg *et al.*, 1959; Conteno and Chiarelli, 1962; Hamtoft and Lindhardt, 1956; Cederlöf *et al.*, 1977); these studies universally find greater concordance among MZ than among DZ twins.

A detailed discussion of these studies is given in Eysenck (1980d); his work deals with much larger samples of MZ and DZ twins than previous studies, and in addition uses the latest model fitting methods of genetic analysis. He also made use of data gathered from adopted children, and from intrafamilial analyses. The general conclusion from this work was that while the *origin* of the smoking habit was not much influenced by genetic factors, but rather was due to peer pressure, the *maintenance* of the smoking habit was strongly influenced by genetic factors. The picture that emerges from these analyses is much more complex than this, of course, but these complexities are of no particular interest in the development of our theme, and will therefore not be detailed here.

As regards the determination of *personality* by genetic factors, a good review of this topic has recently been given by Fulker (1981). As he demonstrates, the major dimensions of personality, in particular extraversion and neuroticism, are strongly determined by genetic factors, to the extent of approximately two-thirds of the total 'true' variance. The genetic architecture of personality differs from that presented by intelligence, in that whereas for intelligence non-additive genetic variance (dominance, assortative mating) play a highly significant part, these non-additive genetic factors are absent in relation to personality. Again, whereas for intelligence between-family environmental factors are about twice as important as within-family environmental factors, for personality between-family environmental factors seem to play little if any part. However that may be, there can be no doubt that genetic factors play a vitally important role in determining individual differences in personality. We may conclude that the relationship between lung cancer, and personality and smoking mediated by genetic factors (i.e. numbers 1, 2 and 3 in Figure 4.1) have received substantial empirical support. Relations between personality and smoking (number 4 in Figure 4.1) have also received considerable support, as reviewed by Eysenck (1980d). The major finding would appear to be that the smoking of cigarettes is correlated significantly with extraversion, neuroticism and psychoticism, in children and adolescents as well as in adults. In addition there are also negative correlations with the L (lie or dissimulation) scale in the Eysenck Personality Questionnaire (Eysenck and Eysenck, 1975), a scale which may often be interpreted as a measure of conformity.

It should be noted that there are certain sex and national differences which are not always easy to interpret. Women for instance seem to show higher correlations between smoking and neuroticism than do males, possibly due to the fact that women have higher neuroticism scores, and tend to smoke in stressful situations to a greater extent than do men (Frith, 1971). Correlations between neuroticism and smoking seem to be found more regularly in the U.S.A. than in the U.K., for reasons that are not immediately obvious. Motivationally, it seems likely that different personality types smoke for different reasons. Thus extraverts may smoke in order to relieve boredom, high N scorers in order to relieve stress, high P scorers in order to express antagonism and rebelliousness, whereas high L scorers may refrain from smoking in order to manifest conformity to social mores. These points are discussed in some detail by Eysenck (1980d).

As regards stress and smoking (number 6 in Figure 4.1) there has been a good deal of research since the early work of Tomkins (1968), Ikard *et al.* (1969), and others, and the work of McKennell and Thomas (1967) and McKennell (1970) classify smokers according to the occasions on which they smoked. A paper by Russell *et al.* (1974) summarises early work and reports a factorial study giving rise to six main factors (stimulation, indulgence, psycho-social, sensory-motor, addictive, and automatic.) Frith (1971), analysing the occasions on which people like to smoke, found strong evidence for the two major factors postulated by Eysenck (1973), namely high arousal situations in which the major purpose of smoking would be to reduce tension or anxiety, and low arousal situations in which the main purpose of smoking would be to combat boredom and increase cortical arousal. Women tend to smoke more in high arousal situations, men in low arousal situations. Other recent studies (Stanaway and Watson, 1980; Best and Hakstian, 1978; O'Connor, 1980) all find evidence for the existence of at least one type of smoker who smoked in stressful situations in order to reduce anxiety, tension and emotional upset.

In a recent study Spielberger *et al.* (in press) has reported the emergence of five major factors related to smoking. The first of these he calls 'emotional arousal'; this corresponds to the relationship implied in Figure 4.1 between stress and smoking. The second factor (restful and relaxing situations) corresponds to Frith's low-arousal situations. The other factors are of less interest here, but it is important to note that the emotional factor in his study correlated significantly with neuroticism, indicating a similarity between the relations marked 4 and 6 in Figure 4.1.

All these well-documented and observed relationships, diagrammed in Figure 4.1, suggest that the relationship between smoking and lung cancer (number 8 in Figure 4.1) may not be a causal one, but may be the product of genetic factors impinging on personality, and partly through personality factors, partly directly, determining the maintenance of the smoking habit, and the onset of lung cancer. Similarly, stress may be related both to smoking and to lung cancer. The precise nature of these relationships, and their quantitative aspects need to be sorted out in great detail on much larger samples than have been used hitherto, and it is obvious that such apparently unidimensional concepts as 'stress' will have to be refined more carefully in terms of chronic and acute stress. Nevertheless, it appears clear that the evidence presented supports an alternative (or supplementary) theory concerning the relationship between smoking and lung cancer to that which implies a direct causal influence of smoking on lung cancer.

6. SUMMARY AND CONCLUSIONS

The theory here developed concerns the various causal relationships involved in the development of lung cancer of stress, personality and smoking. Regardless of whether it is true or not that smoking 'causes' lung cancer, it is perfectly clear that even if there should be a causal effect of this kind, it is neither necessary nor sufficient for the production of carcinomas, and the picture is far more complex than would be suggested by any such simple-minded hypothesis. While the theory here presented, which is diagrammatically illustrated in Figure 4.1, is of course to some degree speculative, there is, as we have shown, considerable evidence for each of the connective links numbered from 1 to 8 in the figure, and it suggests that the theory might be useful in suggesting novel types of research that have not hitherto been done in the absence of a model of this kind.

In our discussion we have made considerable efforts to distinguish between different carcinogenic effects which should be carefully kept apart. In the first place, we have the *initiation* of the neoplastic disorder. Here Burch's (1976) hypothesis appears to be the most relevant, namely that all disorders with reproducible age-dependence effects can be seen to be *initiated* by specific somatic mutations (probably DNA strand-switching events) in stem cells of the central system of growth control; such disorders are described as *autoaggressive*. The random events that initiate natural autoaggressive disorders obey unexpectedly simple stochastic laws, as Burch has shown. It seems unlikely that these random events are influenced to a considerable degree by environmental factors, i.e. either by stress, or smoking, or any other indirect factor.

The second stage is one of *progression*, in which the randomly occurring events which initiate natural autoaggressive disorders fail to be controlled by the immune system. While Burch assumes constant somatic mutations to occur, usually controlled by the immune system, this control fails for various reasons, and then the cancer is allowed to develop. It is at this stage that one might imagine environmental factors (pollution, asbestos, etc.) to have an effect, not so much in enhancing the activity of the cancer itself, but rather by a weakening of the immune system. Stress and stress-related personality factors are likely to exert an influence at this stage.

The third and final stage is that of metastasis, i.e. when the developing tumours are beginning to metastase. Here too the immune reaction presumably plays a vital role, and here too we may imagine that stress and stress-related personality factors may exert a controlling influence.

As Eysenck (1984) points out: 'We thus have four separate factors which may be related to stress and personality, and may be influenced directly or indirectly by genetic factors; the random events that initiate natural autoaggressive disorders, the development of these into neoplastic diseases, the metastasing of the resulting carcinomas, and the immune reaction which may determine the outcome of the second and third stages, and their development. There are suggestions in the literature as to which of these four stages may be involved with stress, personality etc., but it would be premature at the moment to try and give specific details about them. Such detailed exploration must be the task of future experiments.'

The theory here presented has the advantage of being eminently testable. Each of the separate components of it could be falsified by suitable experiment. This is not true of the orthodox 'causal' hypothesis. What the 'causal' hypothesis does is to translate correlation into causation, without specifying the particular mechanisms involved. This of course makes the theory difficult to falsify, and to that extent it is not a scientific theory at all, in Popper's sense. In spite of this objection it may of course be true, at least to some extent, but at the moment the evidence is insufficient to come to any definitive conclusion (Eysenck, 1980d).

Work on the genetic hypothesis here outlined, which in its most general form dates back to Fisher (1958a) has been hampered very much by an ideological climate which finds in cigarette smoking an easy and obvious enemy, and refuses to consider either the evidence contradicting the causal role of smoking, or to take seriously alternative theories. This seems a great pity, as the rather simple-minded advice to give up smoking in order to live longer is not only difficult to follow, but is also unlikely to be found factually correct in the long run (Multiple Risk Factor Intervention Trial Research Group, 1982). The situation is very much more complex than this simplistic theory asserts, and until and unless we take this complexity of nature seriously, we will be grossly hampered in our efforts to conquer what is at the moment a frightening and all too widespread disease. Ultimately it will be found necessary to carry out research in these apparently remote and recondite areas, and while it is of course at present impossible to forecast the nature of the final theory of causation of lung cancer and other carcinomas that will emerge from this research, it seems not impossible that some of the suggestions contained in this paper will find a place, albeit perhaps only a supporting one, in this theory.

REFERENCES

Abse, D. W., Wilkins, M. M., Castle, R., Buxton, W. D., Demars, J., Brown, R. S., and Kirschner, L. G. (1974). Personality and behavioral characteristics of lung cancer patients *Journal of Psychosomatic Research,* **18**, 101–113.

Achterberg, J., Lawlis, G. G., Simonton, O. C. and Simonton, S. M. (1977). Psychological factors and blood chemistries as disease outcome predictors for cancer patients, *Multivariate Experimental Clinical Reaearch*, **3**, 107–122.

Achterberg, J., Simonton, O. C., and Matthews-Simonton, S. (1976). *Stress, Psychological Factors and Cancer*, New Medicine Press, Fort Worth.

Ader, R. (Ed.) (1981). *Psychoneuroimmunology*, Academic Press, New York and London.

Ader, R., and Cohen, N. (1975). Behaviorally conditioned immuno-suppression, *Psychosomatic Medicine*, **37**, 333–340.

Bahnson, C. B., and Bahnson, M. B. (1964a). Cancer as an alternative to psychoses, in *Psychosomatic Aspects of Neoplastic Disease*. (Eds. D. M. Kissen and I. I. LeShan) Lippincott, Philadelphia.

Bahnson, C. B., and Bahnson, M. B. ((1964b) Denial and repression of primitive impulses and of disturbing emotion in patients with malignant neoplasms, in *Psychosomatic Aspects of Neoplastic Disease*(Eds. D. M. Kissen and I. I. LeShan) Lippincott, Philadelphia.

Berndt, H., Günther, H., and Rothe, G. (1980). Persönlichkeitsstruktur nach Eysenck bei Kranken mit Brustrüsen und Bronchialkrebs und Diagnoseverzögerung durch den Patienten, *Archiv für Geschwulstforschung*, **50**, 359–368.

Best, J., and Hakstian, A. (1978). A situation-specific model for smoking behavior, *Addictive Behaviors*, **3**, 79–92.

Binnie-Dawson, J. L. M. (1982). A bio-social approach to environmental psychology and problems of stress, *International Journal of Psychology*, **17**, 397–435.

Bloom, B. L., Asher, J. J., and White, S. W. (1978) Marital disruption as a stressor. A review and analysis, *Psychological Bulletin*, **85**, 867–894.

Bovbjerg, D., Ader, R., and Cohen, N. (1982). Behaviorally conditioned suppression of a graft-versus-host response, *Proceedings of the National Academy of Sciences, U.S.A.* **79**, 583–585.

Brown, R. T., and Wagner, A. R. (1964). Resistance to punishment and extinction following training with shock or nonreinforcement, *Journal of Experimental Psychology*, **68**, 503–507.

Burch, P. R. T. (1976). *The Biology of Cancer. A New Approach*, MTP Press, Lancaster.

Cederlöf, R., Friberg, L., and Lundman, T. (1977). The interaction of smoking, environment and heredity and their implications for disease etiology, *Acta Medica Scandinavia*, Supplement, 612.

Chen, J. S., and Amsel, A. (1977). Prolonged, unsignaled, inescapable shocks increase persistence in subsequent appetitive instrumental learning, *Animal Learning Behaviour*, **5**, 377–385.

Cohen, N., Ader, R., Green, N., and Bovbjerg, D. (1979). Conditioned suppression of a thymus-independent antibody response, *Psychosomatic Medicine*, **41**, 487–491.

Conteno, F., and Chiarelli, B. (1962) Study of the inheritance of some daily life habits, *Heredity*, **17**, 347–359.

Coppen, A., and Metcalfe, M. (1963) Cancer and extraversion, *British Medical Journal*, 1963, July 6, pp. 18–19.

Dohrenwend, B. P., and Dohrenwend, B. S. (1981). Socioenvironmental factors, stress, and psychopathology, *American Journal of Community Psychology*, **9**, 128–59.

Dohrenwend, B. S., and Dohrenwend, B. P. (Eds.) (1974). *Stressful Life Events*, John Wiley & Sons, New York.

Ernster, V. L., Sacks, S. T., Selvin, S., and Petrakis, N. L. (1979). Cancer incidence by marital states: U.S. Third National Cancer Survey, *Journal of the National Cancer Institute*, **63**, 567–585.

Evans, R. B., Stein, E., and Marmorston, J. (1965). Psychological-hormonal relationships in men with cancer. *Psychological Reports*, **17**, 7–15.

Eysenck, H. J. (1967). *The Biological Basis of Personality*, C. C. Thomas, Springfield.

Eysenck, H. J. (1973). Personality and the maintenance of the smoking habit, in *Smoking Behavior: Motives and Incentives*, (Ed. W. L. Dunn), John Wiley & Sons, London.

Eysenck, H. J. (1977). *You and Neurosis*, Maurice Temple Smith, London.

Eysenck, H. J. (1980a) Man as a biosocial animal: comments on the sociobiology debate, *Political Psychology (Journal of the International Society of Political Psychology)*, **2**, 43–51.

Eysenck, H. J. (1980b) The bio-social model of man and the unification of psychology, in *Models of Man*, (Eds. A. J. Chapman and D. M. Jones) The British Psychological Society, Leicester.

Eysenck, H. J. (1980c) The biosocial nature of man, *Journal of Social and Biological Structures*, **3**, 124–134.

Eysenck, H. J. (1980d) *The Causes and Effects of Smoking*, Maurice Temple Smith, London.

Eysenck, H. J. (1981). *A Model for Personality*. Springer Verlag, Berlin & New York.

Eysenck, H. J. (1983a) Classical conditioning and extinction: the general model for the treatment of neurotic disorders, in M. Rosenbaum, C. M. Franks, & Y. Jaffe (Eds.) *Perspectives on Behavior Therapy in the Eighties*, Vol. 9 – *Springer Series on Behavior Therapy & Behavioral Medicine*. Springer Verleg, New York.

Eysenck, H. J. (1983b). Stress, disease, and personality: the 'inoculation' effect, in *Stress Research*, (Ed. C. L. Cooper), pp. 121–146, John Wiley & Sons, New York.

Eysenck, H. J. (1984). Personality, stress and lung cancer, in *Medical Psychology*, Vol. III, (Ed. S. Rachman), Pergamon Press, Oxford.

Eysenck, H. J., and Eysenck, M. W. (in press). *Personality and Individual Differences. A Natural Science Approach*. Plenum Press, New York.

Eysenck, H. J., and Eysenck, S. B. G. (1975). *Manual of the Eysenck Personality Questionnaire*. Edits, San Diego.

Eysenck, H. J., and Wilson, G. D. (1973). *The Experimental Study of Freudian Theories*, Methuen London.

Fisher, R. A. (1958a) Cancer and smoking, *Nature*, **182**, 596.

Fisher, R. A. (1958b) Cigarettes, cancer and statistics, *Centennial Review*, **2**, 157–166.

Fisher, R. A. (1958c) Lung cancer and cigarettes? *Nature,* **182**, 108.

Fox, B. H. (1978). Premorbid psychological factors as related to cancer incidence, *Journal of Behavioral Medicine*, **1**, 45–133.

Friberg, L., Kay, L., Denker, S. J., and Jonsson, E. (1959). Smoking habits of monozygotic and dizygotic twins, *British Medical Journal*, **1**, 1090–1092.

Frith, C. (1971). Smoking behaviour and its relation to the smoker's immediate experience, *British Journal of Social and Clinical Psychology*, **10**, 73–78.

Fulker, D. W. (1981). The genetic and environmental architecture of psychoticism, extraversion and neuroticism, in H. J. Eysenck (Ed.), *A Model for Personality*, (Ed. H. J. Eysenck), Springer Verlag, Berlin and New York.

Garcia, J., Hankins, W. G., and Rusiniak, K. W. (1974). Behavioral regulation of the *milieu interne* in man and rat, *Science* **185**, 824–831.

Goldman, L., Coover, G. D., and Levine, S. (1973). Bidirectional effects of reinforcement shifts on pituitary adrenal activity, *Physiological Behaviour*, **10**, 204–214.

Gray, J. A. (1975) *Elements of a Two-process Theory of Learning*. Academic Press, London.

Gray, J. A., Davis, N., Owen, S., Feldon, J., and Boarder, M. (1981). Stress tolerance: possible neural mechanisms, in *Foundations of Psychosomatics,(Eds. M. J. Christie and P. G. Mellett) John Wiley & Sons, New York.*

Greene, W. A. (1966). The psychosocial setting of the development of leukemia and lymphoma., Annals of the New York Academy of Science, **125**, 794–801.

Greene, W. A., and Swisher, S. N. (1969). Psychological and somatic variables associated with the development and course of monozygotic twins discordant for leukemia, *Annals of the New York Academy of Science*, **164**, 394–408.

Greer, S., and Morris, T. (1975). Psychological attributes of women who develop breast cancer: A controlled study, *Journal of Psychosomatic Research*, **19**, 147–153.

Hagnell, O. (1962). *Svenska Laki-Tidu*, **58**, 4928.

Hamtoft, H., and Lindhardt, M. (1956). Tobacco Consumption in Denmark, II, *Danish Medical Bulletin*, **3**, 150.

Horne, R. L., and Picard, R. S. (1979). Psychosocial risk factors for lung cancer, *Psychosomatic Medicine*, **41**, 503–514.

Ikard, F. F., Green, P. E., and Horn, D. (1969). A scale to differentiate between types of smoking as related to the management of affect, *International Journal of the Addictions*, **4**, 649–659.

Jacobs, T. H., and Charles, E. (1980). Life events and the occurrence of cancer in children.*Psychosomatic Medicine*, **42**, 11–24.

Kasl, S. V. (1983). Pursuing the link between stressful life experiences and disease: A time for reappraisal, in *Stress Research (Ed. C. L. Cooper) pp. 79–102, John Wiley & Sons, New York.*

Kissen, D. M. (1964a). Relationship between lung cancer, cigarette smoking, inhalation and personality, British Journal of Medical Psychology, **37**, 203–216.

Kissen, D. M. (1964b). Lung cancer, inhalation and personality, in *Aspects of Neoplastic Disease, (Eds. D. M. Kissen and C. L. LeShan) Pitman, London.*

Kissen, D. M. (1968). Some methodological problems in clinical psychosomatic research with special reference to chest disease, Psychosomatic Medicine, **30**, 324–335.

Kissen, D. M., and Eysenck, H. J. (1962). Personality in male lung cancer patients, *Journal of Psychosomatic Research*, **6**, 123–137.

Kissen, D. M., and Rowe, L. G. (1969). Steroid excretion patterns and personality in lung cancer., *Annals of the New York Academy of Science*, **164**, 476–482.

Levey, A. B., and Martin, I. (1981). Personality and conditioning, in *A Model for Personality*, (Ed. H. J. Eysenck) Springer Verlag, Berlin and New York.

Krasnoff, A. (1958). Psychological variables in human cancer: a cross validation study, *Psychosomatic Medicine*, **21**, 291–296.

Kreyberg, L. (1962). *Histological Lung Cancer Types*, Norwegian Universities Press, Oslo.

LeShan, L. L. (1966). An emotional life history pattern associated with neoplastic disease, *Annals of the New York Academy of Sciences*, **125**, 780–793.

Levi, R. N., and Waxman, S. (1975). Schizophrenia, epilepsy, cancer, methionine, and folate metabolism. Pathogenesis of schizophrenia, *Lancet*, July 5th, 11–13.

Lewis, D. J. (1960). Partial reinforcement: A selective review of the literature since 1950, *Psychological Bulletin*, **57**, 1–28.

Lombard, H. L., and Potter, E. A. (1950). Epidemiological aspects of cancer of the cervix: hereditary and environmental factors, *Cancer*, **3**, 960–968.

Lynch, H. T. (1976). *Cancer Genetics*. Charles C. Thomas, Springfield, Ill.

McKennell, A. C. (1970). Smoking motivation factors, *British Journal of Social & Clinical Psychology*, **9**, 8–22.

McKennell, A. C., and Thomas, R. K. (1967). *Adults' and Adolescents' Smoking Habits and Attitudes*: *Government Social Survey Report, 353B*, H.M.S.O., London.

Miller, N. E. (1976). Learning stress and systematic symptoms, *Acta Neurobiol*. Exp., **36**, 141–156.

Multiple Risk Factor Intervention Trial Research Group (1982). Multiple Risk Factor Intervention Trial. Risk Factor Changes and Mortality Results, *Journal of the American Medical Association*, **248**, 1465–1477.

Murphy, D. P. (1952). *Heredity in Uterine Cancer., Harvard University Press, Cambridge, Mass.*

O'Connor, K. P. (1980). Individual differences in situational preference amongst smokers, Personality and Individual Differences, **1**, 249–257.

Oeser, von, H. (1979). *Krebs*: *Schicksal oder Verschulden*? Georg Thieme Verlag, Stuttgart.

Peller, S. (1952). *Cancer in Men*, International University Press, New York.

Pettingale, K. W., Greer, S., and Tee, D. H. (1977). Serum IGA and emotional expressions in breast cancer patients, *Journal of Psychosomatic Research*, **21**, 395–399.

Rachman, S., and Wilson, G. T. (1980). *The Effects of Psychological Therapy*, Pergamon Press, Oxford.

Rae, G., and McCall, J. (1973). Some international comparisons of cancer mortality rates and personality: a brief note, *The Journal of Psychology*, **85**, 87–88.

Raine, A., and Venables, P. (1981). Classic conditioning and socialization – a biosocial interaction, *Personality and Individual Differences*, **2**, 273–283.

Riley, A. L., and Clark, C. M. (1977). in *Learning Mechanisms in Food Selection*. (Eds. L. M. Baker, M. R. Best and M. Domjan) pp. 593–616, Baylor University Press, Waco.

Riley, V. (1981). Psychoneuroendocrine influences on immuno-competence and neoplasia, *Science*, **217**, 1100–1109.

Rogers, M. P., Reich, T. B., Strom, T. B., and Carpenter, C. B. (1976). Behaviorally conditioned immuno-suppression: replication of a recent study, *Psychosomatic Medicine*, **38**, 447–452.

Russell, M. A., Peto, J., and Patel, V. A. (1974). The classification of smoking by factorial structure of motives, *Journal of the Royal Statistical Society, Series A*, **137**, 313–346.

Seligman, M. E. P., Maier, S. F., and Solomon, R. C. (1971). Unpredictable and uncontrollable aversive events, in *Aversive Conditioning and Learning, F. R. Brush pp. 347–400, Academic Press, New York.*

Shields, J. (1962). Monozygotic Twins, Oxford University Press, Oxford.

Sklar, L. S., and Anisman, H. (1981). Stress and cancer, *Psychological Bulletin*, **89**, 369–406.

Spence, J. T., and Spence, K. W. (1966). The motivational components of manifest anxiety: drive and drive stimuli, in *Anxiety and Behaviour*, (Ed. C. D. Spielberger) Academic Press, London.

Speilberger, C. D. Jacobs, G., and Warden, T. (in press). Motivational determinants of smoking behavior, *Personality and Individual Differences*, in press.

Stanaway, R. G., and Watson, D. W. (1980). Smoking motivation: a factor analytic study, *Personality and Individual Differences*, **1**, 371–380.

Stavraky, K. M. (1968). Psychological factors in the outcome of human cancer, *Journal of Psychosomatic Research*, **12**, 251–260.

Todd, G. F., and Mason, J. I. (1954). Concordance of smoking habits in monozygotic and dizygotic twins, *Heredity*, **13**, 417–444.

Tokuhata, G. K. (1964). Familial factors in human lung cancer and smoking, *American Journal of Public Health*, **54**, 24–32.

Tokuhata, G. K. (1976). Cancer of the lung: host and environmental interaction, in *Cancer Genetics*, (Ed. H. T. Lynch) pp. 213–232, Charles C. Thomas, Springfield.

Tokuhata, G. K., and Lilienfeld, A. M. (1963a). Familial aggregation of lung cancer among hospital patients, *Public Health Reports, Washington*, **78**, 277–283.

Tokuhata, G. K., and Lilienfeld, A. M. (1963b). Familial aggregation of lung cancer in humans, *Journal of the National Cancer Institute*, **30**, 289–312.

Tomkins, S. (1968). A modified model of smoking behavior, in *Smoking, Health and Behavior*, (Eds. E. F. Boregatta and R. Evans) Aldine, Chicago.

Ure, D. M. (1969). Negative association between allergy and cancer, *Scottish Medical Journal*, **14**, 51–54.

Walshe, W. H. (1846). *Nature and Treatment of Cancer*, London.

Wayner, E. A., Flannery, G. R., and Singer, G. (1978). Effects of taste aversion conditioning on the primary antibody response to sheep red blood cells and *Brucella abortus* in the albino rat, *Physiology and Behaviour*, **21**, *995–1006.*

Weiss, J. M., Glazer, H. I., Pohorecky, L. A., Brick, J., and Miller, N. E. (1975). Effects of chronic exposure to stressors on avoidance-escape behavior and on brain norepinephrine, Psychosomatic Medicine, **37**, 522–534.

Zimel, H., Zimel, A., Petriscu, R., Ghinea, E., and Tasca, C. (1977). Influence of stress and of endocrine imbalance on the experimental metastasis, *Neoplasma*, **24**, 151–159.

Psychosocial Stress and Cancer
Edited by C. L. Cooper

Chapter 5
Methodology in Studies of Life Events and Cancer

E. S. Paykel, Professor of Psychiatry
and
B. M. Rao, Research Assistant
Department of Psychiatry, St. George's Hospital Medical School, London, UK

The concept of psychosocial stress is a wide one including both a variety of external stressors in the social environment and aspects of the subject's internal psychological state. The external and internal aspects are best regarded separately since the second, while they may mediate further consequences to the subject, are often consequences of the first. To employ an engineering model, external stress leads to strain on the structure.

The external social stressors may themselves be of different types. They include persisting situations undergoing little change, such as bad housing, poverty, having a severely handicapped child. Some of these may involve a cluster of features usually thought of as absence of social support: absence of social contacts, lack of someone to confide in or to give the emotional support provided by an intimate relationship, lack of someone to give practical help.

A different kind of social stressor is the life event. In the field of psychiatric disorders a large volume of research in the last 15 years has covered these, and clear findings have been established (Paykel, 1982). There has been an increasing volume of psychosomatic research into somatic consequences of life events (Minter and Kimball, 1978). There are likely to be more studies in the next few years in relation to malignancy.

The concept of a life event has not always been well defined. In this chapter, by a life event we mean a discrete change in the subject's social or personal environment. The event should represent a change, rather than a persisting state, and it should be an external verifiable change, rather than an internal psychological one. One class of internal change which is included is the personal physical illness: it is externally verifiable and shares the characteristics of changes in the external social environment and life pattern which produce subsequent psychological effects. However, in studies of malignancy this must be handled with great care. Cancer itself is a physical illness which may be confounded or confused with others, and the link between a preceding physical illness and subsequent cancer may be by direct induction of malignant change rather than via psychological mechanisms.

This chapter will mainly concern life events and will only peripherally touch on other psychosocial stressors. It will, like most studies, also mainly be limited to life events which are recent. The problems of studying remote events in early life are different and greater, particularly in respect of accurate ascertainment.

The methods for collecting information on life events at first sight appear commonsense and straightforward. However, there are in reality a number of methodological problems which need careful techniques to overcome. Because of these problems a good deal of promising early research in the psychosomatic field will in the long run need to be repeated. The most important of the issues with which we will deal are those of reliable and valid collection of information, exclusion of events which are consequences rather than causes of illness and quantification of the magnitude of events.

DATA COLLECTION

The foremost problem is that of data collection. Prospective studies are difficult. It is possible to collect data prospectively to examine the effects of stress on later outcome of malignancy which is already present (Funch and Marshall, 1983). However, when studying onset of malignancy, prospective studies of life events are rarely feasible. It is easy to identify suitable subjects experiencing a major event and at least in theory feasible to follow them up, but the onset of cancer is infrequent and very large samples are required. This is only possible for record linkage studies between presentation with cancer and major life events which can be identified from official records such as death of the subject's spouse, but it is not feasible for most life events. Therefore most studies involve retrospective collection of event information after the event has happened, usually by comparing subjects with the disorder and controls. Even in prospective studies of outcome, information on recent life events is usually collected retrospectively: one cannot know of the event until it has happened.

Retrospective gathering of information raises problems of incomplete and distorted recall. Psychologists have long been aware of the distortions which can occur in recall of material. Accurate recall of previous life events is difficult. If the reader doubts this he should try to recall accurately the important events which he underwent in the 6 months which finished a year ago. He may be aware of the problem of incomplete recall and forgetting some important ocurrences. He will almost certainly notice how difficult it is to date accurately the events which have occurred. These problems apply to anyone. For the patient with cancer there is an additional problem – what has been called the 'effort after meaning'. With a serious, distressing and life threatening disorder, one will tend to look hard for an explanation, and selectively recall, magnify the nature, or mistake the timing, of events which did occur. This process may not happen to the same extent in a control group.

Self-report questionaires

A major step forward in life events research appeared with the publication of the well-known paper by Holmes and Rahe (1967). A list of 43 life events, the Schedule of Recent Experience, was derived, building on previous work by Thomas Holmes and colleagues, and earlier studies by Hinkle and Wolf (Hinkle, 1974). This list was administered to 394 subjects who were asked to rate the amount of adjustment to life change involved in each, in ratio to marriage, which was assigned a score of 50. Using mean scores a scale was obtained ranging from 100 for death of spouse to 11 for minor violations of the law. The list of life events, set out as a pencil-and-paper questionnaire, was then used in other studies to record the events which had been experienced by subjects in recent time periods: events were assigned the scores obtained in the earlier study and added to give total 'life crisis units', and these scores related to onset of physical illnesses of various kinds (Rahe and Arthur, 1968; Rahe *et al.*, 1967, 1974).

This method gave the impetus for a large amount of research into somatic and psychiatric disorders, using the same questionnaire (Lundberg *et al.*, 1975; Bruhn *et al.*, 1972; Garrity *et al.*, 1978; Jacobs and Charles, 1980; Hendrie *et al.*, 1975; Isherwood *et al.*, 1982; Thomson and Hendrie, 1972). A number of other similar self-report life event questionnaires have been devised and have been used in studies (Cochrane and Robertson, 1975; Grant *et al.*, 1974; Tennant and Andrews, 1976).

In due course, as often happens with innovations, the technique of Holmes and Rahe has come in for criticism (Brown, 1981; Dohrenwend and Dohrenwend, 1981). Some of this concerns the method of quantification and will be dealt with later. Some concerns the specific life event list, which has deficiencies, particularly in that some of the items, such as change in sleep pattern, are more like symptoms than events (Hudgens, 1974). Later life event lists have tended to be more selective in this regard, although more comprehensive overall.

A more basic criticism concerns the self-report method, and this applies more generally to pencil-and-paper life event questionnaires. There is a crucial dichotomy in data collection methods for life events: between self-report questionnaires and interviews. The self-report checklist is appealing;

it can be clearly set out and administered on a large scale, with comparatively little research effort.

However, the realities must make this method of data collection suspect. It is quite difficult to define an event. For instance, in assessing an argument with someone close, one needs to define the relationship, together with the magnitude and persistence of a dispute which will cross the threshold to be an event worth recording, rather than a trivial occurrence. Such a definition is feasible, but it is too cumbersome to be incorporated in a short questionnaire. Added to this is the difficulty in recalling time of occurrence. Our own experience is that it takes frequent reminders, and anchoring by clear dates such as Christmas, to avoid a tendency by subjects to report events occurring well outside the time period specified in a study.

Some of the difficulties are exemplified by a study of children with cancer and controls attending a paediatric clinic with minor illnesses (Jacobs and Charles, 1980). Using the Holmes – Rahe questionnaire completed by parents, much more stress was reported in the families of the cancer patients prior to first manifestation of the cancer. However, there must be a very real risk that parents who are very upset and concerned by the diagnosis of cancer will report on a pencil-and-paper questionnaire in a very different way to those whose children have minor illness.

Life event interviews

A much better alternative is to use some kind of interview. This should still be based on a list of life events so as to cover the field. A completely unstructured interview would run serious risk of sporadic reporting. One study (Lipman *et al.*, 1965) asking patients simply to volunteer events found evidence that reports were secondary to mood change. The interview format allows use of a subsidiary lexicon to define each event in detail, and as much probing as necessary to ascertain the precise details of the event. Factual material can largely be separated from perception and effects of heightened distorted recall. Adequate judgements can also be made of independence of the event from illness and of the qualities important in quantifying it, as will be discussed in later sections.

There are a number of published interviews for life events which have been used extensively, tested for reliability and validated. The most detailed and probing is that of Brown and colleagues (Brown *et al.*, 1973, Brown and Harris, 1978). It is based on an extensive list of 38 types of event falling into eight groups. Administration may take up to half a day, with the content of the interview tape recorded and later rating judgements made on the tape recorded material, of independence of events from psychiatric illness, and the degree of threat to the subject which they involve. The method has produced major findings in psychiatric disorders (Brown and Harris, 1978) and has been used in studies of physical illness (Murphy and Brown, 1980; Creed, 1981). Specific training from Brown's group is required for its use. A very large amount of work has gone into its development, with careful formulation of definitions and testing of reliability. A correspondingly large investment in time for interview and rating, and in research costs, is required for its proper use.

Our own method, the Interview for Recent Life Events (Paykel, 1983) was originally derived in New Haven, Connecticut, in 1967. The list of 61 life events was subsequently expanded and modified in London to 64, to cover fairly comprehensively most major life changes. Each event is defined, the definitions being much longer than the short-hand labels reported in tables for publication. The list is organised for interview convenience into nine areas: work, education, finance, health, bereavement, migration, courtship, legal, family and social relationships, marital. At the end the interviewer enquires for any other major occurrences which may not have been covered, but these are infrequent. An extract is shown in Figure 5.1.

MARITAL
55. *Marriage*.
56. *Serious argument* with spouse
'Serious argument' is defined as a one-way or interactive altercation adversely affecting behaviour of one or both parties for a minimum of five days.
57. *Marital separation of one month not due to argument*. Do not code if some regular contact maintained or spouse working away but home for weekends, spouse or interviewee in hospital but visited regularly.

Figure 5.1: Extract from Marital Section of Recent Life Events

The instrument is administered as a semi-structured interview. Each event is enquired for unless it cannot apply: e.g. marital events for the unmarried. Wording may be modified appropriately for the subject. If an event has occurred there is further probing to ascertain the precise circumstances and timing. Ratings are made of independence of the events from psychiatric illness, and of their objective negative impact. The interview is shorter and less detailed than Brown's, taking between half an hour and one and a quarter hours including time for coding, depending on the capacities of the subject and the number of events. Good reliability has been found (Paykel, 1983). The instrument has been used in a number of studies of psychiatric and physical illness (Paykel *et al.*, 1969, 1975; Paykel and Tanner, 1976; Paykel, 1974; Paykel *et al.*, 1980; Jacobs *et al.*, 1974; Kennedy *et al.*, 1983) and events have been scaled in Britain and the U.S.A. (Paykel *et al.*, 1976, 1971). Where studies of psychiatric patients have been studied we have usually postponed the interview until acute disturbance has subsided, to facilitate accurate interview and reporting: there is a case for similar precautions in studies of physical illness.

A third inventory has been developed by Dohrenwend *et al*. (1978). The Psychiatric Epidemiology Research Interview (PERI) contains a list of 102 life events with wide coverage over areas of school, work, love and marriage, children, family, residence, crime and legal matters, finance, social activities, health and miscellaneous. Although it has been used as a self-report (Monroe, 1982) it is intended as a structured interview for use in epidemiology studies, with life event content particularly relevant to New York City. For this purpose, short event definitions and a structured interview technique with little probing are useful. These characteristics render the instrument somewhat less ideal for clinical studies, but its basic format is suitable.

Tennant and Andrews (1976) have described a life event inventory intended either for interview or self-report questionnaire and incorporating 67 events. Definitions are brief. The instrument has been used in epidemiological studies as a self-report questionnaire (Tennant and Andrews, 1978), with, in a second study, limited supplementation by interview (Steele *et al*., 1981). It lacks definitions and ratings for more detailed interview.

We strongly recommend use of an interview method rather than a self-report questionnaire in studies of life events and cancer. Standards adopted by journals may make questionnaire studies less acceptable for publication in future. The available interviews vary in their length and in their degree of structure. A completely standardised interview with items asked in specified wording with no additional probing has little advantage over a self-report questionnaire. We believe that a semi-structured interview with some probing and flexibility is best.

EVENTS RESULTING FROM ILLNESS

Events tend to be regarded as objective occurrences coming from outside. However, clearly this is not necessarily the case. We all to some extent may create the events from which we suffer. In particular illness itself may produce new events – inability to work, loss of job, financial problems, secondary worsening in relationships and arguments in the house.

It is important in studies of aetiology to eliminate the events which are consequences of illness. There are two main approaches and it is better to use both and combine them. The first is to confine attention to time periods antedating the onset of illness. In the field of cancer it is not easy to date onset but at least some attempt should be made to date appearance of first manifestations if one is seeking to relate the event to the development of the disorder. The time period covered by interview may depend on the study. It is reasonable to cover 6 months or a year before onset, but covering any earlier than 2 years before the date of interview magnifies problems of recall considerably.

A second way of tackling the problem is the separation of the 'independent' event, an important concept introduced by Brown and colleagues (Brown *et al.*, 1973). This is the idea that on detailed scrutiny certain events can be isolated which would be unlikely to have been brought about by illness, if it were present. The technique involves scrutiny of the individual circumstances of the event occurrence to make this rating. Job loss due to closure of the whole factory is likely to be independent of illness, but job loss where very few people have been laid off may well in part be due to the inefficiency of the subject.

Tennant and Andrews (1977) have atempted to derive consensus judgements for a list of events in this way so as to avoid judging individual occurrences. Although some events, such as deaths of other persons, are almost always independent of the subject, there are many events which depend on particular circumstances, so that the judgement is better an individual one.

A shortened version of Brown's judgement is incorporated in the current version of our own procedure. Reliability in our hands is not as high as for recording of event occurrence (Paykel, 1983), but it is acceptable. The concept applies whether the subject is actually ill or not, the test being whether the occurrence could have resulted from an illness, had one been present. By using the judgement one can also seek to relate events after onset to worsening: the possibility that stress may affect not the genesis of cancer but the rate at which it progresses is a real one (Funch and Marshall, 1983).

QUANTIFICATION OF LIFE EVENT STRESS

A third major issue is that of quantification. It is obvious that all life events are not equal. Simply determining whether a subject has had any event, or counting the number of events experienced, are a very limited approaches. We need somehow to distinguish the more stressful events.

The techniques which have been used, listed from the more general to the more individual are: consensus scaling; categorisation of events into groups; contextual judgements of threat; personal subjective judgements made by the subject who experienced the event. We will deal briefly with each of these issues. The generalised techniques are less sensitive, but the individualised methods are more prone to bias.

Holmes and Rahe (1967) in their pioneering study, asked subjects to scale the adjustment to life change involved for each event in their list, in ratio to marriage. Remarkable consensus was obtained for different social and ethnic groups (Rahe, 1969). We (Paykel *et al.*, 1971, 1976) carried out similar studies, first in the U.S.A., later in London, using a different scaling technique. We also used a different scaling concept of how upsetting the event was, with connotations of distress and undesirability. There is evidence that this concept relates more closely to the development of psychiatric disorder than does life change, irrespective of desirability (Paykel and Uhlenhuth, 1972; Ross and Mirowswky, 1979). The issues and problems in the use of consensus scales have been discussed by Dohrenwend and Dohrenwend (1981). Assigning a standard weight by agreement must be a blunt tool, missing the particular circumstances of individual event occurrences. On the other hand it can be done externally, without any possibility that knowledge of who became ill may produce rater bias in the individual judgement. Surtees has described a technique for weighting more highly the more recent event occurrences (Surtees and Ingham, 1980).

Holmes and Rahe added the weights for individual event occurrences to derive a total stress score. Brown and Harris (1978) have argued that events are not aditive, but that once a single major event has been experienced, the others do not matter much. This contention has not been critically tested in empirical studies but the evidence suggests that additional events do make a contribution. There are other problems with total weighted scores since empirically they often correlate highly with the number of events reported (Skinner and Lei, 1980). The variation in event weights is limited by omission of trivial events and infrequency of the most severe events such as deaths. There is considerable variation in the number of events within a fairly narrow range of moderate stress, and this accounts for most of the variation in the total score. Weighted total scores are an improvement on event counts, but only to a limited degree. Their main value is where some kind of continuous score is needed for parametric analyses. It is unwise to depend entirely on them.

An alternative approach, which also involves using group rather than individual judgements so as to avoid bias, is to categorise events on some logical or agreed basis based on the general event, not the particular occurrence. We have found this a most useful approach. In several studies of depression, schizophrenia, suicide attempters (Paykel *et al.*, 1969, 1975, 1976, 1980; Paykel, 1979), we divided events into general classes which were found to behave differently in regard to the onset of illness. Table 5.1 illustrates findings from a study of depression (Paykel *et al.*, 1969) involving 185 depres-

Table 5.1 Depression and life event categories. Number of depressives and general population controls reporting one or more event occurrences in specific classes in 6 months before onset*

Event category	Depressivies (*N*=185)	General population (*N*=185)	Significance difference
Exits	46	9	<.01
Entrances	21	18	NS
Undesirable	82	31	<.01
Desirable	6	10	NS

*Modified from Paykel *et al.*, (1969).

sives and 185 matched general population controls, interviewed regarding events in a 6 month period prior to onset. Based on the event definition rather than individual occurrences we divided events into exits (involving departure of someone from the immediate field of the respondent) and entrances (involving introduction of someone into the immediate social field). Exits included events such as deaths, marital separation, departures of children from the home; entrances such events as birth of a child, having a lodger in the home. Separately we also divided events into those which would generally be regarded as undesirable, such as demotion, going to gaol, and those which were desirable, such as marriage, promotion. Events which could not be categorised clearly were omitted from the specific analyses. In comparison with general population controls depressives had experienced a considerable excess of exits and undesirable events, but no excess of entrances or desirable events, indicating that events behaved selectively in relation to the genesis of clinical depression.

Another method of quantifying is Brown's judgement of contextual threat. Based on the detailed circumstances of the individual event occurrence, but ignoring the subjective reaction of the patient, raters make a judgement of the expected stressfulness of the event. Death of mother, although always stressful to some degree, might be relatively mild for a middle-aged male with his own children and for a long time living distant from his parents; it might be extremely stressful for an adolescent girl at home. As usually employed the judgement is a fairly global one depending on long-term implications of the event, although Brown and others (Miller and Ingham, 1983) have explored use of finer judgements of different qualities. The rating of contextual threat has been widely used and found reliable in various hands (Brown *et al.*, 1973; Tennant *et al.*, 1979; Parry *et al.*, 1981). We have incorporated a shorter variant which we call objective negative impact and have found it useful (Paykel *et al.*, 1980). The judgement has intuitive appeal as a sensitive measure. However, it does have one disadvantage: it requires a good deal of interviewing to get all the information so that in spite of all precautions, it is possible that a sympathetic interviewer, knowing that the subject became ill after the event, will exaggerate the circumstances.

A last procedure is to ask the subject himself whether the event was stressful. This seems the obvious method and it is probably the most sensitive, since in the long run it is the perception of the individual which counts. However, it should be avoided if studies are to convince the sceptic. It may be acceptable in studies of outcome which are truly prospective but in the usual retrospective studies, there is too much risk that the subject, having become ill after the event, will retrospectively perceive it as stressful.

Thus there is a series of methods, in which increasing sensitivity is accompanied by increasing risk of bias and retrospective falsification due to illness onset. Each method is legitimate in appropriate circumstances; each has some problems. It is best to use more than one method in any study, and probably the best compromise is to analyse independently by a bias free method such as categorising events, and a more sensitive one such as judgement of contextual threat. The evidence which exists suggests that different methods tend to produce the same results (Paykel, 1983).

RELIABILITY AND VALIDITY

There have been a moderate number of studies of reliability and validity of life event data collection, derived both from studies of psychiatric and of physical illness. These are reviewed more fully elsewhere (Paykel, 1983). Table 5.2 lists findings from studies of reliability, mainly test – retest. In this and subsequent tables, where possible, percent concordance is given, based on proportion of events reported on either occasion which are reported on both, but in many of the studies only a correlation is reported. The studies are divided into those using a self-report method, most commonly the Holmes – Rahe questionnaire, and those using an interview method. A few studies have used intermediate methods, such as interviewing only for events listed as present on a self-report questionnaire, or a very standardised interview with no probing. Some simplification of complex findings has been necessary. As can be seen from the table, although there is some variation, self-report checklists tend to have low reliabilities: interview or intermediate methods acceptably high reliabilities.

Table 5.2 Studies of reliability of life event reporting*

	Test–retest Interval	Concordance		
Self-report				
Casey *et al.* (1967)	9 months		0.74†	
Thurlow (1971)	2 weeks		0.78†	
	2 years	0.07	—	0.34†
McDonald *et al.* (1972)	6 months	0.48	—	0.60†
Jenkins *et al.* (1979)	9 months	0.38	—	0.45†
Horowitz *et al.* (1977)	6 weeks	0.71	—	0.90†
Intermediate				
Steele *et al.* (1980)	10 days			
	Total score	0.89	—	0.94†
	Specific events		70%	
Interview				
Paykel (1983)	Inter-rater			
	Specific event		95%	
	Month of occurrence		85%	

*Modified from Paykel (1983); reproduced by permission of the *Journal of Psychosomatic Research*.
†Correlation

Another test is to examine the fall-off in mean number of events reported in the general population as time periods extend back into the past. In ill subjects some recent peaking of events is to be expected, if events cluster before illness. In the general population events should be randomly distributed in time. Table 5.3 shows the results of some studies. The self-report studies have found substantial fall-off of 4–5% per month. The interview studies have found acceptably low rates of fall-off, usually around 1% per month. The exception is a study by Schmid *et al.* (1981) using Brown's interview, but without his training (Brown and Harris, 1982).

Table 5.3 Studies of fall-off of event recall in general population*

	Time period	Fall-off	Fall-off per month
Self-report			
Jenkins *et al.* (1979)	9 months	34%–46%	4%–5%
Uhlenhuth *et al.* (1977)	18 months	66%	4%
Monroe (1982)	8 months	36%	5%
Intermediate			
Henderson *et al.* (1981)	12 months	32%	3%
Interview			
Paykel (1980)	6 months	9%	1%
Schmid *et al.* (1981)	6 months	62%	10%
Brown and Harris (1978)	6 months	8%	1%
Brown and Harris (1982)	1 year	34%	3%

*Modified from Paykel (1983), reproduced by permission of the *Journal of Psychosomatic Research*.

An approach to validity is comparison of information provided by the subject with that provided by another informant. Studics arc summarised in Table 5.4. Most have reported percent agreement. Again concordances have been low with self-report questionnaires, reasonably high with interview methods. There are some exceptions. The study of Hudgens *et al.* was an early one using only briefly and broadly specified life events. The method used by Neugebauer (1983) does appear to have been adequate. The subjects were schizophrenics with at least two previous hospitalisations, and the report does not make clear whether they were currently ill. These subjects are often uncommunicative and difficult to interview and would be expected to be at the lower end of reliability.

Overall it can be seen that when self-report checklists are used, there are serious deficiencies in data collection. Methods which are intermediate between interview and self-report produce intermediate results. Careful interviews do produce data of adequate reliability and validity and should be the preferred method of data collection.

Table 5.4 Studies of patient-informant concordance for life events*

	Agreement for individual events
Self-report	
Rahe (1974)	0.07 — 0.75†
Yager *et al.* (1981)	35%
Intermediate 4	
Schless and Mendels (1978)	43%
Interview	
Hudgens *et al.* (1970)	57%
Brown *et al.* (1973)	
Schizophrenics 3 months	81%
Depressives 1 year	79%
Brown and Harris (1982)	78%
Neugebauer (1983)	22%

*Modified from Paykel (1983), reproduced by permission of the Journal of Psychosomatic Research.
†Correlations of total scores.

SELECTION OF CONTROLS

The need for control groups in studies of life events is obvious, since the events which occur in patients also occur not uncommonly in non-patients and the general population. Matching of controls on demographic variables is important. The type of event which may occur will be influenced by the background situation of the subject, including age (adolescents experience somewhat different events to the elderly), sex, whether or not married, and whether the subject has children. What is less obvious and not fully explained, is a consistent general tendency for younger subjects to report more events than older subjects, both among patients and the general population. It may be that old age does bring tranquility, or at least relative stability, or there may be some bias in the events included in most event schedules. On the other hand the more threatening events with greater impact, such as death and serious illnesses of family members, retirement, tend to be reserved for middle and old age.

It is not always easy to control for circumstances of interview: patients who are under medical care may be more motivated to report embarrassing and painful personal events than are subjects in the general population visited with little warning by an interviewer. There is a good case for having two comparison groups: general population subjects and subjects with another physical disorder, both to control for the reporting phenomena, and to test whether any association found with life events is a specific one. The strategy of interviewing potential cancer patients before the results of biopsy are known (Katz *et al.*, 1970), with subsequent comparisons between those found positive and negative is an elegant one to deal with reporting effects due to awareness of having a malignancy.

SOCIAL SUPPORT AND CHRONIC DIFFICULTIES

More recent studies on life events have increasingly tended also to incorporate measures of longer-term problem situations and absence of social support. Brown and Harris (1978) have found that certain longer-term situations which they term 'difficulties' may precipitate depression, while other background factors, including presence of young children in the home, not working outside the home, and absence of a confidant, render women more likely to become depressed after the occurrence of life events. A large literature suggests that these and other factors reflecting absence of social support, are associated with depression and other disorders.

Assessment of chronic difficult problems and social support is not as well established as is that of life events. It remains for some of the methodological difficulties to be solved and reliability and validity to be firmly established. A number of interviews have been incorporated in studies. The same general problems arise as for life events. Careful interview is necessary for information gathering. It is difficult to separate internal perception from external reality, in determining for instance whether a work situation is really unsatisfying or whether a marriage without open hostility is poor. It is even more difficult to establish whether a problem situation is truly independent rather than a consequence of personality and maladaptive behaviour on the part of the subject. The general area may be less appropriate to studies of life event and malignancy; the first task is to establish whether life events play a role, before studying factors which modify them.

REMOTE EVENTS

The problems which arise in studying recent life events are magnified when remote events are studied. The techniques described earlier are probably only reliable over 2 years or so prior to interview, and are better reserved for periods more recent than that.

Study of early events in childhood involve different methodological traps (Granville-Grossman, 1968). There have been many studies of early loss and psychiatric disorder (Paykel, 1982). Particular care must be undertaken in matching controls. Rates of childhood bereavement tend to be higher in older subjects, born in earlier decades, as death rates in young adults have declined progressively throughout this century, except for periods of war. Divorce rates on the other hand, have risen. Death rates also tend to be higher in lower social classes, and in certain areas. Higher rates of childhood bereavement will also be found in conditions associated with greater parental age, and in genetic conditions with fatal outcome from which both parent and child may suffer. Loss by death must be distinguished from loss by other causes, such as marital separation: the latter may be mediated in part by personality and the general social milieu.

Qualitative aspects of early family environment, parent – child relationships and early upbringing, studied retrospectively in adults, are particularly problematic because of the large possibilities for distortion by current state and the limited possibilities for validation. In an elegant recent study Wolkind and Coleman (1983) showed that recollections of the quality of relationships between parents in childhood varied with mood state at the time of the interview; reports of significant separation from parents in childhood did not do so.

CONCLUSIONS

This chapter has dealt with methodology for assessing life events in studies of malignancy. There are three major issues. The first and most important concerns reliable data collection. Self-report event questionnaires are inadequate; some form of interview method should be used, preferably one permitting enough probing to establish detail. The second issue concerns events which are consequences of illness. Events should be documented in relation to the time of illness onset, and those events likely to be caused by illness should be eliminated. The third issue is quantification. There are alternative methods, ranging from concensus scaling, to event categorisation and contextual judgements regarding individual event occurrences, and it is better to use more than one. Careful selection of matched control samples is also necessary. Assessment of persisting stressful situations and of remote events is more difficult. For recent life events careful attention to interview methods allows reliable and valid collection of information.

REFERENCES

Brown, G. W. (1981). Life events, psychiatric disorder and physical illness., *J. Psychosom. Res.*, **25**, 461–473.

Brown, G. W., and Harris, T. (1978). *The Social Origins of Depression: a study of Psychiatric Disorder in Women*, Tavistock, London, Free Press, New York.

Brown, G. W., and Harris, T. (1982). Fall-off in the reporting of life events, *Soc. Psychiat.*, **17**, 23–28.

Brown, G. W., Sklair, F., Harris, T. O., and Birley, J. L. T. (1973). Life-events and psychiatric disorders. Part I: Some methodological issues, *Psychol. Med*, **3**, 74–87.

Bruhn, J. G., Philips, B. U., and Wolf, S. (1972). Social readjustment and illness patterns: comparisons between first, second and third generation Italian-Americans living in the same community, *J. Psychosom. Res*, **16**, 387–394.

Casey, R. L., Masuda, M., and Holmes, T. H. (1967). Quantitative study of recall of life events, *J. Psychosom. Res*, **11**, 239–247.

Cochrane, R. and Robertson, A. (1975). Stress in the lives of parasuicides, *Soc. Psychiat.*, **10** 161–171.

Creed, F. (1981). Life events and appendicectomy, *Lancet*, 1381–1385.
Dohrenwend, B. S., and Dohrenwend, B. P. (1981). Life stress and illness: formulation of the issues, in *Stressful Life Events and Their Context*, (Eds. B. S. Dohrenwend and B. P. Dohrenwend, Prodist, New York.
Dohrenwend, B. S., Krasnoff, L., Askenasy, A. R., and Dohrenwend, B. P. (1978). Exemplification of a method for scaling life events: the PERI life events scale, *J. Health & Soc. Behav.*, **19**, 205–229.
Funch, D. P., and Marshall, J. (1983). The role of stress, social support and age in survival from breast cancer. *J. Psychosom. Res.*, **27**, 77–83.
Garrity, T. F., Marx, M. B., and Somes, G. W. (1978). The relationship of recent life change to seriousness of later illness, *J. Psychosom. Res.*, **22**, 7–12.
Grant, I., Kyle, G. C., Teichman, A., and Mendels, J. (1974). Recent life events and diabetes in adults, *Psychosom. Med.* **36**, 121–128.
Granville-Grossman, K. L. (1968). The early environment in affective disorder, in *Recent Developments in Affective Disorders*. (Eds. A. Coppen and A. Walk) Royal Medico-Psychological Association, London.
Henderson, S., Byrne, D. G., and Duncan-Jones, P. (1981). *Neurosis and the Social Environment*, Academic Press, Sydney.
Hendrie, H. C., Lachar, D., and Lennox, K. (1975). Personality trait and symptom correlates of life change in psychiatric population, *J. Psychosom. Res*, **19**, 203–208.
Hinkle, L. E. (1974). The effect of exposure to culture change, social change, and changes in interpersonal relationships on health, in *Stressful Life Events: Their Nature and Effects*, (Eds. B. S. Dohrenwend and B. P. Dohrenwend), pp. 9–44, John Wiley & Sons, New York.
Holmes, T. H., and Rahe, R. H. (1967). The social readjustment rating scale, *J. Psychosom. Res.*, **11**, 231–218.
Horowitz, M., Schaefer, C., Hiroto, D., Wilner, N. and Levin, B. (1977). Life event questionnaires for measuring presumptive stress, *Psychosom. Med.*, **39**, 413.
Hudgens, R. W. (1974). Personal catastrophe and depression: a consideration of the subject with respect to medically ill adolescents, and a requiem for retrospective life-event studies, in *Stressful Life Events: Their Nature and Effects*, (Eds. B. P. Dohrenwend, and B. S. Dohrenwend, John Wiley & Sons, New York.
Hudgens, R. W., Robins, E., and Delong, W. B. (1970). The reporting of recent stress in the lives of psychiatric patients, *Brit. J. Psychiat.*, **117**, 635.
Isherwood, J., Adam K. S., and Hornblow, A. R. (1982). Life event stress, psychosocial factors, suicide attempt and auto-accident proclivity, *J. Psychosom. Res.*, **26**, 371–383.
Jacobs, T. J., and Charles, E. (1980). Life events and the occurrence of cancer in children, *Psychosom. Med.*, **42**, 11–25.
Jacobs, S. C., Prusoff, B. A., and Paykel, E. S. (1974). Recent life events in schizophrenia and depression, *Psychol. Med.* **4**, 444–453.
Jenkins, C. D., Hurst, M. W., and Rose, R. M. (1979). Life changes. Do people really remember? *Arch. Gen. Psychiat.*, **36**, 379.
Katz, J. L., Weiner, H., Gallagher, T. F., and Hellman, L. (1970). Stess, distress and ego defences, *Arch. Gen. Psychiat.*, **23**, 131–142.
Kennedy, S., Thompson, R., Stancer, H. C., Roy, A., and Persad, E. (1983). Life events precipitating mania, *Brit. J. Psychiat.* **142**, 398–403.
Lipman, R. S., Harvey, M., Hammer, M. D., Bernardes, J. F., Park, L. C., and Cole, J. O. (1965). Patient report of significant life situation events, *Dis. Nerv. Syst.*, **26**, 580–591.
Lundberg, U., Theorell, T., and Lind, E. (1975). Life changes and myocardial

infarction: individual differences in life change scaling, *J. Psychosom. Res*, **19** 27–32.

McDonald, B. W., Pugh, W. M., Gunderson, E., and Rahe, R. H. (1972). Reliability of life change cluster scores, *Brit. J. Soc. clin. Psychol.*, **11**, 407.

Miller, P. McC., and Ingham, J. G. (1983). Dimentions of experience, *Psychol. Med.*, **13**, 417–429.

Minter, R. E., and Kimball, C. P. (1978). Life events and illness onset: a review, *Psychosomatics*, **19**, 334–339.

Monroe, S. M. (1982). Assessment of life events, *Arch. Gen. Psychiat.*, **39**, 606–610.

Murphy, E., and Brown, G. W. (1980). Life events, psychiatric disturbance and physical illness, *Brit. J. Psychiat.*, **136**, 326–338.

Neugebauer, R. (1983). Reliability of life event interviews with outpatient schizophrenics, *Arch. Gen. Psychiat.*, **40**, 378–383.

Parry, G., Shapiro, D. A., and Davies, L. (1981). Reliability of life-event ratings: an independent replication, *Brit. J. Clin. Psychol*, **20**, 133–134.

Paykel, E. S. (1974). Recent life events and clinical depression, in *Life Stress and Illness*, (Eds. E. K. Gunderson and R. H. Rahe) Ch. 9, pp. 134–163, Charles C. Thomas, Springfield, Illinois.

Paykel, E. S. (1979). Causal relationships between clinical depression and life events, in *Stress and Mental Disorder*, (Ed. E. J. Barrett), pp. 71–86, Raven Press, New York.

Paykel, E. S. (1980). Recall and reporting of life events (Letter), *Arch. Gen. Psychiat.*, 485.

Paykel, E. S. (1982). Life events and early environment, in *Handbook of Affective Disorders*, (Ed. E. S. Paykel) Churchill Livingstone, Edinburgh.

Paykel, E. S., (1983). Methodological aspects of life events research, *J. Psychosom. Res.*, **27**, 341–352.

Paykel, E. S., Emms, E. M., Fletcher, J., and Rassaby, E. S., (1980). Life events and social support in puerperal depression, *Brit. J. Psychiat.* **136**, 339–346.

Paykel, E. S., McGuiness, B., and Gomez, J. (1976). An Anglo-American comparison of the scaling of life events, *Brit. J. Med. Psychol.*, **49**, 237–247.

Paykel, E. S., Myers, J. K., Dienelt, M. N., Klerman, G. L., Lindentha, J. J., and Pepper, M. P. (1969). Life events and depression: a controlled study, *Arch. Gen. Psychiat.*, **21**, 753–760.

Paykel, E. S., Prusoff, B. A., and Myers, J. K. (1975). Suicide attempts and recent life events: a controlled comparison, *Arch. Gen. Psychiat.*, **32**, 327–333.

Paykel, E. S., Prusoff, B. A., and Uhlenhuth, E. (1971). Scaling of life events, *Arch. Gen. Psychiat.*, **25**, 340–347.

Paykel, E. S., and Tanner, J. (1976). Life events, depressive relapse and maintenance treatment, *Psychol. Med.*, **6**, 481–485.

Paykel, E. S., and Uhlenhuth, E. H. (1972). Rating the magnitude of life stress *Canad. Psychiat. Assn. J.*, **17**, 93–100.

Rahe, R. H. (1969). Multi-cultural correlations of life change scaling: American Japan, Denmark and Sweden, *J. Psychosom. Res.*, **13**, 191–195.

Rahe, R. H. and Arthur, R. J. (1968). Life-change patterns surrounding illnes experience, *J. Psychosom. Res.* **112**, 341–345.

Rahe, R. H., McKean, J. D., and Arthur, R. J. (1967). A longitudinal study of life change and illness patterns, *J. Psychosom. Res.*, **10**, 355–366.

Rahe, R. H., Romo, M., Bennett, L., and Siltanen, P. (1974). Recent life changes myocardial infarction, and abrupt coronary death, *Arch. Inten. Med.*, **133**, 221–228

Ross, C. E., and Mirowsky II, J. (1979). A comparison of life-event weightin schemes: change, undesirability, and effect-proportional indices, *J. Health & Soc. Behav.*, **20**, 166–177.

Schmid, I., Scharfetter, C., and Binnder, J. (1981). Lebensereignisse in Abhangfigkeit von soziodemographischen variablen, *Soc. Psychiat.*, **16**, 63–68.

Schless, A., and Mendels, J. (1978). The value of interviewing family and friends in assessing life stressors, *Arch. Gen. Psychiat.*, **35**, 565–567.

Skinner, H. A., and Lei, H. (1980). Differential weights in life change research: useful or irrelevant? *Psychosom. Med.*, **42**, 367–370.

Steele, G. P., Henderson, S., and Duncan-Jones, P. (1980). The reliability of reporting adverse experiences, *Psychol. Med.*, **10**, 301–306.

Surtees, P. G., and Ingham, J. G. (1980). Life stress and depressive outcome: application of a dissipation model to life events, *Soc. Psychiat.*, **15**, 21–31.

Tennant, C., and Andrews, G. (1976). A scale to measure the stress of life events, *Aust. New Zeal. J. Psychiat.*, **10**, 27–32.

Tennant, C., and Andrews, G. (1977). A scale to measure the cause of life events, *Aust. New Zeal. J. Psychiat.*, **11**, 163–167.

Tennant, C., and Andrews, G. (1978). The pathogenic quality of life event stress in neurotic impairment, *Arch. Gen. Psychiat.*, **35**, 859–863.

Tennant, C., Smith, A., Bebbington, P., and Hurry, J. (1979). The contextual threat of life events: the concept and its reliability, *Psychol. Med.*, **9**, 525–528.

Thomson, K. C., and Hendrie, H. C. (1972). Environmental stress in primary depressive illness, *Arch. Gen. Psychiat.*, **26**, 130–132.

Thurlow, H. J. (1971). Illness in relation to life situation and sick-role tendency, *J. Psychosom. Res.*, **15**: 73.

Uhlenhuth, E. H., Haberman, S. J., Balter, M. D., and Lipman, R. S. (1977). Remembering life events, in *The Origins and Course of Psychopathology: Methods of Longitudinal Research*. (Eds. J. S. Strauss, H. M. Babigian and M. Roff, Plenum Press, New York.

Wolkind, S., and Coleman, E. (1983). Adult psychiatric disorder and childhood experiences. The validity of retrospective data, *Brit. J. Psychiat.*, **143**, 188–191.

Yager, J., Grant, I., Sweetwood, H. L., and Gerst, M. (1981). Life event reports by psychiatric patients, non-patients, and their partners, *Arch. Gen. Psychiat.*, **38**, 343.

Section Three
Psychophysiological Processes

Psychosocial Stress and Cancer
Edited by C. L. Cooper

Chapter 6
Stress and Pathology: Immunological and Central Nervous System Interactions

Jill Irwin and Hymie Anisman
Department of Psychology, Carleton University, Ottawa, Canada

It is commonly believed that an individual's emotional state can profoundly influence physical well-being. Indeed it has been demonstrated that certain personality traits and adverse psychological conditions are correlated with the onset and increased incidence of various psychosomatic disorders (e.g. asthma, ulcers), cardiovascular disease, as well as immunologically related illnesses and neoplasia (see reviews by Ader, 1980, 1981; Locke, 1982; Rogers *et al.*, 1979; Solomon and Amkraut, 1981; Stein, 1981). Although stressful events were traditionally related exclusively to the psychosomatic disorders, they have recently been implicated in the provocation or exacerbation of pathological conditions in which dysfunction of the immune system plays a significant role. This group of disorders includes infectious diseases, autoimmune disorders, allergy and cancer. Although the role of the immune system in cancer is less well understood, psychological factors have been suspected of influencing malignancies (Fox, 1981; Sklar and Anisman, 1981). However, it is beyond the scope of the present discussion to review in detail that rather extensive literature (see reviews in Fox, 1978; Sklar and Anisman, 1981).

When a pathogen invades an organism the various elements of the immune system are mobilized to arrest its progress. Thus, disease is not an inevitable outcome, but rather, occurs when the host defence system is compromised or is unable to recognize the foreign material. At birth neither of the two major systems of immunity – cellular and humoral – is fully developed and immunocompetence increases during childhood and adolescence. In senescence, however, immune regulation is impaired and this period of life is associated with higher incidences of autoimmune diseases (e.g. rheumatoid arthritis) and malignancies (Kay, 1980; Weksler, 1981). Similarly, when nutritional status is deficient the incidence of infectious diseases increases, and direct measures of immunologic function indicate decreased immunocompetence (Fudenberg *et al.*, 1980; Richter, 1982).

Psychological factors, and in particular stressors, may compromise the host defence system as well. A number of studies have shown an association between life stress events and increased susceptibility to respiratory infections, autoimmune diseases and allergic conditions. Moreover, there is a large body of data indicating that stressors profoundly alter neurotransmitter and neuroendocrine activity. The way in which the immune systems and central neuronal systems interact so that psychological variables could influence pathogenesis has been the focus of considerable recent interest. As a framework for a discussion of this interaction the model shown in Figure 6.1 is proposed.

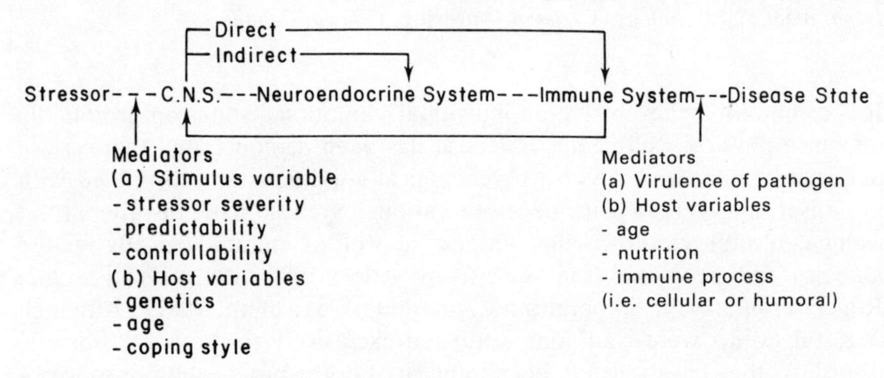

Figure 6.1: Stressors result in alterations of neurotransmitters which may influence disease states either by directly acting on target tissues of the immune system, or by influencing neuroendocrine activity which in turn affects immune processes. Furthermore, the immune system provides information about pathogenic activity to the central nervous system. The reaction of the organism to stressor application is mediated by such factors as stimulus severity and controllability, as well as the age and genetic and stress history of the host. Likewise, these variables mediate the ability of the host to mount an immune response to pathogenic stimulation.

Whether a disease state is manifested following the introduction of a pathogen depends upon the integrity of the immune system. This will depend upon such factors as age and genetically determined vulnerability (Fudenberg *et al.*, 1980). In addition, stressors may play a role by activating the CNS, which may act either directly or indirectly upon the immune system (see Besedovsky and Sorkin, 1981; Fabris, 1973; Ganong, 1976; Gisler, 1974, Hall and Goldstein, 1981). Consequently, discussion of the relationship between psychological events and illness must *per force* consider the effects of stressors on central nervous system activity. In the following sections evidence that psychological factors can influence the course of immunological disorders in humans will be presented. This will be followed by a discussion of animal models of stress-induced immune dysfunction, and finally, mechanisms of CNS – immune system interactions will be explored.

CLINICAL STUDIES

Several approaches have been used to investigate the influence of psychological variables upon immunocompetence, including case studies, as well as clinical and epidemiological analyses. Although attempts have been made to relate psychological factors and life-event changes to the occurence of immunologically related disorders using prospective and prognostic analyses, the greatest attention has been devoted to retrospective analyses. Evaluations of the individuals' recent life changes have revealed that a high incidence of stressful events is associated with depression (Brown, 1979; Paykel *et al.*, 1969), infectious disease (Boyce *et al.*, 1977); Meyer and Haggerty, 1962), arthritis (Rimon *et al.*, 1979; Solomon, 1981), multiple sclerosis (Warren *et al.*, 1982); and various forms of cancer (Bahnson and Bahnson, 1969; Fox, 1981; Horne and Picard, 1979).

Although considerable research into the relationship between previous life stress and illness has been undertaken, the validity of such data has been repeatedly challenged (Cohen, 1981; Monroe, 1982; Rabkin and Streuning, 1976; Yager *et al.* 1981). Among other things, retrospective data may be influenced by factors such as unreliable recall and altered cognitive functioning due to the current illness (see aforementioned critical reviews for further details). Moreover, in the absence of strict diagnostic criteria, it may be the case that people respond to stressful situations by reporting more illness and taking on the sick role (Minter and Kimball, 1978). Despite the difficulties with such research, clinical data are suggestive of a relationship between stress and various forms of immunologically mediated illness. There exist a few prospective as well as prognostic studies, and these data are far more compelling than those based exclusively on retrospective analyses.

Infectious Disorders

Infectious disorders constitute a large heterogeneous group of illnesses caused by viral, bacterial and fungal microorganisms which can affect virtually every organ system of the body. Depending on the nature of the pathogen (e.g. viral versus bacterial), either humoral or cell mediated processes will be induced to defend against infection. Several of the more commonly occurring infectious diseases have been investigated with respect to the role of psychological factors in compromising host defence systems.

Tuberculosis, a bacterial infection of the lungs, was among the first disorders for which a psychological component was postulated. As early as 1919 Ishigami observed that among TB patients phagocytic activity was diminished during phases of emotional excitement (Ishigami, in Locke, 1982). This is significant since macrophages and granulocytes provide the main line of defence against the tubercule bacillus and this is supplemented by T-cell immune processes (Bellanti, 1978).

Employing an early version of the schedule of recent events (SRE), it was reported that a significant increase in stressors such as job and residential changes occurred during the 2 years preceding the onset of TB symptoms (Holmes *et al.*, 1957). Moreover, where greater social supports were available in the form of job security, freedom from financial worries and strong family ties, the prognosis for recovery from TB was enhanced (Holmes *et al.*, 1961). This finding is consistent with reports that such buffering mechanisms are effective in decreasing vulnerability to psychological pathologies as well (see Brown, 1979).

Several studies have linked adverse psychological conditions with the onset of minor upper respiratory tract infections. In a series of studies conducted by Hinkle *et al.* (1974), a greater number of colds were reported by telephone company employees who rated their work as unsatisfying, than were reported by workers satisfied with their jobs. Likewise, Meyer and Haggerty (1962) found that individuals who reported a high degree of family stress were four times more likely to develop streptococcal respiratory infections than moderately stressed individuals. It was also noted that the incidence of stress was highest during the 2 weeks immediately preceding the onset of symptoms. Consistent results were reported for a group of children followed over a 1 year period (Boyce *et al.*, 1977). For those experiencing the highest stress levels, more severe and protracted symptoms were reported and this was confirmed in the analysis of throat cultures. Taken together, these data suggest that in both severe and minor respiratory infections psychological factors contribute to the prognosis. To what extent these factors exert their influence by directly acting on the tissues involved (e.g. increased mucous secretion, vasodilation) or by a generalized immunosuppressive action remains to be determined.

Evaluation of the role of psychological variables in the course of infectious mononucleosis have yielded conflicting results. This infection is caused by the Epstein – Barr virus, a variant of herpes, and the body's defence against it depends upon both humoral and cell-mediated processes. In retrospective studies of the role of stressful life events, Roark (1971) found higher stress levels among men with mononucleosis, but not among women. In contrast, Wilder *et al.* (1971) failed to detect a relationship between stress and mononucleosis for either gender. Still other investigations revealed that psychological factors influence both the incidence and duration of this illness under some conditions. That is, in a group of military cadets the incidence of illness, and the amount of time necessary for recuperation, were highest among those who were highly motivated to achieve and yet exhibited poor academic ability, and were therefore presumed to be experiencing the greatest stress (Kasl *et al.*, 1979). A more rapid rate of recovery from mononucleosis has been positively correlated with ego strength, leading to the suggestion that the ability to cope with stressors may be an important mediator of infection (Greenfield *et al.*, 1959). The discrepancies in these reports may be due to (1) the different criteria for determining stress levels and (2) retrospective (Wilder *et al.*, 1971) versus prospective (Kasl *et al.*, 1979) data gathering techniques.

Unlike mononucleosis, infections due to herpes simplex virus may recur and the frequency of these recurrences may be influenced by psychological factors. Type I herpes simplex virus results in fever blisters or cold sores, whereas Type II causes genital lesions and is one of the most prevalent sexually transmitted infections (Fudenberg *et al.*, 1980). Although anecdotal accounts indicate that both types of herpes may be subject to emotional influences, few clinical or experimental studies have been undertaken to investigate this issue. In a prospective study of Type I herpes it was found that during the 4 days preceding an outbreak, ratings of negative mood were increased among patients, but this trend was not significant (Luborsky *et al.*, 1976). More positive evidence for an interaction between stress and herpes manifestation is found in experimental studies of the Epstein – Barr virus and these results will be discussed in a later section.

Allergic Disorders

Allergy or hypersensitivity constitutes a significant health problem since 15 to 20% of the population experiences at least one form of allergic disorder (Mathews, 1982) and it is commonly held that the hypersensitivity may be influenced by psychological factors. The most common form of allergy is due to a Type I immediate hypersensitivity reaction which results in symptoms of hay fever, asthma or urticaria (hives). This reaction is mediated by antibodies that cause an immediate inflammatory response which may be either localized (e.g. rhinitis) or systemic (e.g. anaphylaxis) (Bellanti, 1978). Following the introduction of an allergen to the body via inhalation or ingestion, B lymphocytes divide and form IgE producing cells. The IgE molecules attach themselves to mast cells in the lung, skin or nasal tissue for several weeks. Upon re-exposure the allergen binds to the mast cell resulting in the release of histamine and other mediators, consequently producing symptoms of allergy within minutes of exposure. Symptoms of allergy due to delayed hypersensitivity reactions may take hours or days to appear and unlike immediate reactions, this process is cell mediated.

Bronchial asthma has long been considered to be associated with family conflicts, dependency states and heightened emotional arousal (Weiner, 1977). For example, Purcell *et al.* (1962) reported that asthmatic attacks among children were precipitated by laughing, crying and both pleasurable and unpleasant states such as anger and anxiety. Moreover, separation from a parent or spouse or the anticipation of such an event contributes to the onset of an atack in up to 50% of patients (Weiner, 1977). The reaction to these stressful events is mediated by, among other things, an individual's coping style. De Araujo *et al.* (1972) reported that asthmatic patients with lower coping ability required higher doses of medication to control their symptoms than did those who coped well.

The symptoms of asthma displayed by predisposed individuals may be precipitated by allergic stimulation, together with exercise, infection and psychosocial factors (Weiner, 1977). Similarly, clinical studies have indicated that hay fever and rhinitis may be triggered or exacerbated by stressful events (Holmes *et al.* 1961). However, it has not been satisfactorily demonstrated whether symptoms are intensified as a result of the stressor directly affecting the immune system or by some other parasympathetic activity (Stein, 1981). It seems paradoxical that stressors apparently have an immunosuppressive effect leading to increased susceptibility to infectious states, whereas in the case of allergy, aggravated symptoms may reflect enhanced immune functioning. However, it has been postulated that allergy may result from an inhibition of suppressor T-cells, which under normal circumstances may act as a damper of antibody production (Katz, 1978). Stressors could therefore exacerbate allergic symptoms by depressing suppressor T-cell activity and consequently enhancing the IgE antibody response. Alternatively, non-immunologic processes such as neurotransmitter release may contribute to the observed effects via a direct influence on mast cells. Indeed, acetylcholine, epinephrine and norepinephrine influence the release of histamine from mast cells, and it has been postulated that a beta-adrenergic defect may be responsible for symptoms of allergy in some individuals (Barnes *et al.*, 1983; Frick, 1980).

Autoimmune Diseases

The principle of 'horror autotoxicus' first described by Ehrlich in 1900, states that, in general, an organism cannot immunologically respond to the chemical groupings of its own body (Rose, 1981). That is, under most circumstances the body does not produce autoantibodies and is therefore tolerant of its own tissues. However, it has recently been recognized that in some instances the body does begin to attack its own cells, both by the production of autoantibodies and by cell mediated processes, resulting in autoimmune disease. It is generally agreed that the autoimmune disorders include rheumatoid arthritis, myasthenia gravis and lupus erythematosus, and further, autoimmunity has been implicated in the aetiology of multiple sclerosis and Grave's disease, a disorder involving the thyroid (Bellanti, 1978; Rose, 1981).

Systemic lupus erythematosus (SLE), considered to be the prototype of systemic autoimmune diseases, is a multisystem disorder involving the production of autoantibodies to many tissues and may involve damage to the skin, joints, kidney and blood-producing tissues. Rheumatoid arthritis similarly involves multiple autoantibody production and the major target organ is the synovial lining of the joints. Rather than reflecting a generalized hyperactivity of the immune system, these disorders may be due to reduced activity or dysfunction of suppressor T-cells and a consequent increase in B lymphocyte activity (Kohler and Vaughan, 1982). Interestingly, autoimmune disorders are accompanied by a relative state of immunodeficiency such that patients are more susceptible to various infections. Although the reason for this has not been determined it may be due to regulatory T-cell or granulocyte dysfunction (Heise, 1982).

Retrospective studies of patients suffering from SLE have reported that they show compulsive traits and increased needs for independence and activity (McClary *et al.*, 1957). Moreover, women with SLE reported more stress in the months preceding illness onset than did controls (Otto and McKay, 1967). The illness is characterized by cycles in which symptoms vary in their severity, and in a recent survey of 19 SLE patients, 12 reported deterioration in their conditions following acute stress (Hall *et al.* 1981). This study lent some support to the notion that coping style is an important factor in the course of the disease. Patients in this survey who were members of patient support groups or other social clubs reported a mean of 3.5 episodes of exacerbated symptoms per year, compared to 7 episodes per year experienced by patients who lacked these social supports.

Numerous studies reported a relationship between rheumatoid arthritis (RA) and personality traits such as compulsiveness, hostility, introversion and restricted emotional expression (Solomon and Amkraut, 1981). The most consistent data are derived from studies employing the M.M.P.I., which indicated that a typical RA profile reflects a high degree of bodily concern and depression (Achterberg-Lawlis, 1982). This is not particularly surprising given the chronic and debilitating nature of arthritis, and this profile might be consistent with any number of chronic disease states. Indeed Spergel *et al.* (1978) compared M.M.P.I. profiles of arthritics with those of patients with ulcers, low back pain and multiple sclerosis, and found no significant differences between these groups. However, M.M.P.I. scores differed from normal controls leading to the conclusion that there is a chronic illness profile rather than an arthritic profile *per se*.

Few studies have examined the role of stressful life events in the aetiology of RA; however, patients with this illness frequently attribute symptoms to recent stressful events (Solomon, 1981). Among patients who exhibited a rapid onset and progression of the illness, exacerbation of symptoms was associated with increased stress, but apparently stress was not a contributing factor in more insidious rheumatoid arthritis (Rimon *et al.*, 1979). A relationship between stress and juvenile rheumatoid arthritis was found in 37% of cases, and this group also exhibited elevated levels of viral antibodies, indicating that there may be subsets of this disorder or that individuals are differentially reactive to stressors (Rimon *et al.*, 1977, 1979). It seems that although there are valid reasons to suspect psychosocial influences on rheumatoid arthritis, the data concerning such a relationship have been inconclusive and often contradictory. Unfortunately, since the onset of RA cannot be predicted, retrospective studies must be relied upon, despite the problems associated with this research strategy.

Clinical studies have tended to support anecdotal accounts which suggest that psychological states influence the course of multiple sclerosis (MS), a progressive neuromuscular disorder. Mei-Tal, *et al.* (1970) reported that of 32 MS patients in their sample, 28 indicated that the disease was preceded by a stressful event. However, since no control cases were reported, this retrospectively reported pattern may be attributable to emotional states associated with chronic illness or hospitalization. In a recent study comparing MS patients with acutely ill controls, the MS patients reported the occurrence of three times as many stressful events (e.g. personal illness, financial, marriage and interactional problems), for the 2 years preceding symptom onset than did controls (Warren, *et al.*, 1982). Bereavement, which is thought to represent one of the major forms of stress, was identified as a contributing factor to MS on the basis of case reports (e.g. Adams *et al.*, 1950); however, this was not substantiated in the survey conducted by Warren *et al.* (1982). It is conceivable that rather than precipitating illness onset, stressors exacerbate the symptoms of MS (McAlpine and Compston, 1952), in much the same fashion as they exacerbate the symptoms of lupus erythematosus and other autoimmune diseases.

Summarizing, it appears that psychosocial factors may play a role in the onset and exacerbation of symptoms of SLE, rheumatoid arthritis and multiple sclerosis. Moreover, a few reports are available which provisionally suggest that stressful events may also contribute to other disorders with an autoimmune component such as Grave's disease, ulcerative colitis and diabetes mellitus (Linn, *et al.*, 1983; Solomon and Amkraut, 1981; Stein, 1981; Weiner, 1977). The difficulty with such studies, as in those previously described, is the reliance upon retrospectively reported events, and the fact that the autoimmune disorders tend to be chronic debilitating diseases. The possibility must therefore be entertained that the significant stress – illness relationships reported are actually reflections of psychological factors associated with chronic illness.

Cancer

The contribution of psychosocial influences to the course of neoplastic disease has received considerable attention (see reviews by Fox, 1981; Riley, 1981;

Sklar and Anisman, 1981). As in the case of other immune diseases, data derived from clinical investigations are often contradictory and difficult to interpret. However, results of retrospective, prospective and prognostic investigations have frequently demonstrated a relationship between psychosocial factors and cancer.

Rather than a single entity, cancer actually represents a large heterogeneous group of diseases characterized by the uncontrollable proliferation of cells. In order for cancer to develop, essentially two changes must occur. First, normal cells must be transformed to malignant ones, as a result of genetic coding, spontaneous mutation, or exposure to a carcinogen. Secondly, there must be a failure of the host's defences against this cellular proliferation (Penn, 1981). Additionally, malignant cells may break away from the main tumor mass, and travel either via the blood or lymphatic systems, ultimately lodging at a distant site, and provoking the appearance of secondary tumors. Owing to the unpredictability of the metastitic processes, the development of secondary tumors has proven to be the greatest difficulty in the clinical control of neoplasia (Fidler, 1978).

Although much remains to be determined about the nature of host defences, immune functions are thought to play a major role. In particular, cytotoxic T-cells, macrophages, antibodies and NK cells can suppress the rate of proliferation or destroy cancer cells. Failure of the immune system to defend against the development of malignancy may be attributable to deficiencies of helper T-cells, the presence of antibodies which enhance the growth of tumor cells, or inadequate NK cell activity (Broder and Whitehouse, 1968; Kamo and Friedman, 1977). According to the immune surveillance hypothesis, one of the functions of cytotoxic T-cells is to recognize and destroy mutant cells which have the potential to form tumors (Burnet, 1971). Consequently, suppression of immunosurveillance results in the progression of neoplastic disease. Although this model is widely accepted, it has been criticized on a number of grounds. For instance, neither athymic mice (which lack T-cells) nor mice administered immunosuppressant drugs necessarily exhibit increased rates of neoplasia (Stutman, 1975). Similarly, among patients with immunodeficiency disorders an increased incidence of malignancies has not been noted (Penn, 1981). Furthermore, spontaneous tumors apparently lack tumor specific transplantation antigens which are required for identification by cytotoxic cells (Prehn, 1974). It is possible that the immune system does not respond uniformly to all types of cancer, and indeed in some forms of neoplasia the immune system may not be involved.

In order for a malignancy to develop, there must be a dysfunction of the host's defence system, and it is this aspect of the cancer process that may be particularly vulnerable to the influence of psychological factors. Based on retrospective investigation, breast cancer patients have been described as masochistic, emotionally constricted, and unable to deal with anger or hostility (Bahnson and Bahnson, 1969; LeShan, 1966, Voth, 1976). In contrast, in prospective studies these patients were not found to differ from controls with respect to hostility or neuroticism, although they did experience difficulty in expressing strong emotions, and in particular, anger (Greer and Morris, 1975; Morris *et al.*, 1981). Similarly, women with gynaecological cancers have described themselves as more controlled, less aggressive and more perfectionistic than controls (Mastrovito *et al.*, 1979; Schmale and Iker, 1966). Restricted emotional expression has also been associated with lung cancer, and patients with pancreatic cancer scored higher than controls on the depression scale of the M.M.P.I. (Fras *et al.*, 1967; Kissen, 1967). It has been suggested that the blockade of emotional expression, which seems to be characteristic of cancer patients, represents a state of chronic stress, and as such the course of the neoplasia may be influenced by endogenous immunological, hormonal and transmitter alterations that are associated with stressful events (Grossarth-Maticek, *et al.*, 1982).

Consistent with the association of particular personality traits with neoplasia, increased incidence of stressful life events including the illness or death of a family member have been found to precede the onset of cervical, pancreatic and lung cancer (Ernster *et al.*, 1979, Fras *et al.*, 1967; Horne and Picard, 1979; Lehrer, 1980; Schmale and Iker, 1966). Furthermore, the increased incidence of cancer seems to be related specifically to the inability to cope with the loss, accompanied by a pervading sense of hopelessness (Greene, 1966).

Although patients with malignant tumors may differ from controls on some dimensions of personality, a relationship between breast cancer and stressful life events was not observed in either retrospective or prospective studies (Greer and Morris, 1975; Muslin *et al.*, 1966). As Blaney (1983, in press) has noted, however, the lack of an association may be due, in part, to the use of patients with benign breast disease as controls. That is, patients with benign tumors have been reported to have higher stress levels than non patients (Kosch, 1981). Consequently, potential relationships between stressful events and malignancy may not have been detected. Moreover, benign tumors may become transformed into malignant tumors, hence making comparisons between benign and malignant tumor groups at any specific time an inappropriate procedure.

Of particular interest are prospective studies which demonstrated an association between psychosocial factors and cancer. Thomas and associates have assessed a group of former medical students since the 1940's, and recent follow-up studies revealed a significant relationship between the lack of closeness to parents in adolescence and subsequent development of cancer (Thomas *et al.*, 1979). Moreover, an individual's emotional history as reflected by such attitudes was more closely related to disease states than the incidence of stressful events *per se* (Cox and MacKay, 1982). Horne and Picard (1979) used a composite index based on ratings of childhood instability, job and marriage stability and recent significant loss in order to predict lung cancer incidence. The index correctly identified 61% of those with malignancies, the single best predictor being the loss of a significant relationship during the preceding 5 years (Horne and Picard, 1979). Interestingly, a diagnosis of depression, which has been associated with increased life stress, was associated with a two-fold increase in cancer incidence over a period of 17 years following initial assessment (Shekelle *et al.*, 1981).

Finally, attempts have been made to form prognoses on the basis of coping styles. Increased survival times for various forms of cancer have been observed among cancer patients who were able to express anger and hostility openly (Blumber, *et al.*, 1954; Derogatis *et al.*, 1977; Stavrakay, 1968). Poor prognoses were noted among patients who maintained destructive interpersonal relationships and who had a history of alienation from others (Weisman and Worden, 1975). Reactions to the disease itself may be an important indicator of prognoses, since it has been observed that denial and a sense of being physically unable to fight the disease characterize patients with short survival times (Achterberg *et al.*, 1977). Moreover, patients who rated the adjustment to a diagnosis of malignant melanoma as particularly difficult were less likely to relapse than patients who rated the adjustment as less taxing (Rogentine *et al.*, 1979). Although the significance of the difference in attitude between the patient groups is not clear, this outcome may reflect an inappropriate lack of concern among patients that relapsed.

Summarizing, many clinical investigations have demonstrated that psychosocial factors may influence the course of various immunologically mediated diseases. The extent to which stressors exert a significant influence may depend upon the coping style of an individual and the resources or social supports available. It should be emphasized, however, that not all disorders appear to be equally susceptible to the influence of stressors. For example, as opposed to other forms of cancer, a positive association between stress and breast cancer has not been adequately demonstrated (Blaney, 1983). Furthermore, the data suggesting a positive relationship between illness and stressful events should be interpreted with caution since the validity of many studies has encountered considerable scepticism. First, on scales such as the SRE, stressors are conceived of as a series of additive changes rather than events which can be ranked as positive or negative by the individual. For example, according to the SRE, divorce has a high stress ranking, although for some individuals taking such a step may serve to reduce anxiety and stress. By viewing stress as life change, chronic conditions such as physical disability or job dissatisfaction would not be rated as stressful. Secondly, some events are confounded with existing illness states. For example, a change in sleeping habits may be ranked as a stressor when in fact it may be symptomatic of illness (Brown, 1979; Cohen, 1981; Rankin and Streuning, 1976). Finally, since clinical detection of cancer may occur years after the initial presence of malignant cells, evaluation of stress history during the 6 to 12 month period preceding illness identification may be of dubious value (Fox, 1978).

STRESS AND DIRECT MEASURES OF IMMUNE FUNCTION – HUMAN STUDIES

Phagocytic Processes

The phagocytic cells of the immune system provide the frontline defence against various pathogens, and several recent reports have suggested that phagocytic functions are subject to the influence of stressors. In a series of experiments, Palmblad and his associates (Palmblad *et al.*, 1976; 1979a; b) subjected volunteers to sleep deprivation, and required them to complete various questionnaires and vigilence tasks. During a 72 hour deprivation period, the ability to phagocytize staphylococcus bacteria was diminished compared to pretest levels, and following recovery, the rate of phagocytosis was increased beyond baseline (Palmblad *et al.*, 1976). In a later study, differences in granulocyte adherence were not detected during 48 hrs of sleep deprivation (Palmblad *et al.*, 1979a). This discrepancy may indicate that diminishment of phagocytosis is dependent upon the duration of the stressor, or it may be due to the different techniques employed to assess granulocyte function.

Granulocyte adherence has been assessed among healthy individuals undergoing minor surgery, an event which is both physically and psychologically stressful. Compared to presurgical levels, adherence was diminished 24 hours following surgery (Palmblad *et al.*, 1979b). When granulocyte function was measured 5 days after minor surgery, it did not differ from baseline, indicating that this phenomenon may be rather transient (Linn and Jensen, 1983). In comparison to healthy infants, newborns in states of physical distress owing to respiratory problems of Caesarean delivery, have been shown to have depressed granulocyte function (Wright, *et al.*, 1975).

There have been reports associating the stress of space flight with imunological functioning. Relative to preflight levels, the total white blood cell (WBC) counts of Apollo astronauts were increased immediately following splashdown and recovery, and they returned to normal within a few days (Fischer, *et al.*, 1972). In a subsequent report it was noted that following prolonged periods in space (59 days), returning Skylab astronauts exhibited marked elevations in WBC counts, and further analysis indicated this was due to increased numbers of granulocytes (Kimzey *et al.*, 1976).

Antibody Reactions

Limited evidence is available concerning alterations of immunoglobulin levels in response to acute stress. Strenuous physical activity (Tomasi, *et al.*, 1982), and exam stress (Jemmott *et al.*, 1983) are associated with depressed IgA levels in saliva, rendering subjects more susceptible to respiratory infections. The paucity of data is not altogether surprising, given the stability of antibody levels under adverse conditions (Palmblad, 1981).

Under long-term stressful conditions, which have been assessed by life events scales, antibody responses are relatively resistant to change. Locke and Heisel (1977) reported that there was no association between retrospectively reported stressful life events scores and individuals' antibody response to viral inoculation; an observation which has been confirmed in subsequent investigations (Greene *et al.*, 1979; Roessler *et al.*, 1979). However, among subjects who reported high stress levels in the two weeks following viral challenge, antibody titers were depressed (Locke, *et al.*, 1979). Although stress levels *per se* may not be strongly linked to alterations in immunoglobulin levels, it has been reported that ego strength is positively correlated with antibody responses (McClelland *et al.*, 1980), suggesting that coping style may be an important factor in mediating antibody reactions to stress (Locke, 1982). Elevated levels of IgA were also seen among women ranked high in anger suppression, while they were awaiting cancer biopsy. This relationship was seen regardless of whether the ultimate diagnosis was malignant or benign (Pettingale *et al.*, 1977).

Lymphocyte Activity

Although some alterations of the immune response may be detected, stressors do not produce dramatic changes in total white blood cell counts, phagocytic function, or antibody responses. However, alterations of the functional capacity of the immune system may be better assessed by measuring the rate of lymphoblast transformation.

T-cell transformation was depressed among Skylab astronauts on the day of splashdown, and gradually returned to preflight levels over several days (Kimzey *et al.*, 1976). Minor surgery also led to depressed T-cell transformation (possibly suppressor T-cells) when measured on the fifth day following the operation (Lin and Jensen, 1983). This response was only seen among older patients (60 yrs and over), and yet these individuals recovered as well as those who were younger. Finally, Palmblad *et al.* (1979a) reported that during and after a 48 hour sleep deprivation schedule, subjects exhibited a decreased response to phytohemagglutinin (PHA) stimulation, indicating depressed T lymphocyte function.

The stress of preparing and taking exams was shown to depress lymphocyte function (Dorian *et al.*, 1981). Compared to a control group of physicians, both B and T lymphoblast transformation were decreased among individuals who were studying for professional exams, and returned to normal in the weeks following. It has recently been demonstrated that although there is apparently no relationship between cytotoxic activity of natural killer (NK) cells and the number of stressful events encountered, coping ability does have an effect. That is, among students rated as poor copers on the basis of MMPI scores, NK cell activity was significantly diminished (see Locke, 1982).

Bartrop *et al.* (1977) assessed a group of 26 adults over several weeks following the death of their spouses. At none of the intervals investigated were any differences from control subjects found with respect to immunoglobulin levels, total lymphocyte counts or levels of pituitary and adrenocortical hormones. However, T-cell responses to mitogen were significantly depressed at 6 weeks, but not at 2 weeks following bereavement. Similarly, Scheifer, *et al.*, (1983) prospectively investigated the responses of a group of men whose wives were in the advanced stages of breast cancer. Compared with pre-bereavement data, total numbers of lymphocytes and the relative proportion of T- and B-cells did not change 5 to 7 weeks following bereavement. However, the responses to both the T-cell mitogen PHA and the B-cell mitogen pokeweed were significantly depressed at that time.

Together, these data suggest that as bereavement continues, the functional capacity of T- and B-cells is depressed. This alteration may reflect the gradual response of the immune system to a state of chronic stress. Alternatively, the stresses experienced immediately following the loss of a spouse are qualitatively different from those encountered in later weeks and months, and are therefore associated with different immunological status. It is also conceivable that the inception of a traumatic stressor stimulates an active process which serves to blunt the emotional impact that would otherwise be elicited. Thus, soon after the trauma immune functioning would not be depressed, but with the passage of time, and the resultant diminuation of the emotional blunting, expression of the reduced immune functioning would be evident. Irrespective of the processes involved, it is of interest that immunological changes can be detected following bereavement, given the numerous reports indicating that this a period associated with increased rates of illness, hospital admission and mortality (Parkes and Brown, 1972; Jacobs and Ostfeld, 1977).

ANIMAL STUDIES

Data from human experimental reports indicate that the suppression of lymphocyte and monocyte activity associated with states of stress may be responsible for the exacerbation of symptoms of various illnesses. Limited information is available, however, concerning the conditions wherein stressors provoke alterations in immune functioning, and the nature of clinical investigation precludes invasive analyses of immune processes. Consequently, most of the available data concerning the stress/immune relationship have come from infrahuman studies.

Disease Susceptibility

Studies employing various animal species have confirmed that stressors increase susceptibility to infectious disorders. Avoidance training (6 hr per day) for 2 or 4 weeks prior to viral inoculation increased susceptibility to herpes simplex (Rasmussen *et al.*, 1957), poliomyelitis (Johnsson and Rasmussen, 1965) and Coxsackie B viruses (Johnsson, *et al.*, 1963). Likewise, susceptibility to herpes simplex was increased by physical restraint (Friedman, *et al.*, 1965), and the rate of morbidity due to Coxsackie B was increased by exposure to unavoidable footshock (Rasmussen *et al.*, 1957). However, the response to influenza and respiratory viruses was unaltered by stressors (Johnsson and Rasussen, 1965).

Social conditions may also alter susceptibility to infection among animals. Mice infected with a cardiac virus (encephalomyocarditis, EMC) had much shorter life spans if they were housed individually than if they were housed in groups of 5 to 20 (Friedman *et al.*, 1970). In contrast, mice housed in large groups were highly susceptible to mortality from *Plasmodium berghei*, a malarial parasite, compared to animals housed alone (Plaut, *et al.*, 1969). Consistent with these results, mortality following the administration of *Salmonella typhinium* was increased among mice housed in groups of 30 – 60, compared with those housed in smaller groups (Edwards and Dean, 1977). Because none of the animals were isolated in this study, it is not clear whether susceptibility to salmonella varies as a linear function of group size (as in the case of the malarial and EMC viruses), or whether both isolation and overcrowding could increase susceptibility to this pathogen. Although the reasons for the differential effects of isolation on susceptibility to the malarial and cardiac viruses remains to be determined, it may be that these pathogens are differentially affected by the hormonal and neurochemical milieu created by such stressors (see later discussion).

Clinical studies have shown that autoimmune disorders, such as multiple sclerosis and arthritis, are subject to the influence of stressors. Although these particular disorders have not been studied in infrahuman species, adjuvent induced arthritis has been employed as an animal model of autoimmune disease. Typically, animals are injected with a derivative of cartilage, and Freund's adjuvent, an emulsion which magnifies the antigenicity of the cartilage tissue (Rose, 1981). Using such a procedure, it was demonstrated that joint inflammation in rats subjected to overcrowding was intensified, although the rate of recovery was accelerated in this stressed group (Amkraut, *et al.*, 1971). In contrast, repeated stress (exposure to a predator) reduced the incidence of experimental arthritis (Rogers, *et al.*, 1979).

Experiments that investigated the role of stress in the exacerbation of neoplastic disease have supported the contention that psychological or physical insults may contribute to the course of the illness. Moreover, factors such as stress severity, duration and controllability were found to influence the rate of tumor development (see reviews by LaBarba, 1970; Fox, 1981; Sklar and Aniskan, 1981). Acute physical stressors, such as footshock, whole body irradiation, or surgical trauma have been found to enhance the growth of transplanted tumors (Jamasbi and Nettesheim, 1977; Peters, 1975; Peters and Kelly, 1977; Sklar and Anisman, 1979). Moreover, the incidence of tumor development after transplantation of a single lymphosarcoma cell could be enhanced by whole body irradiation (Marayuma and Johnson, 1969). In addition to increasing the rate of tumor development the latter study suggests that stress may enhance the probability of metastases (i.e. the formation of secondary neoplasms). Indeed, following intravenous administration of malignant cells, increased pulmonary and liver tumors were evident in animals that had been exposed to stressors such as restraint, tumbling or surgery (Fisher and Fisher, 1959; Saba and Antikatzides, 1976; Van den Brenk *et al.*, 1976). Surgical stress also increased the occurrence of secondary neoplasms in spontaneously metastasizing tumors (Hattori *et al.*, 1982; Lundy *et al.*, 1979), and this effect was attenuated if animals were treated with immunopotentiating drugs prior to tumor innoculation (Hattori *et al.*, 1982).

Whether an animal can exert control over the aversive stimulation is fundamental in determining whether tumor growth will be enhanced. When mice were exposed to a single session of escapable shock 24hr following tumor cell transplantation, the rate of tumor growth did not differ from control animals. In contrast, an equivalent amount of inescapable shock resulted in earlier tumor appearance and an increase in tumor size (Sklar and Anisman, 1979). In the same fashion, inescapable but not escapable shock significantly reduced the incidence of rejection of transplanted non-syngeneic tumor cells (Visintainer *et al.*, 1982).

Although the acceleration of tumor growth prompted by stressors might be a result of a large variety of variables, the possibility has been entertained that suppression of the immune system provoked by aversive stimulation was responsible for the tumorigenic changes (Riley, 1981; Riley *et al.*, 1981). According to Riley and his associates (Riley and Spackman, 1977; Riley *et al.*, 1979), stressors will only enhance tumor development if the tumor is under partial or complete control of the immune system. The release of corticosterone induced by a stressor is thought to result in immunosuppression (see later), thereby permitting the augmentation of tumor development, provided that the immune system ordinarily limits the growth of this particular tumor type. In accordance with this position, it was demonstrated that in two substrains of C3H mice, exposure to rotation stress enhanced the growth of a lymphosarcoma that was nonhistocompatible with the host, but this treatment had little effect when the two were histocompatible. In a second study, it was shown that stress in the form of viral challenge accelerated the growth of a non-pigmented melanoma in the C57B1/6 line of mouse, but had no effect on the development of a pigmented melanoma, which is more histocompatible (Riley, 1981). While these data are certainly impressive, it should be emphasized that alternative interpretations of these experiments are possible. For instance, the pigmented melanoma in the latter study develops more rapidly than the non-pigmented one, and hence any further enhancement of growth that could potentially be induced by the stressor was precluded. In the former study, the possibility exists that differences in the two substrains of mice (e.g. reactivity to the aversive stimuli, differences in endogenous chemical status other than immune functioning, etc.) could have accounted for the differences observed. Moreover, it has been demonstrated that manipulations such as adrenalectomy do not prevent the effects of stressors on tumor development (Peters and Kelly, 1977), and stress-induced enhancement of tumor growth has been seen using syngeneic tumors (i.e. where the cell line and host are compatible), and this effect could not be reversed by reconstitution of syngeneic spleen cells (Jamasbi and Nettesheim, 1977). These caveats notwithstanding, the date presented by Riley and his associates certainly are consistent with the view that stressors may influence the course of neoplastic growth.

Unlike acute stress, repeated application of restraint (Bhattacharyya and Pradhan, 1979), footshock (Kalisnik, *et al.*, 1979; Newberry and Sengbusch, 1976; Pradhan and Ray, 1974) and sound stress (Monjan, 1981), inhibited the growth of various carcinogen-induced and transplanted tumors. Unfortunately, only a limited number of studies have compared the effects of acute and chronic stressors on tumor development within a single experiment. Nevertheless, using a carcinogen induced tumor it was found that little change in growth was evident after 25 days of shock stress, but both 40 and 85 days of this treatment inhibited tumor development (Newberry and Sengbusch, 1976). Likewise, Nieburgs *et al.*, (1979) reported that when animals were exposed to a brief duration shock every 4 days for 90 days, the rate of tumor growth was accelerated, whereas the growth rate declined if shocks were applied for 150 days. Employing a transplanted tumor Sklar and Anisman (1979) demonstrated that the enhancement in growth ordinarily seen after acute shock was eliminated in chronically stressed mice. Anisman and Sklar (1982) suggested that in addition to an adaptive response to the stressor, the attenuation in tumor growth observed following chronic stress may be due to some type of active process (possibly neurochemical) which inhibits the proliferation of malignant cells.

As in the case of infectious disorders, social condions may influence the course of neoplastic development. In particular, housing mice in isolation increased the incidence and growth rate of spontaneous, carcinogen-induced and transplanted tumors (Dechambre, 1981; DeChambre and Gosse, 1973; Sklar and Anisman, 1980). It has been suggested that rather than isolation *per se*, a change in environmental conditions may have been responsible for the observed effects. That is, if mice were raised in isolation from the time of weaning, the growth rate of transplanted tumors was the same as for mice raised in groups. If group housed mice were placed in isolation following transplantation, however, a marked increase in the growth rate was noted (Dechambre, 1981; Sklar and Anisman, 1980).

Although some of the variables which determine the way in which stressors will influence tumor development have been identified, inconsistent data have been reported (see review in Sklar and Anisman, 1981). In part, some of the divergent results may stem from the differences in tumor lines employed or the variations in methods of inducing tumors. Additionally, investigators have employed different types of stressors, as well as varied stressor regimens. If nothing else, the abundance of data do suggest that stressor controllability and chronicity influence the course of tumor development. The mechanisms underlying the source for these particular effects have not been identified. However, speculations as to the critical factors that might play a role in determining the effects of these variables will be discussed in ensuing sections.

Phagocytic Processes

Paralleling the human investigations, experiments with animals have indicated that various aspects of immunocompetence are altered by stressful manipulations. Following exposure to signalled escapable shock, animals previously injected with the inflammatory agent glycogen, exhibited impaired phagocytic functions (Bassett and Tait, 1981). The numbers of polymorphonuclear cells (PMN) in the bloodstream and at the injection site were significantly reduced when measured 6 to 36 hours following the end of the stress session. Monocytes, the precursors of macrophages, were also reduced at the injection site, and together these data indicate that migration of phagocytic cells to an antigen was interrupted by stress. Both restraint and overcrowding also significantly disrupted the response of macrophages to antigenic stimulation (Gisler, 1974; Teshima *et al.*, 1982), and restraint impaired the ability of macrophages to destroy leukemia cells *in vitro* (Pavlidis and Chirigos, 1980).

Humoral Processes

Depressed antibody levels have been noted in animals subjected to the stress of changed environmental conditions such as overcrowding (Solomon, 1969); Gisler, 1974; Edwards and Dean, 1977), isolation (Glenn and Becker, 1969), and housing in food-restricted activity cages (Hara *et al.*, 1981). Antibody titers were also lowered among mice that were chronically isolated and then subjected to attack by a dominant mouse (Beden and Brain, 1982). Conversely, elevated antibody levels were seen in dominant mice (Vessey, 1964). Other indices of the humoral response, such as white blood cell counts and the intensity of antigen inflammatory responses, have also revealed that immunosuppression occurs as a consequence of both short-term and long-term overcrowding (Gisler, 1974; Boranic *et al.*, 1982).

As in the case of social stressors, exposure to physical insults, such as combined noise and light (Hill *et al.*, 1967) or immobilization (Gisler, 1974; Boranic *et al.*, 1982) also attenuated humoral reactivity as indicated by lowered antibody titers. Antibody levels were more resistant to change, however, following exposure to footshock stress (Rasmussen, 1969; Solomon, 1969).

Cell Medited Immunity

As with phagocytic and humoral processes, cellular immunity is subject to change by a variety of environmental manipulations. For example, depressed T-cell responses were reported in infant monkeys following maternal separation (Laudenslager *et al.*, 1982). Increases in noise level as a consequence of building construction (Folch and Waksman, 1974), and weekly reversals of the light – dark cycle (Kort and Weijma, 1982) also resulted in depressed T-cell activity. In contrast, enhancement of T-lymphocyte responsiveness was detected after chronic exposure to the stress of overcrowding (Joasoo and McKenzie, 1976).

Consistent with the observation that alterations in environmental conditions influence immune processes, it was reported that daily sessions of inescapable shock diminished lymphocyte responsiveness to stimulation by both concanavalin A (Con A) and PHA (Solomon *et al.*, 1974). Shock coupled with intense noise, likewise suppressed cell-mediated immunity (Teshima *et al.*, 1982). In particular, T-cell cytotoxicity of mice injected with chicken red blood cells was decreased regardless of whether the stressor was administered before or after the injection. Moreover, it has been reported that a single prolonged shock session (intermittent shock over 20 to 24 hrs), in addition to reducing the total number of lymphocytes (Nieburgs *et al.*, 1979) also depressed the T-cell response to PHA (Keller *et al.*, 1981). In a subsequent report it was demonstrated that although adrenalectomy influenced the stress induced lymphopenia, it did not affect mitogen responsivity (Keller *et al.*, 1983). Thus it seems that although corticosteroids are probably not responsible for the alteration in the functional capacity of T-cells following stress exposure, multiple mechanisms account for the wide range of immune alterations associated with aversive stimuli.

It has been demonstrated that the response to mitogens was depressed in animals exposed to intermittent footshocks over a 20 min period, but with a continuous less protracted exposure, no alteration was noted (Shavit *et al.*, 1982). Furthermore, if the mitogen response was assessed 24 hr following the end of the stress session, a slight elevation was observed, indicating that both stressor severity and timing of stressor application are important determinants of the lymphocyte response. Parenthetically, in the latter study, the depression of the mitogen response was detected with stress parameters previously shown to induce opioid analgesia, leading Shavit *et al.*, 1982) to suggest that opioids may be involved in tumor development. Indeed, in rats injected with a mammary ascites tumor, administration of naltrexone, an opiate antagonist, prevented the tumor enhancing effect of this type of stressor (Lewis *et al.*, 1983a, b in press) Likewise, naltrexone administration delayed the appearance of a neuroblastoma, which is known to have opiate receptors (Zagon and McLaughlin, 1983).

In addition to the variations of T-cell responsivity, physical insults will apparently influence NK activity. In particular, depression of NK cell activity was observed following surgical stress (Toge *et al.*, 1981) and the stress of transportation (Herberman and Holden, 1978). Intermittent inescapable footshock likewise suppressed the activity of NK cells in spleen tissue, and this effect could be mimicked by the administration of high doses of morphine (Shavit *et al.*, 1983). Moreover, mild shock application suppressed NK cell activity in animals that had previously been exposed to inescapable shock; however, the shock reexposure was without effect on animals that had received escapable shock (Lewis, Shavit, Terman, Nelson *et al.*, 1983). Thus, the experience with inescapable shock may have sensitized the animals so that a mild stressor provoked an exagerated immunological response in much the same fashion as animals may be sensitized to stress-induced neurochemical alterations (Anisman and Sklar, 1979; Irwin *et al.*, 1982).

Factors Influencing Immune System Responses to Stress

Data from a variety of experimental paradigms have shown that humoral, cell-mediated and phagocytic activities, just like susceptibility to infectious and neoplastic diseases, are altered by stressor application. These immunological alterations appear to be subject to host, pathogenic and environmental variables. Indeed, a great deal of the variance in data observed across laboratories may be accounted for on the basis of such factors as the controllability and chronicity of stressors, temporal relationships, and the social environment onto which stressors are superimposed.

It has repeatedly been shown that behavioral and neurochemical responses to stress are mediated by the controllability of aversive stimuli, and the data derived from immunological studies tentatively support the hypothesis that controllability influences immune responsivity. Although there are few studies which have explicitly examined this factor, it has been demonstrated that contrary to the lack of observable effects of escapable shock, an equivalent amount of inescapable shock promoted tumor growth (Sklar and Anisman, 1979; Visintainer *et al.*, 1982). More recently it was shown that in animals exposed to shock from which escape was possible, a slight facilitation of responsiveness to Con A occurred. However, when mice were exposed to an equivalent amount of inescapable shock, reactions to both Con A and PHA stimulation were significantly suppressed (Laudenslager *et al.*, 1983). Given the parallel effects of stressors on neoplasia, it is tempting to speculate that the differential effects of escapable and inescapable shock on tumor development are related to the altered immune status engendered by the stressors.

It will be recalled that in contrast to acute stress, repeated application of physical stressors inhibited the growth of tumors. This dichotomy is not as readily apparent, however, when susceptibility to infectious disease or discrete changes in immunoreactivity are considered. Both acute and chronic shock treatments have been shown to result in immunosuppression as indicated by depressed T-cell functions (Laudenslager *et al.*, 1983; Teshima *et al.*, 1982), and increased susceptibility to Coxsackie B viruses (Friedman *et al.*, 1965). Although it might be said that acute changes in environmental conditions result in immunosuppression whereas chronic conditions result in enhancement, this very much depends on the definition of 'chronic'. For instance, Monjan and Collector (1977) reported that intermittent noise stress for 2 weeks (acute) depressed T and B lymphocyte activity; however, with more protracted stress (2 months, chronic) mitogen responsivity was enhanced. Similarly, noise and water deprivation schedules for 5 days resulted in T-cell depression, but after 2 to 3 weeks enhancement was noted (Folch and Waksman, 1974). In both examples the acute phases were nearly as long as those defined as chronic in paradigms involving other forms of aversive stimuli (e.g. Sklar and Anisman, 1979). Therefore, in the absence of experiments which have investigated the effects of single and repeated applications of the same stressor with consistent parameters, it is premature to make definitive conclusions about the effects of chronic versus acute physical stress. Nevertheless, the available data strongly suggest that this variable may be critical in determining the immunological alterations associated with aversive stimulation (Monjan, 1981), just as it is fundamental in determining pathological and neurochemical variations.

Social stressors also alter immune responsivity, and with a few exceptions, it has been reported that following both acute and chronic isolation or overcrowding, immune activity is suppressed, and susceptibility to infectious disorders and neoplasia is enhanced (Beden and Brain, 1982; Friedman *et al.*, 1970; Sklar and Anisman, 1980). However, it should be noted that depending upon genetic predisposition and the type of pathogen under investigation, animals may be rendered more or less susceptible to the influence of social stressors. For example, CD-1 mice are more resistant to malaria virus when housed alone rather than in small groups, whereas several other strains of mice are apparently unaffected by this manipulation (Friedman and Glasgow, 1973). Various strains of mice are also differentially susceptible to alterations of neuroendocrine or neurotransmitter status as a consequence of stress exposure (see Anisman, 1978), and this in turn may influence immune responsiveness.

Another issue to be considered is the nature of the environment onto which stressful conditions were superimposed. It will be recalled that Sklar and Anisman (1980) demonstrated that a change from group to individual housing exacerbated tumor growth. Alterations in housing conditions likewise contributed to mortality resulting from inoculation with EMC virus (Friedman *et al.*, 1973), and resulted in suppressed antibody responses to bovine serum albumim (Edwards *et al.*, 1980). In contrast, mortality from malaria virus was higher among grouped mice regardless of pre-infection housing conditions (Plaut *et al.*, 1969). Without sufficient time for the organism to adapt to altered environmental conditions, the effects of other stressors may be masked (Plaut and Friedman, 1982; Riley, 1981). Parenthetically, social conditions may not only have immediate repercussions with respect to immunological status, but may also have long-term effects. For instance, early handling of animals was found to contribute to enhanced antibody responses measured in adulthood (Solomon *et al.*, 1968). Conversely, daily handling of newborn mice prior to weaning increased mortality to subsequent *E. coli.* injection (Schlewinski, 1976). Likewise, early nutritional deprivation apparently resulted in, or contributed to, depressed phagocytic and cell-mediated responses in adulthood (Dutz *et al.*, 1976).

With respect to temporal factors, the time of stressor application in relation to the introduction of a pathogen appears to be an important determinant of tumor development. For example, as noted earlier, when shock was administered for several days following the injection of Maloney sarcoma virus, the rate of tumor growth was enhanced (Amkraut and Solomon, 1972). Conversely, smaller tumors were noted among mice shocked prior to inoculation. The time of stressor application in relation to injection with streptozotocin, which induces diabetes, also influenced resistance to this disease. That is, exposure to a combined light – shock stimulus increased resistance to diabetes when applied on the same day as inoculation, but had no effect when applied 2 days later (Huang *et al.*, 1981). However, in response to a noise – shock stimulus, T-cell cytotoxicity was depressed regardless of the time of stressor application (Teshima *et al*, 1982). The discrepancies in these reports may be a consequence of the type of antigen administered, the strain of mouse employed, or the intensity of the aversive stimuli.

Conditioned Immunosuppression

Evidence in support of the argument that psychological variables can influence disease susceptibility is derived not only from stress paradigms, but has also resulted from a series of innovative behavioral conditioning experiments conducted by Ader and his associates (Ader and Cohen, 1975, 1981, 1982; Ader *et al.*, 1982; Bovjberg *et al.*, 1982). In these experiments a novel saccharin flavoured solution was used as a conditioned stimulus (CS), which was paired with an injection of cyclosphosphamide (CY), an immunosuppressant drug. Several days after the pairing of these stimuli, animals were injected with antigen, the CS alone was presented, and immunoreactivity was assessed thereafter. Using such a procedure it was found that upon re-exposure to the CS, antibody titres to sheep red blood cells (SRBC) were depressed (Ader and Cohen, 1975).

Subsequent studies demonstrated that cell mediated as well as humoral processes are subject to behavioral conditioning. Rats re-exposed to the saccharin CS plus a single injection of CY 7 weeks after conditioning exhibited suppression of a graft versus host (GvH) response that equalled that seen among naive mice that received three injections of the immunosuppressant drug (Bovjberg *et al.*, 1982). Along the same line, Gorczynski *et al.* (1982) reported that presentation of cues associated with a skin grafting procedure (in this case, sham grafting was employed as the CS) resulted in an increase of cytotoxic T-cell precursors in blood. Moreover, pairing saccharin with injection of rabbit anti-rat lymphocyte serum (ALS), a biologic immunosuppressant, resulted in suppression of T-lymphocyte activity upon CS re-exposure (Kusnecov *et al.*, 1983).

The conditioned immunosuppression technique was successfully employed to delay development of autoimmune disease in experimental animals. Between the ages of 8 and 14 months, female New Zealand mice spontaneously develop various symptoms of lupus erythematosus, including glomerulonephritis, a lethal kidney inflammation. Regular administration of CY has been shown to delay onset of glomerulonephritis, and so in this experiment weekly injections of CY were paired with the saccharin CS according to several schedules. In mice that received CS – CY pairings each week, symptom onset was delayed. For animals that were presented with the CS each week, but only received CY injections every second week, symptom onset was also retarded compared to untreated controls, as well as compared to a third group that received the same number of injections in the absence of saccharin pairings (Ader and Cohen, 1982). Evidently, the conditioning procedure coupled with immunosuppressant treatment was effective in delaying the onset of symptoms. In a similar manner, it was recently demonstrated that the presentation of several saccharin – cyclophosphamide pairings attenuated the spreading of swelling ordinarily observed following the onset of adjuvent induced arthritis (Klosterhalfen and Klosterhalfen, 1983).

Consistent with animal experiments, it has been demonstrated that immunological responses in humans may be subject to behavioral conditioning. Once a month for 5 months, a group of individuals who exhibited positive reactions to a tuberculin skin test (delayed hypersensitivity reaction) were given a tuberculin scratch test on one arm, and saline on the other arm. The skin tests were always conducted under the same stimulus conditions (i.e. same time, place, etc.). On the sixth test day, unbeknowns, to the subject, the saline and tuberculin were reversed, and the delayed hypersensitivity reaction (i.e. test that subject believed was saline) was substantially depressed (Smith and McDaniel, 1983). Taken together, such experiments provide further evidence for the hypothesis that immunological functions may be influenced by psychological factors (see Table 6.1).

CONTRIBUTION OF THE CENTRAL NERVOUS SYSTEM

The fact that stressful events may come to influence immunoresponsivity and susceptibility to various illnesses is consistent with the belief that regulation of the immune system is influenced either directly or indirectly by central nervous system function, or peripheral neurotransmitters and hormones. The precise mechanisms that are operative in this respect remain to be identified, although several promising candidates have recently been suggested. This literature has been reviewed by several investigators (Fauman, 1982; Hall and Goldstein, 1981; Spector and Korneva, 1981; Stein *et al.*, 1981), and it seems reasonable to suppose that among other brain regions, the hypothalamus may play a fundamental role in immunoregulation, and conversely, variations of immune activity will come to influence activity in the central nervous system.

C.N.S. Lesions and Immune Function

In their review, Spector and Korneva (1981) revealed several sources of evidence indicating C.N.S. and immune system interactions. For example, electrolytic lesions of various brain regions suppress immune, inflammatory,

Table 6.1 Effects of Stressors on Immune Functions in Infrahuman Experiments

Stressor		Phagocytic	Humoral	Cellular	Disease Susceptibility
Avoidance/Escape					
	Acute	—		0 T	0 Herpes
				+ T	+ Coxsackie B
					+ Poliomyelitis
					0 Tumor
	Chronic				− Leukemia virus
Footshock					
	Acute		0 ab	− T	+ Coxsackie B
					+ Tumor
				− NK	0 Influenza
					0 Respiratory Infection
					− Tissue rejection
	Chronic			− T	− Tumor
					+ Coxsackie B
Noise					
	Acute		− ab	− T	
			− B		
	Chronic		+ B	+ T	
Restraint		—	− ab		+ Herpes
Isolation			− ab		+ EMC
					0 Malaria
					+ Tumor
Overcrowding					
	Acute	—	− ab		0 EMC
			− WBC		+ Malaria
					+ Salmonella
					+ Adjuvent Arthritis
	Chronic			+ T	
Surgical Stress		—	(+)*	− T	+ Tumor
				− NK	+ Metastases

+ indicates an increase, − indicates a decrease, 0 indicates no change, * transient effect, ab = antibody, B = B-lymphocyte, T = T-lymphocyte, NK = Natural Killer cell.

and allergic reactions (Jankovic and Isakovic, 1973; Hall et al., 1979; Spector *et al.*, 1975; Szentivanyi and Filipp, 1958), while electrical stimulation of brain sites enhanced both humoral and cell mediated immune responses (Baciu, 1978; Jankovic *et al.*, 1979; Korneva, 1976). In particular, lesions of the anterior, but not the median or posterior regions of the hypothalamus resulted in inhibition of anaphylactic reactions in the rat, indicating that humoral responses were depressed (Luparello *et al.*, 1964). Indeed, such an effect has been noted in several species including the rabbit and guinea pig (Macris, *et al.*, 1970; Szentivanyi and Filipp, 1958).

In addition to the effects of hypothalamic lesioning on anaphylaxis, such manipulations have been shown to suppress other facets of humoral immunity. In particular, Macris *et al.* (1970) found that hypothalamic lesions altered levels of circulating antibodies in response to antigenic challenge, but these effects were restricted to the anterior portion of the hypothalamus.

Ovalbumin antibody production was also found to be depressed in rats that sustained anterior hypothalamic lesions (Tyrey and Nalbandov, 1972). Ado and Goldstein (1973) in contrast, found that neither lesions of the anterior, medial, nor posterior hypothalamic nuclei influenced antibody response to ovalbumin. However, other investigators reported that variations of antibody titers were induced in animals that had sustained posterior and/or medial hypothalamic damage (Filipp and Szentivanyi, 1958; Korneva, 1976; Korneva and Khai, 1964; Paunovic *et al.*, 1976; Tsypin and Maltsev, 1967, cited in Stein *et al.*, 1981). The source for these divergent outcomes has yet to be determined, but it was suggested that the variable procedures employed across laboratories may have contributed to the inconsistent results (e.g. use of different animal species, different types and test dosages of antigen; diverse time schedules and lesions) (Stein *et al.*, 1981).

The variations of the humoral immune response engendered by hypothalamic manipulations are not restricted to suppression, but immunofacilitation can be elicited as well. While lesions of the hypothalamus inhibited the Arthus reaction (an *in vivo* measure of hypersensitivity), electrical stimulation of the hypothalamus had the opposite effect (Jankovic and Isakovic, 1973; Jankovic *et al.*, 1979). Likewise, stimulation of the posterior hypothalamus facilitated antibody production (Korneva, 1976).

Not only have hypothalamic manipulations been found to affect humoral immunity, but cell-mediated processes are influenced as well. Whereas anterior hypothalamic lesions suppressed delayed hypersensitivity reactions, lesions of the medial and posterior hypothalamus had no effect (Macris *et al.*, 1970). Lesions of the anterior hypothalamus also diminished the delayed cutaneous reponse to antigen challenge by tuberculin purified protein derivative (PPD), and lymphocyte responses to PHA mitogen in samples of whole blood (Keller *et al.*, 1980; Warejcka and Levy, 1980). Consistent with these results, bilateral lesions of the anterior hypothalamus were shown to result in decreased numbers of splenocytes, thymocytes and lymphocytes, as well as decreased responses to mitogenic stimulation with Con A (Brooks *et al.*, 1982).

In contrast to the effects of hypothalamic manipulations, lesions of the hippocampus resulted in increased numbers of thymocytes and increased responses to Con A in thymus and spleen tissue These effects were maximal 4 days following ablation and returned to control levels within 14 days. On the basis of these findings Brooks *et al.* (1982) suggested that the hypothalamus is not the only important site for immunoregulation, but rather several brain areas may contribute in this respect. In a second series of experiments, it was shown that the effects of lesions of the hippocampus and amygdala, which enhanced mitogenic responses of thymus lymphocytes, could be attenuated by hypophysectomy (Cross *et al.*, 1982), sugggesting that the pituitary is an important mediator of the central and the immune system interaction.

Cross *et al.* (1982) offered the suggestion that alteration of C.N.S. activity may have resulted in neuroendocrine changes, which in turn, altered immunoresponsivity. Stein *et al.* (1981) posited that anterior hypothalamic lesions may interfere with antibody binding, alter release of histamine or diminish the responsiveness of target tissues to pharmacological agents that are released by antigen – antibody reaction.

There are a variety of ways in which the activity of the C.N.S. may come to influence the immune system. For example, corticotropin releasing factor (CRF) is secreted in the median eminence of the hypothalamus and is transported via the hypophyseal portal system to the pituitary. There it stimulates the release of adrenocorticotropic hormone (ACTH), which in turn causes the release of hormones (i.e. corticosteroids) from its target gland, the adrenal. At least nine such releasing factors have been identified, which may have either excitatory (e.g. CRF) or inhibitory (e.g. Somatostatin) effects upon the release of the putuitary hormones, including thyroid hormone (TH), leutinizing hormone (LH), prolactin, and growth hormone (GH) (see reviews in Guillemin, 1978; Muller *et al.*, 1978).

Neurotransmitters, released in the hypothalamus, may exert either an inhibitory or excitatory effect upon the releasing factors. Generally, norepinephrine (NE) appears to inhibit CRF release (and consequently the release of ACTH and corticosteroids), both *in vivo* (Ganong, 1976) and *in vitro* (Edwardson and Bennett, 1974). Conversely, there is evidence that NE has an excitatory effect upon the release of GSH (Durand *et al.*, 1977), TSH (Reichlin *et al.*, 1978), and prolactin (Terry and Martin, 1978). Dopamine has also been implicated in hormonal regulation and like NE it seems to inhibit ACTH release (Ganong, *et al.*, 1976) and facilitate GH secretion (Durand *et al.*, 1977). However, unlike NE, the administration of DA precursors may antagonize prolactin release (Terry and Martin, 1978). In contrast to the catecholamines, both acetylcholine (ACh) and serotonin (5HT) stimulate ACTH activity (Edwardson and Bennett, 1974); however, the influence ACh may exert on other hormones remains to be determined. Although it is likely that other transmittter systems mediate hormonal regulation, it is significant that the catecholamines are involved since these amines are particularly sensitive to stressors, and may thus be responsible for the hormonal alterations noted following stress exposure (see later discussion).

It is conceivable that the hypothalamic induced alterations of immune functioning described earlier were a consequence of a number of hormonal alterations produced by the lesions. It has been demonstrated that in large doses corticosteroids depress lymphocytes, monocytes and polymorphonuclear cells, and consequently they are used clinically to treat inflammatory conditions and to prevent graft reject (Fauci *et al.*, 1976; Fudenberg *et al.*, 1980). In small, physiological doses however, they may have a stimulant effect (Comsa *et al.*, 1982).

Consistent with the immunosuppression evident following the administration of large amounts of corticosteroids, adrenalectomy generally leads to enhancement of immune functioning. For example, adrenalectomy results in elevated antibody titers, increased susceptibility to anaphylaxis and increased intensity of delayed hypersensitivity reactions, indicating augmentation of both humoral and cell mediated processes (Ahlqvist, 1976; Streng and Nathan, 1973; Van Dijk *et al.*, 1976). However, it seems that the immunoenhancing effects of adrenalectomy may depend upon the organ and cellular process under investigation. It was reported that although increased lymphocyte responses to the mitogens Con A and PHA occurred in spleen cells following adrenalectomy, lymphocytes in the lymph nodes were depressed by this procedure. Furthermore, adrenalectomy also resulted in depression of antibody dependent cellular cytotoxicity and the activity of NK cells (Calvano *et al.*, 1982).

Upon secretion of growth hormone releasing factor (GRF) from the hypothalamus, the pituitary is stimulated to release growth hormone (GH), which acts at various sites including liver, thymus, muscle, and adipose tissues. Unlike corticosteroids, GH has an enhancing effect upon immune functions. Snell – Bagg mice, a strain with congenital hypoactivity of the pituitary, and consequently low levels of growth hormone, exhibit various indices of immunodeficiency. These mice display decreased antibody responses to SRBC and deficient rejection of transplanted tissue, both of which can be reversed with the administration of growth hormone and thyroxine (Fabris, *et al.*, 1971; Pierpaoli, *et al.*, 1969). Likewise, the suppression of humoral responses to SRBC following the administration of corticosteroids was restored with GH (Gisler, 1974).

Paralleling the influence of growth hormone on immune responses, the thyroid hormones apparently have an immunoenhancing effect. Removal of the thyroid from rats at birth inhibited the plaque forming cell response in spleen tissue, which could be restored by daily thyroxine (thyroid hormone) injections (Fabris, 1973). Similarly, thyroidectomy in rats depressed the graft rejection response, which could also be restored by administration of thyroxine. However, if thyroid damage was accompanied by removal of the thymus and adrenals, thyroxine did not reverse the delayed graft rejection response, indicating that immune responses may be mediated by interactions of these organs (Comsa *et al.*, 1975). Consistent with these observations, protection from lethal anaphylaxis afforded by hypothalamic lesions was antagonized by thyroxine administration (Filipp and Mess, 1969). Although experiments with human populations are lacking, it is significant that among individuals injected with various antigens, relatively high antibody titers were evident in patients with Grave's disease (hyperthyroidism), and low titers in those with hypothyroidism (Torgyan, 1972, cited in Comsa *et al.*, 1982).

In addition to TH, GH and corticosteroids, other hormones have been implicated in immunoregulation. Receptors for both estrogen and testosterone have been isolated in lymphoid tissue (Abraham and Buga, 1976; Gillette and Gillette, 1979), and preliminary data suggest that these hormones may exert an immunosuppressive effect, possibly by producing thymic atrophy (see Comsa *et al.*, 1982; Fauman, 1982). Moreover, prostaglandins, which mimic the effects of several pituitary hormones, may have an inhibitory role in immune regulation (Fauman, 1982).

Neurotransmitter Regulation of the Immune System

The aforementioned data are consistent with the notion that the central nervous system may influence the activity of the immunological processes via neuroendocrine pathways. Alternatively, neurotransmitter pathways may directly mediate immunological activity, since it is known that lymphocytes carry receptors on their surface membranes that are sensitive to several transmitters, including epinephrine, norepinephrine, acetylcholine, enkephalin (and other opiates), as well as hormones and steroids (see for example Besedovsky and Sorkin, 1981; Bourne 1974; Hall and Goldstein, 1981; Spector and Korneva, 1981; Williams *et al.*, 1976; Wybran *et al.*, 1979). Moreover, it has been demonstrated that various tissues of the immune system including lymph nodes, thymus, spleen and appendix receive innervation from noradrenergic fibres (Felten, *et al.*, 1981; Giron *et al.*, 1980; Williams and Felten, 1981; Williams *et al.*, 1981). Hence, alterations of hypothalamic activity, which are known to influence peripheral neurotransmitters (Kvetnansky, 1981) may alter binding to receptors located on the lymphocyte surface, thereby affecting immune responsivity.

In support of such a position, it has been demonstrated that variations of central neurotransmitters will come to affect immune function. Generally, treatments that reduce central 5HT increase antibody production (e.g. Bliznakov, 1980; Devoino *et al.*, 1970). Additionally, the latent phase of antibody production in rabbits that had been immunized with typhoid vi-antigen was associated with decreased hypothalamic 5HT concentrations. It might be noted as well that neuroendocrine functioning may subserve the effects of 5HT reactivity on immunoresponsitivity, since hypophysectomy prevented the immunological consequences ordinarily engendered by the 5HT precursor, 5-hydroxytryptophan (Devoino *et al.*, 1970).

Variations of dopamine neuronal activity apparently influence immune functioning as well. Stimulation of dopamine receptors induces immunofacilitation (Cotzias and Tang, 1977; Tang and Cotzias, 1977; Tang *et al.*, 1974), while catecholamine depletion induced by reserpine resulted in immunosuppression (Dukor *et al.*, 1966). Indirect evidence supporting DA effects on immunological processes is also derived from the finding that individuals suffering from neurological disturbances associated with reduced DA activity exhibit suppressed lymphocyte functioning (see Hall and Goldstein, 1981). Moreover, catecholamine stimulating drugs, such as L-DOPA and amphetamine, have been shown to inhibit DMBA induced tumors and transplanted syngeneic tumors (Driscoll *et al.*, 1978; Quadri *et al.*, 1973; Wick, 1977, 1978, 1979), whereas catecholamine reductions resulted in exacerbation of tumor development (Lacassagne and Duplan, 1959; Lapin, 1978; Welsch and Meites, 1970; Sklar and Anisman, 1981). Consistent with these data, Sarkar *et al.*, (1982) reported that prolactin secreting pituitary tumors (in aged female rats and in younger rats chronically treated with estrogens) were accompanied by damage to tuberinfundibular DA neurons. It should be noted that although the bulk of evidence supports the contention that DA reductions exacerbate tumor development, contradictory results have been reported in that administration of DA receptor blockers attenuated tumor growth in some instances. Considering that in some of these studies either very high doses of drug, or chronic administration were used, DA receptor blockade *per se* may not have been responsible for tumor reduction. Rather, these treatments may have resulted in receptor supersensitivity, and consequently reduction of tumor development (see discussion in Sklar and Anisman, 1981).

There are some data to suggest that central norepinephrine (NE) modulates immunological function as well as tumor development. Several of the drugs that influence DA neuronal activity, also modify NE neuronal functioning. Thus, the observed outcomes may have been related to changes of NE rather than DA activity. Moreover, it has been demonstrated that β-adrenergic agonists and antagonists can alter the lymphocyte response to mitogen stimulation. In particular, NE receptor blockers reduce the response of lymphocytes to the T cell mitogen Con A (Johnson *et al.*, 1981), and chemical sympathectomy by systemic administration of 6-hydroxydopamine, depressed antibody production (Hall *et al.*, 1980; Kasahara *et al.*, 1977), and reduced mitogenic responsivity (Hall and Goldstein, 1981).

The discovery of opiate receptors on elements of the immune system including granulocytes, monocytes and lymphocytes, coupled with observations of the pharmacological action of opioids on tumor growth, indicate opiate involvement in immune regulation. For example, it was demonstrated that morphine administration depressed rosette formation of T-lymphocytes *in vitro* (Wybran *et al.*, 1979). It will be recalled that shock parameters which induced opiate analgesia suppressed lymphocyte responsivity (Shavit *et al.*, 1982). In an analogous fashion, administration of high doses of morphine suppressed the activity of NK cells and enhanced the growth of a mammary ascites tumor (Lewis et al, in press). Moreover, opiate antagonist administration reversed these effects. It was suggested that the accelerated growth rate of the tumor resulted from opiate influences on pituitary – adrenal activity, or from the suppression of NK functioning (Lewis *et al.*, in press). In contrast to these findings, heroin administration inhibited the growth of a neuroblastoma in A/J mice (Zagon and McLaughlin, 1981). The reason for these discrepancies is not clear; however, in light of the fact that neuroblastoma cells have opiate receptors, heroin may have had a direct non-immunological influence on tumor growth.

Influence of Immune System on C.N.S. Activity

Clearly, communication between the nervous system and the immune system is a complex process involving interactions between an enormous array of neurotransmitter and neuroendocrine pathways. Although the data presented to this point demonstrate the potential for communication from the CNS to components of the immune system, there is also evidence to suggest that the immune system can influence central processes. Besedovsky and his associates (Besedovsky, *et al.*, 1977; Besedovsky and Sorkin, 1981; Besedovsky *et al.*, 1983) demonstrated that peripheral immune responses are followed by changes in central nervous system activity. In an initial series of experiments, animals were inoculated with SRBC and at various intervals afterwards electrical activity in the ventromedial nucleus of the hypothalamus was recorded (Besedovsky *et al.*, 1977). On the first day following inoculation, when plaque forming cells were not yet detected, electrical activity of the hypothalamus did not differ from baseline. However, during the peak phase of plaque formation in response to antigen, a two-fold increase in electrical activity was noted. In animals in which an immune response to antigen was apparently not mounted, firing rates of hypothalamic neurons did not differ from baseline values.

It was recently suggested that noradrenergic neurons in particular respond to immunological activity (Besedovsky *et al.*, 1983). In animals that mounted a strong PFC response to SRBC (high responders), the time of peak immunological response was accompanied by a marked decrease in norepinephrine turnover in the hypothalamus. In a second experiment, supernatant containing products of an *in vitro* reaction to Con A (i.e. lymphokines, monokines) was administered to a group of rats. Two hours following injection, hypothalamic NE was significantly reduced, again suggesting that a relationship exists between peripheral immune activity and central processes (Besedovsky *et al.*, 1983). Because the alterations in electrical activity and NE were not observed until 4 days following antigenic challenge, these effects were not attributed to a stress effect. However, the possibility that physiological alterations associated with the immunological response to inoculation may have caused distress to the organism should be considered. Nonetheless, these data offer considerable support for the notion that an afferent pathway exists to provide the brain with information about invading pathogens.

Neurochemical Consequences of Stressors

There is compelling support for the suggestion that alterations of central neurotransmitters may directly, or indirectly, come to modify immune functioning. Accordingly, environmental conditions which favour variations of central neurotransmitters might be expected to alter these functions, thereby affecting vulnerability to illness. Infrahuman studies have revealed that stress alters central neurochemical activity (see reviews in Anisman *et al.*, 1981; Stone, 1975; Weiss *et al.*, 1979). For instance, both physical and social stressors alter norepinephrine (NE) turnover in a number of brain regions. Following exposure to a brief stressor, synthesis of NE increases, and elevations of amine concentrations are evident. If stressor application continues, synthesis may fail to keep pace with a further increase of utilization, and a net decline of NE may ensue (Anisman and Sklar, 1979; Kvetnansky *et al.*, 1976; Thierry, 1973; Weis *et al.*, 1976). Stressor-induced changes of NE turnover have been observed in whole brain homogenates and in various regions including the hypothalamus, locus coeruleus, hippocampus and cortex (e.g. Anisman *et al.*, 1980; Iimori *et al.*, 1982; Weiss *et al.*, 1980). In the periphery, concentrations of epinephrine and norepinephrine (released from the adrenal and sympathetic nerves), increase rapidly during the application of a stressor and return to baseline shortly after stressor termination (DeTurck and Vogel, 1980; Keim and Sigg, 1976). In light of the finding the adrenergic and noradrenergic fibres innervate peripheral lymphoid tissues, the possibility should be considered that immunological changes observed following exposure to adverse stimuli (see preceding sections) may be due, in part, to peripheral transmitter variations, which in turn may result from direct communication with the central nervous system.

Experiments involving determination of dopamine (DA) in discrete brain regions have shown stressors to appreciably alter activity of this amine. Substantial reductions of DA were noted in the arcuate nucleaus of the hypothalamus (Kobayashi *et al.*, 1976) and in the lateral septal nucleus (Saavedra, 1982) following stress exposure. Moreover, in response to physical stressors, such as footshock, increases in DA turnover have been detected in the nucleus accumbens and the frontal mesolimbic cortex, whereas substantia nigra DA was unaffected by stressors (Blanc *et al.*, 1980; Fekete *et al.*, 1981., Herman *et al.*, 1982). Given the inhibitory influence of DA on ACTH release, and the excitatory effect of this amine on both GSH and TSH in the median eminence, it is significant that stress-induced alterations were detected in proximal hypothalamic nuclei.

Unlike other monoamines, relatively intense aversive stimulation is apparently required to produce alterations of 5HT turnover (Thierry, 1973; Palkovits *et al.*, 1976). In general, stressor application increases 5HT turnover without significantly altering concentrations of the amine (Kennett and Joseph, 1981), although in some instances net increases have been detected

(Anisman and Sklar, 1981; Morgan *et al.*, 1975) and biphasic variations of 5HT concentrations were noted over time following stressor application (Palkovits *et al.*, 1976). There may be important regional variations in serotonergic responses, since reductions of 5HT were detected in the septum and anterior cortex following footshock stress (Petty and Sherman, 1982). The significance of serotonergic responses for immune functioning is not yet clear; however, as noted in an earlier section, increased 5HT concentrations have been associated with immunosuppression (Bliznakov, 1980).

Acetylcholine (ACh) may be implicated in immunoregulation since it mediates the release of various pituitary hormones, and because muscarinic and nicotinic receptors have been detected on lymphoid tissues (Gordon *et al.*, 1978; Maslinski *et al.*, 1980; Richman and Arnason, 1979). Whether ACh changes occur depends on the nature of the stressor employed. Whereas ACh turnover was reduced in response to cold exposure (Costa *et al.*, 1980; Brunello *et al.*, 1981), increased turnover was noted following footshock (Schmidt *et al.*, 1980). Immobilization stress, which produces alterations in catecholaminergic and immune activity, was without effect on ACh turnover (Brunello *et al.*, 1981). The source for the differential effects of these stressors on ACh turnover remains to be determined. It is conceivable that the diverse outcomes may have been due to the differential severities of the stressors employed. Alternatively, the time at which ACh activity was determined may have been responsible for the observed effects. Indeed, there is reason to believe that the effects of stressors on ACh concentration are not evident immediately after exposure to a stress, but are maximal some time (approximately 40 min–1 hr) after stressor termination (Zajaczkoska, 1975; see Anisman, 1975).

Variations of endogenous opioids have been detected following exposure to physical insults. Aversive stimuli result in increased endorphin secretion from the anterior pituitary, thus leading to decreased concentrations in this region (Baizman *et al.*, 1979; Vuolteenaho *et al.*, 1982; Przewlocki *et al.*, 1982) coupled with increased concentrations in plasma (Przewlocki *et al.*, 1982). In the hypothalamus endogenous opioid concentrations increase following various forms of aversive stimulation (Barta and Yashpal, 1981; Przewlocki *et al*, 1982), the extent of the increase varying with stressor severity. Barta and Yashpal, (1981), for instance, reported that the increasing hypothalamic endorphin concentrations became more pronounced as stress severity was accentuated; however, the reduction of pituitary endorphin concentrations was minimized with the application of a more intense stressor.

Factors Influencing Stressor-Induced Neurochemical Alterations

It will be recalled that stressor controllability is an important factor in determining the immune system's response to aversive stimulation. This variable also appears to be an important determinant of stress-induced NE reduction. It has repeatedly been demonstrated that while exposure to escapable shock did not result in measurable change of NE levels, application of an equivalent amount of uncontrollable shock produced a significant reduction of this amine (Anisman *et al.*, 1980; Weiss *et al.*, 1976). Consistent with these data, it was reported that the elevations of peripheral NE and E which accompanied stress exposure, were more pronounced among rats exposed to inescapable footshock than among animals that could control shock offset (Swenson and Vogel, 1983).

Few experiments have assessed the influence of coping factors on DA activity in brain regions where stressors are known to alter turnover or concentrations of this amine. It has been reported that while escapable shock was without effect, repeated sessions of yoked inescapable shock altered DA receptor sensitivity in the mesolimbic frontal cortex (Cherek *et al.*, 1980). Similarly, serotonin reductions were noted in the lateral septal nucleus of the hypothalamus following uncontrollable, but not controllable shock application (Petty and Sherman, 1982). Although alterations of ACh activity have not been examined in experiments specifically designed to address the issue of controllability, it has been demonstrated that following inescapable footshock ACh concentrations were elevated, whereas in a separate experiment, no alterations were detected following avoidable/escapable shock (Karczmar *et al.*, 1973). Finally, while comparisons of escapable and inescapable shock on endorphin concentrations have yet to be reported, data are available which suggest that this variable may be an important one in determining the activity of endogenous opioids (Lewis *et al.*, 1982).

When confronted with a stressor, animals will alter their behavior in an effort to minimize the aversiveness of the situation, and these behavioral attempts will be accompanied by alterations of neuroendocrine and neurotransmitter activity. Animals exposed to footshock, for example, will attempt to escape by running or jumping, or by adopting postures which minimize the aversiveness of the shock. It has been postulated that if behavioral attempts to cope are unsuccessful, a compensatory increase of neurochemical activity will occur in order to meet the environmental demands placed on the organism. The increased neuronal activation may be essential for the organism to emit defensive responses, they may minimize or eliminate the aversiveness of the stimuli, or they may blunt the psychological impact associated with the adverse stimuli. However, it is possible that when the stressor cannot be dealt with through behavioral means, neurochemical systems may become overly taxed. In the case of biogenic amines, utilization rates may increase to a point that exceeds synthesis, producing a net amine reduction and thus leave the organism more vulnerable to pathology (Anisman and Sklar, 1982; Anisman *et al.*, 1981). Additionally, the directed mobilization of resources at a given period of time may also leave the organism more susceptible to pathology upon subsequent encounters with another form of stress (or encounters with an antigen) at a time when recovery from the initial transmitter alterations had not occurred (see discussion in Sklar and Anisman, 1981).

In an earlier discussion of the consequences of stressful events, it was noted that the context in which a stressor was applied was a significant determinant of immunocompetence. Environmental and experiential factors likewise appear to influence neurochemical responsivity. Just as isolated housing altered susceptibility to infection, such a treatment altered turnover of NE (Modigh, 1976) and increased the organism's susceptibility to further amine depletion upon exposure to other forms of stress (Anisman and Sklar, 1979). Similarly, social housing conditions have been shown to influence the DA variations induced by stressors in limbic forebrain regions (Blanc *et al.*, 1980).

Neurochemical consequences of stressors, like the immunological alterations, are dependent upon prior experience. In particular, exposure to uncontrollable stressors such as inescapable footshock, increases vulnerability to subsequent stressors so that even relatively mild aversive stimulation will come to provoke reductions of brain NE (Anisman and Sklar, 1979). Presentation of cues previously paired with shock were also found to result in increased turnover of NE (Cassens *et al.*, 1980), enhance mesolimbic DA activity (Herman *et al.*, 1982) and increase ACh concentrations (Hingtgen *et al.*, 1976). In effect, experience with stressful events may predispose animals to exaggerated neurochemical responses upon re-exposure to stressors, or to the cues with which they are associated (Anisman *et al.*, 1982; Anisman and Sklar, 1982). It will be recalled that immunological changes associated with stressors (in a conditioned taste aversion paradigm) are similarly influenced by conditioning or sensitization processes (e.g. Ader and Cohen, 1981). Albeit speculative, thc possibility should be considered that one or more of the transmitter alterations seen upon stress re-exposure (or exposure to cues that had been paired with aversive stimuli) may be causally related to the conditioned immunological alterations.

The profile of neurochemical responses to acute physical stressors may be altered in animals that had been exposed to a chronic stress regimen. Following repeated stressor application over several days or weeks, the reductions of NE ordinarily induced by acute stressors may be absent (Roth *et al.*, 1982; Weiss *et al.*, 1976; 1981). Although absolute amine levels may not differ from baseline, Kvetnansky (1981) has noted that chronic stressors increase the activity of both tyrosine hydroxylase and dopamine-B-hydroxylase thereby preventing amine depletion. In addition, it seems that utilization rates vary with time following a chronic stress regimen. Immediately following the last of 14 daily sessions of inescapable footshock, concentrations of amine were not found to differ from control levels, but utilization of NE was increased. Interestingly, within 24 hr of stressor termination (in a chronic paradigm) NE concentrations exceeded those of nonstressed mice and utilization of the transmitter was appreciably lower than that of mice that received either no treatment or exposure to stress. In the face of sustained environmental demands (i.e. during shock), synthesis is increased in order to keep pace with amine utilization. The enhanced synthesis persists for some time following stressor termination, while utilization rates actually decline upon stressor termination. Consequently, the net concentrations of the amine are substantially increased, thereby leaving the organism better prepared to deal with impending threats.

It will be recalled that following chronic stressor application the tumor enhancing effects of stressors are eliminated, and a reduction of tumor growth (relative to nonstressed animals) may be engendered. In effect, the chronic stress effect is not simply a reflection of adaptation (habituation) to the effects of the stressor, but rather represents an active process that may function to inhibit tumor enhancement (see Anisman and Sklar, 1982; Monjan, 1981). If central neurotransmitters are involved in the tumor enhancement associated with acute shock, then the altered neurochemical activity which follows chronic stress may contribute to the tumor suppression evident after such a stressor regimen.

Hormonal Changes and Stress

Variations of pituitary hormone activity have been associated with alterations in the capacity of an organism to mount a response to pathogenic stimulation. Consequently, the alterations of hormonal activity that occur under stressful conditions may contribute to the variations of immune responsivity seen following psychological or physical insults. In particular, it has been shown that secretion of corticosteroids, which have immunosuppressant properties, was elevated among animals following extreme cold exposure (Hendley *et al.*, 1977), immobilization, and footshock (Keim and Sigg, 1976; Weiss *et al.*, 1975). Furthermore, in animals that had control over shock offset, or that could predict shock onset, the elevations of corticosteroids ordinarily engendered by footshock stress were diminished (Swenson and Vogel, 1983; Weiss, 1970, 1971). Human subjects exposed to physical stressors such as surgery or exercise, or to psychological stresses such as hospital admission or exam taking, also exhibited elevated plasma corticosteroid levels (Sachar *et al.*, 1980). It is of interest that other reports have shown that these same stressors are associated with suppression of various immune responses (see earlier discussion).

Consistent with reports of neurochemical adaptation to chronic stress, some degree of corticosteroid adaptation has been reported. Whereas acute shock stress resulted in significantly elevated corticosteroid levels, following 15 daily sessions concentrations approached, but did not reach baseline levels (Weiss *et al.*, 1977). Moreover, repeated sessions of immobilization stress attenuated the corticosterone response provoked by acute exposure to this stressor (Keim and Sigg, 1976). In contrast, such adaptation has not been observed following the stress of cold exposure (Weiss *et al.*, 1977; Vernikos *et al.*, 1982).

Varied data have been reported with respect to the response of other hormones to stressful conditions. Although increases in both GH and TSH levels have been observed following the application of physical stressors such as restraint or footshock (Mason *et al.*, 1976), other reports have indicated that such stressors tend to reduce TSH and consequently the thyroid hormones (Bennett and Whitehead, 1983). Among both humans and infrahumans, cold exposure results in rapid elevation of TSH, and following chronic exposure, levels return to baseline (Martin, 1974). Likewise, adaptation to restraint-induced GH release has been reported (Mason *et al.*, 1976). Given the limited data available, it is difficult to assess the contribution of such factors as controllability, chronicity and stress history to the GH and TSH changes associated with stressors. However, given the striking influence of such factors upon central neurotransmitter activity and the role of neurotransmitters on hormonal regulation, it would not be surprising to find that these variables have a significant impact upon neuroendocrine responses to stress.

Table 6.2 Effects of Stressors on Neurotransmitter Activity

	Norephrine			Dopamine			Serotonin		
	L	S	U	L	S	U	L	S	U
Footshock									
Acute	−	+	+	0		+	− 0	+	+
Chronic	0	+	0 −	0	+				
Avoidance/Escape	0	+	+	0		+	− 0		
Restraint	-	+	+	−	(−)	−	− +		+
Noise	+ 0			0			0		
Isolation	− 0		−	−			−		
Overcrowding		− 0		0					
Surgical Stress						−			

L = Level; S = Synthesis; U = Utilization.
Stressor effects on neurochemical activity depend on factors such as stressor severity and duration, as well as brain region examined. Alterations of dopamine activity have been detected in regions such as the arcuate nucleus, the nucleus accumbens and the mesolimbic frontal cortex. Likewise, alterations in serotonin concentrations depend on the brain region examined.

SUMMARY

Clinical studies have supported the notion that emotional and psychological factors can render individuals more susceptible to illness, and furthermore, laboratory investigations have confirmed that various facets of the immune system may be compromised by stressful experiences. Both the nature and magnitude of stress to which an individual is exposed are important determinants of alterations in immunocompetence. Moreover, coping style and the buffering systems available to an individual are of considerable significance in this respect.

Investigations of infrahuman populations have confirmed and extended this hypothesis. It has been shown for instance, that phagocytic, humoral and cell-mediated immune processes may all be altered to some extent by stressor application. When animals are able to control or to predict the onset of stressor application, the deleterious effects of the stressor are substantially diminished. Likewise, there are indications that with repeated exposure, the immunosuppressive effects of stressors may be attenuated.

As seen in Table 6.2, alterations of neuroendocrine and neurotransmitter activity resulting from aversive stimulation have been documented, and these parallel the immunological changes associated with stressors. Again, such factors as controllability, chronicity and stressor severity are important modifiers of the organism's response to such stimuli. Moreover, transmitters and hormones involved in the stress response have the capacity to alter, either directly or indirectly, humoral and cell-mediated immune processes. Conversely, it appears that the immune system may influence central nervous system activity.

Taken together, these data suggest that psychological variables associated with stressful events may influence pathology owing to the effects of such factors on immunological activity. Moreover, variations in the activity of central nervous system transmitters may contribute to the alterations of immunocompetence. To be sure, there exist substantial interindividual differences in neuroendocrine, neurochemical and immunological activity following stressor application. A more compelling analysis of the relationship between stress and the induction of pathology will ultimately require the identification of those variables which maximize stressor-provoked alterations of endogenous elements.

REFERENCES

Abraham, and Buga, G. (1976). 3H-testosterone distribution and binding in rat thymus cells *in vivo*., *Mol. Cell. Biochem.*, **13**, 157–163.

Achterberg, J., Lawlis, G. F., Simonton, O. C., and Mathews-Simonton, S. (1977). Psychological factors, blood factors and blood chemistries as disease outcome predictors for cancer patients, *Multivar. Exp. Clin. Res.*, **3**, 107–122.

Achterberg-Lawlis, J. (1982). The psychological dimensions of arthritis, *J. Consult. Clin. Psychol.*, **50**, 984–992.

Adams, D. K., Sutherland, J., and Fletcher, W. (1950). Early clinical manifestations of multiple sclerosis, *Brit. Med. Journ.*, **2**431–437.

Ader, R. (1980). Psychosomatic and psychoimmunologic research, *Psychosom. Med.*, **42**, 307–321.

Ader, R. (1981). *Psychoneuroimmunology*, Academic Press, New York.

Ader, R., and Cohen, N. (1975). Behaviorally conditioned immunosuppression, *Psychosom Med.*, **37**, 333–340.

Ader, R. A., and Cohen, N. (1981). Conditioned immunopharmacologic responses, in *Psychoneuroimmunology* (Ed. R. Ader) Academic Press, New York.

Ader, R. A., and Cohen, N. (1982). Behaviorally conditioned immunosuppression and murine systemic lupus erythematosus, *Science*, **215**, 1534–1535.

Ader, R. A., Cohen, N., and Bovjberg, D. (1982). Conditioned suppression of humoral immunity in the rat, *J. Comp. Physiol. Psych.*, **96**, 517–520.

Ado, A., and Goldstein, M. M. (1973). The primary immune response in rabbits after lesion of different zones in the medial hypothalamus, *Ann. Allergy*, **31**, 585–589.

Ahlqvist, J. (1976). Endocrine influences on lymphatic organs, immune responses, inflammation and autoimmunity, *Acta Endocrinol. (Copenhagen)*, Suppl. **206**.

Amkraut, A., and Solomon, G. F. (1972). Stress and murine sarcoma virus (Maloney)-induced tumors, *Cancer Res.*, **32**, 1428–1433.

Amkraut, A. A., Solomon, G. F., and Kraemer, H. C. (1971). Early experience and adjuvent-induced arthritis in the rat, *Psychosom. Med.*, **33**, 203–214.

Anisman, H. (1975). Time-dependent variations in aversively motivated behaviors: Nonassociative effects of cholinergic and catecholaminergic activity, *Psych. Rev*, **82**, 359–385.

Anisman, H. (1978). Neurochemical changes elicited by stress, in *Psychopharmacology of Aversively Motivated Behavior* (Eds. H. Anisman and G. Bignami), Plenum Press, New York.

Anisman, H., Kokkinidis, L., and Sklar, L. S. (1981). Contribution of neurochemical change to stress-induced-induced behavioral deficits, in *Theory in Psychopharmacology*, Vol. 1, (Ed. S. J. Cooper), Academic Press, London.

Anisman, H., Pizzino, A., and Sklar, L. S. (1980). Coping with stress, norepinephrine depletion and escape performance, *Brain. Res.*, **191**, 583–588.

Anisman, H., and Sklar, L. S. (1979). Catecholamine depletion upon re-exposure to stress: Mediation of the escape deficits produced by inescapable shock, *J. Comp. Physiol. Psychol.*, **93** 610–625.

Anisman, H., and Sklar, L. S. (1982). Stress provoked neurochemical changes in relation to neoplasia, in *Biological Mediators of Behavior and Disease: Neoplasia* (Ed. S. M. Levy), Elsevier Biomedical, New York.

Baciu, I. (1978). Physiologie normale et pathologique: La physiologie due systeme phagocytaire, *Arch. Union Med. Balk.*, **16**, 473–477.

Bahnson, C. B., and Bahnson, M. B. (1969). Role of ego defenses: Denial and repression in the etiology of malignant neoplasm, *Ann. N. Y. Acad. Sci.*, **164**, 346–359.

Baizman, E. R., Cox, B. M., Osman O. H., and Goldstein, A. (1979). Experimental alterations of endorphine levels in rat pituitary, *Neuroendocrinology*, **28**, 402–424.

Barnes, P. J., Brown, M. J., Silverman, M., and Dollery, C. T. (1983). Circulating catecholamines in exercise and hyperventilation induced asthma, *Thorax*, **36**, 435–440.

Barta, A., and Yashpal, K. (1981). Regional redistribution of B-endorphin in the rat brain: The effect of stress. *Prog. Neuropsychopharmacol.*, **5**, 595–598.

Bartrop, R. W., Lazarus, L., Luckhurst, E., Kiloh, L. G., and Penny, R. (1977). Depressed lymphocyte function after bereavement, *Lancet*, **1**, 834–836.

Bassett, J. R., and Tait, N. N. (1981). The effect of stress on the migration of leukocytes into the peritoneal cavity of rats following injection of an inflammatory agent. *Austral. J. Exp. Biol. Med. Sci.*, **59**, 651–666.

Beden, S. N., and Brain, P. F. (1982). Studies on the effect of social stress on measures of disease resistance in laboratory mice, *Agressive Beh.*, **8**, 4126–129.

Bellanti, J. (1978). *Immunology II*, W. B. Saunders, Philadelphia.

Bennett, G. W., and Whitehead, S. A. (1983). *Mammalian Neuroendocrinology*, Croom Helm, London.

Ben-Sira, Z. (1981). Stress and illness: A revised application of the stressful life events approach, *Res. Commun. Psychol. Psychiat. Behav.*, **6**, 317–327.

Besedovsky, H., Del Rey, A., Sorkin, E., Da Prada, M., Burri, R., and Honegger, C. (1983). The immune response evokes changes in brain noradrenergic neurons, *Science*, **221**, 564–566.

Besedovsky, H. O., and Sorkin, E. (1981). Immunologic – neuroendocrine circuits: Physiological approaches, in *Psychoneuroimmunology* (Ed. R. Ader), Academic Press, New York.

Besedovskly, H. O., Sorkin, E., Felix, D., and Haas, H. (1977). Hypothalamic changes during the immune response, *Eur. J. Immunol.*, **7**, 325–328.

Bhattacharya, A. K., and Pradhan, S. N. (1979) Effects of stress on DMBA-induced tumor growth, plasma corticosterone and brain biogenic amines in rats, *Res. Commun. Chem. Pathol. Pharmacol.*, **23**, 107–116.

Blanc, G., Hervé, D., Simon, H., Lisoprawski, A., Glowinski, J., and Tassin, J. P. (1980). Response to stress of mesocortico-frontal dopaminergic neurons in rats after long-term isolation, *Nature*, **284**, 265–267.

Blaney, P. H. (1983, in press). Psychological considerations in cancer, in *Behavioral Medicine: A Multi-Systems Approach* (Eds. N. Schneiderman and J. T. Tapp), Erlbaum, New York.

Bliznakov, E. G. (1980). Serotonin and its precursors as modulators of the immunological responsiveness in mice, *J. Med.*, **11**, 81–105.

Blumber, E. M., West, P. M., and Ellis, F. W. (1954). A possible relationship between psychological factors and human cancer, *Psychosom. Med.*, **16**, 277–288.

Boranic, M., Pericic, D., Radacic, M., Poljak-Blazzi, Sverko, V., and Miljenovic, G. (1982). Immunological and neuroendocrine response of rats to prolonged or repeated stress.

Bourne, H. R., Lichtenstein, L. M., Melmon, K. L., Heney, C. S., Weinstein, Y., and Shearer, G. M. (1974). Modulation of inflammation and immunity by cyclic AMP, *Science*, **184**, 19–28.

Bovjberg, D., Ader, R., and Cohen, N. (1982). Behaviorally conditioned suppression of a graft-vs-host response *Proc. Nat. Acad. Sci. U.S.A..*, **79**, 583–585.

Boyce, W. T., Cassel, J. C., Collier, A. M., Jensen, E. W., Ramey, C. T., and Smith, A. H. (1977). Influence of life events and family routines on childhood respiratory tract illness, *Pediatrics*, **60**, 609–615.

Broder, S., and Whitehouse, F. Jr. (1968). Immunologic enhancement of tumor xenografts by pepsin-degraded immunoglobulin, *Science*, **162**, 1494.

Brooks, W. H., Cross, R. J., Roszman, T. L., and Markesbery, W. R. (1982). Neuroimmunomodulation: Neural anatomical basis for impairment and facilitation, *Ann Neurol.*, **12**, 56–61.

Brown, G. W. (1979). The social etiology of depression – London studies, in *The Psychobiology of the Depressive Disorders* (Ed. R. A. DePue), Academic Press, New York.

Brunello, N., Tagliomonte, A., Cheney, D. L., and Costa, E. (1981). Effects of immobilization and cold exposure on the turnover rate of acetylcholine in rat brain areas, *Neuroscience*, **6**, 1759–1764.

Burnet, F. M. (1971). Immunological surveillance in neoplasia, *Transplant. Rev.*, **7**, 3–25.

Calvano, S. E., Mark, D. A., Good, R. A., and Fernandes, G. (1982). In vitro assessment of immune function in adrenalectomized rats, *Immunopharmacology*, **4**, 291–302.

Cassens, G., Roffman, M., Kuruc, A., Ursulak, P. J., and Schildkraut, J. J. (1980). Alterations in brain norepinephrine metabolism induced by environmental stimuli previously paired with inescapable shock, *Science*, **209**, 1138–1140.

Cherek, D. R., Lane, J. D., Freeman, M. E., and Smith, J. E. (1980). Receptor changes following shock avoidance, *Soc. Neurosci. Abstr.*, **6**, 543.

Cohen, F. (1981). Stress and bodily illness, *Psychiat. Clin. North Amer.*, **4**, 269–286.

Comsa, J., Leonhardt, H., and Schwarz, J. A. (1975). Influence of the thymus – corticotropin – growth hormone interaction on the rejection of skin allografts in rats, *Ann. N. Y. Acad. Sci.*, **249**, 387.

Comsa, J., Leonhardt, H., and Wekerle, H. (1982). Hormonal coordination of the immune response, *Rev. Physiol. Biochem. Pharmacol.*, **92** 115–191.

Costa, E., Tagliomente, A., Brunello, N., and Cheney, D. L. (1980). Effect of stress on the metabolism of acetylcholine in the cholinergic pathways of extrapyramidal and limbic systems, in *Catecholamines and Stress: Recent Advances* (Eds. E. Usdin, R. Kvetnansky and I. J. Kopin) pp. 59–68, Elsevier-North Holland, New York.

Cotzias, G. C., and Tang, L. (1977). An adenylate cyclase of brain reflects propensity for breast cancer in mice, *Science*, **197**, 1094–1096.

Cox, T., and MacKay, C. (1982). Psychosocial factors and psychophysiological mechanisms in the aetiology and development of cancers, *Soc. Sci. Med.*, **16**, 381–396.

Cross, R. J., Brooks, W. H., Roszman, T. L., and Markesbery, W. R. (1982). Hypothalamic – immune interactions, *J. Neurol. Sci.*, **53** 557–566.

de Araujo, G., Dudley, D. L., and van Asdel, P. P. Jr. (1972). Psychological assets and severity of chronic asthma, *J. Allergy Clin. Immunol.*, **50**, 257.

Dechambre, R. P. (1981). Psychosocial stress and cancer in mice, in *Stress and Cancer* (Eds. K. Bammer and B. H. Newberry), Hogrefe, Toronto.

Dechambre, R. P., and Gosse, C. (1973). Individual versus group caging of mice with grafted tumors, *Cancer Res.*, **33**, 140–144.

Derogatis, L. R., Abeloff, M. D., and Melisaratos, N. (1979). Psychological coping mechanisms and survival time in metastatic breast cancer, *J. Am. Med. Assoc.*, **242**, 1504–1508.

DeTurck, K., and Vogel, W. H. (1980). Factors influencing plasma catecholamine levels in rats during immobilization, *Pharmacol. Biochem. Behav.*, **13**, 129–131.

Devoino, L. V., Eremina, O. F. N., and Ilyutchenok, R. Y. (1970). The role of the hypothalarmopituitary system in the mechanism of action of reserpine and 5-hydroxytryptophan on antibody production, *Neuropharmacology*, **9**, 67–72.

Dorian, B. J., Keystone, E., Garfinkel, P. E., and Brown, G. M. (1981). Immune mechanisms in acute psychological stress, *Psychosom. Med.* **43**, 84 (Abstr.).

Driscoll, J. S., Melnick, N. R., Quinn, F. R., Davignon, J. P., Ing, R., Abbott, B. J., Congleton, G., and Dudeck, L. (1978). Psychotropic drugs as potential antitumor agents: A selective screening study, *Cancer Treat. Rep.*, **62**, 45–73.

Dukor, P., Salvin, S. B., Dietrich, F. M., Glezer, J., Hess, R., and Loustalot, P. (1966). Effect of reserpine on immune reactions and tumor growth, *Eur. J. Cancer*, **2**, 253–261.

Durland, D., Martin, J. B., and Brazeau, P. (1977). Evidence for a role of β-adrenergic mechanisms in regulation of episodic growth hormone secretion in rats, *Endocrinology*, **100**, 722–728.

Dutz, W., Kohout, E., Rossipal, E., and Vessal, K. (1976). Infantile stress, immune modulations and disease patterns, *Pathol. Annu.*, **11**, 415–454.

Edwards, E. A., and Dean, L. M. (1977). Effects of crowding of mice on humoral antibody formation and protection to lethal antigenic challenge, *Psychosom. Med.*, **39**, 19–24.

Edwards, E. A., Rahe, R. A., Stephens, P. M., and Henry, J. P. (1980). Antibody response to bovine serum albumin in mice: The effects of psychosocial environmental change, *Proc. Soc. Exp. Biol. Med.*, **164**, 478–81.

Edwardson, J. A., and Bennett, G. W. (1974). Modulation of corticotropin releasing factor (CRF) release from hypothalamic synaptosomes, *Nature*, **251**, 425–427.

Ernster, V. L., Sacks, S. T., Selvin, S., and Petrakis, N. L. (1979). Cancer incidence by marital status: U.S. Third National Cancer Survey, *J. Natl. Cancer Inst.*, **63**, 567–585.

Fabris, N. (1973). Immune depression in thyroidectomized animals, *Clin. Exp. Immunol.*, **15**, 601.

Fabris, N., Pierpaoli, W., and Sorkin, E. (1971) Hormones and the immunological capacity III. The immunodeficiency disease of the hypopituitary Snell-Bagg dwarf mouse, *Clin Exp. Immunol.*, **9**, 209–225.

Fauci, A. S., Dale, D. C., and Balow, J. E. (1976). Glucorticosteroid therapy: Mechanisms of action and clinical considerations, *Ann. Internal Med.*, **84**, 304–315.

Fauman, M. A. (1982). The central nervous system and the immune system, *Biol. Psychol.*, **17**, 1459–1481.

Fekete, M. I. K., Szentendrei, T., Kanyicska, B., and Palkovits, M. (1981). Effects of anxiolytic drugs on the catecholamine and DOPAC (3, 4-dihydroxyphenylacetic acid) levels in brain cortical areas and on corticosterone and prolactin secretion in rats subjected to stress, *Psychoneuroendocrinology*, **6**, 113–120.

Felten, D. L., Overhage, J. M., Felten, S. Y., and Schmedtje, J. F. (1981). Noradrenergic sympathetic innervation of lymphoid tissue in the rabbit appendix: Further evidence for a link between the nervous and immune systems, *Brain Res. Bull.*, **7**, 595–612.

Fidler, I. J. (1978). Tumor heterogeneity and the biology of cancer invasion and metastasis, *Cancer Res.*, **38**, 2651–2660.

Filipp, G., and Mess, B. (1969). Role of the adrenocortical system in suppressing anaphylaxis after hypothalamic lesion, *Ann. Allergy*, **27**, 607–610.

Filipp, G., and Szentivanyi, A. (1958). Anaphylaxis and the nervous system. Part III, *Ann. Allergy*, **16**, 306–311.

Fischer, C. L., Daniels, J. C., Levin, S. L., Kimzey, S. L., Cobb, E. K., and Ritzman, W. E. (1972). Effects of the spaceflight environment on man's immune system: II. Lymphocyte counts and reactivity, *Aero. Med.*, 1122–1125.

Fisher, B., and Fisher, E. R. (1959). Experimental studies of factors influencing hepatic metastases: II. Effect of partial hepatectomy, *Cancer*, **12**, 929–932.

Folch, H., and Waksman, B. H. (1974). The splenic suppressor cell, *J. Immunol.*, **113**, 127–139.

Fox, B. H. (1978). Premorbid psychological factors as related to cancer incidence, *J. Behav. Med..*, **1**, 45–133.

Fox, B. H. (1981). Psychosocial factors and the immune system in human cancer, in *Psychoneuroimmunology*, (Ed. R. Ader), Academic Press, New York,

Fras, I., Litin, E. M., and Pearson, J. S. (1967). Comparison of psychiatric symptoms in carcinoma of the pancreas with those in some other intra-abdominal neoplasms, *Am. J. Psychiat.*, **123**, 1553–1561.

Frick, O. L. (1980). Immediate hypersensitivity, in *Basic and Clinical Immunology* (Eds. H. H. Fudenberg, D. P. Stites, J. L. Caldwell and J. V. Wells), Lange Medical, Los Altos.

Friedman, S. B., Ader, R., and Glasgow, L. A. (1965) Effects of psychological stress in adult mice inoculated with Coxsackie B virus, *Psychosom. Med.*, **27**, 361–368.

Friedman, S. B., Ader, R., and Grota, L. J. (1973). Protective effect of noxious stimulation in mice infected with rodent malaria, *Psychsom. Med.*, **35** 535–537.

Friedman, S. B., and Glasgow, L. A. (1973). Interaction of mouse strain and differential housing upon resistance to *Plasmodium berghei*, *J. Parasitol.*, **59**, 851–854.

Friedman, S. B., Glasgow, L. A., and Ader, R. (1970). Differential susceptibility to a viral agent in mice housed alone or in groups, *Psychosom. Med..*, **32**, 285–299.

Fudenberg, H. H., Stites, D. P., Caldwell, J. L., and Wells, J. V. (1980). *Basic and Clinical Immunology* 3rd Edn., Lange Medical, Los Altos.

Ganong, W. F. (1976). The role of catecholamines and acetylcholine in the regulation of endocrine function, *Life Sci.*, **15**, 1401–1414.

Ganong, W. F., Kramer, N., Reid, I. A., Boryczka, A. T., and Shackelford, R. (1976). Inhibition of stress-induced ACTH secretion by norepinephrine in the dog: Mechanisms and site of action, in *Catecholamines and Stress* (Eds. E. Usdin, R. Kvetnansky and I. J. Kopin), Pergamon Press, Oxford.

Gillette, S., and Gillete, R. W. (1979). Changes in thymic estrogen receptor expression following orchidectomy, *Cell. Immunol.*, **42**, 194–196.

Giron, L. T. Jr., Crutcher, K. A., and Davis J. N. (1980). Lymph nodes – A possible site for sympathetic neuronal regulation of immune responses, *Ann. Neurol*, **8** 520–525.

Gisler, R. H. (1974). Stress and the hormonal regulation of the immune response in mice, *Psychotherapeut, Psychosom.*, **23**, 197–208.

Glenn, W. G., and Becker, (1969). Individual versus group housing in mice: Immunological response to time and phase injections, *Physiol. Zool.*, **42**, 41–416.

Gorczynski, R. M., Macrae, S., and Kennedy, M. (1982). Conditioned immune response associated with allogeneic skin grafts in mice, *J. Immunol.*, **129**, 704–709.

Gordon, M. A., Cohen, J. J., and Wilson, I. B. (1978). Muscarinic cholinergic receptors in murine lymphocytes: Demonstration by direct binding, *Proc. Nat. Acad. Sc. U.S.A..*, **75**, 2902–2904.

Greene, W. A. (1966). The psychosocial setting of the development of leukemia and lymphoma, *Ann. N.Y. Acad. Sci.*, **125**, 794–801.

Greenfield, N. S., Roessler, R., and Crosley, A. P. (1959). Ego strength and recovery from infectious mononucleosis, *J. Nerv. Ment. Dis.*, **128**, 125.

Greer, S., and Morris, T. (1975). Psychological attributes of women who develop breast cancer: A controlled study, *J. Psychosom. Res.*, **19**, 147–153.

Greene, W. A., Betts, R. F., Ochitill, H. N., Iker, H. P., and Douglas, R. G. (1979). Psychosocial factors and immunity: Preliminary report, *Psychosom. Med.*, **40**, 87, (Abstract).

Grossarth-Maticek, R., Kanazir, D. S., Schmidt, P., and Vetter, H. (1982). Psychosomatic factors in the process of cancerogenesis, *Psychoter. Psychosom.*, **38**, 284–302.

Guillemin, R. (1978). Peptides in the brain: The new endocrinology of the neuron, *Science*, **202**, 390–402.

Hall, N. R., and Goldstein, A. L. (1981). Neurotransmitters and the immune system, in *Psychoneuroimmunology* (Ed. R. Ader), Academic Press, New York.

Hall, N. R., Lewis, J. K., Smith, R. T., and Zornetzer, S. F. (1979). Effects of locus coeruleus and anterior hypothalamic brain lesions on antibody formation in mice, *Soc. Neurosci. Abstr..*, **5**, 511.

Hall, N. R., McClure, J. E., Hu, S. H., Tick, N. T., Seales, C. M., and Goldstein, A. L. (1980). Effects of chemical sympathectomy upon thymus dependent immune responses, *Soc Neurosci. Abstr.*, **26**, 4.

Hall, R. C. W., Stickney, S. K., and Gardner, E. R. (1981). Psychiatric symptoms in systemic lupus erythematosus, *Psychosomatics*, **22**, 15–28.

Hara, C., Ogawa, N., and Imada, Y. (1981). The activity – stress ulcer and antibody production in rats, *Physiol. Behav.*, **27**, 609–613.

Hattori, T., Hamai, Y., Ikeda, T., Takiyama, W., Hirai, T., and Miyoshi, Y. (1982). Inhibitory effects of immunopotentiators on the enhancement of lung metastases induced by operative stress in rats, *Gann*, **73**, 132135.

Heise, E. R. (1982). Diseases associated with immunosuppression, *Environ. Health Perspect.*, **43**, 9–19.

Hendley, E. D., Burrows, G. H. Robinson, E. S., Heidenreich, K. A., and Bulman, C. A. (1977). Acute stress and the brain norepinephrine uptake mechanism in the rat, *Pharmacol. Biochem. Behav.*, **6**, 197–202.

Herberman, R. B., and Holden, H. T. (1978). Natural cell-mediated immunity, in *Advances in Cancer Research*, Vol. 27 (Eds. G. Klein and S. Weinhouse), Academic Press, New York.

Herman, J. P., Guillonneau, D., Dantzer, R., Scatton, B., Semerdjian-Rouquier., and Le Moal, M. (1982). Differential effects of inescapable footshock and stimuli previously paired with inescapable footshocks on dopamine turnover in cortical and limbic areas of the rat, *Life Sci.*, **30**, 2207–2214.

Hill, C. W., Green, W. E., and Felsenfeld, O. (1967). Psychological stress, early response to foreign protein, and blood cortisol in vervets, *Psychosom. Med.*, **29**, 279–283.

Hingtgen, J. N., Smith, J. E., Shea, P. A., Aprison, M. H., and Gaff, T. M. (1976). Cholinergic changes during conditioned suppression in rats, *Science*, **193**, 332–334.

Hinkle, L. E. (1974). The effect of exposure to cultural change, social change, and changes in interpersonal relationships on health, in *Stressful Life Events: Their Nature and Effects* (Eds. B. S. Dohrenwend and B. P. Dohrenwend), John Wiley, New York.

Holmes, T. H., Hawkins, N. G., Bowerman, C. E., Clarke, E. R., and Joffe, J. R. (1957). Psychological and physiological studies of tuberculosis, *Psychosom. Med.*, **19**, 134–143.

Holmes, T. H., Joffe, J. R. Ketcham, J. W., *et al.* (1961). Experimental study of prognosis. *J. Psychosom. Res.*, **5**, 235–252.

Horne, R. L., and Picard, R. S. (1979). Psychosocial risk factors for lung cancer, *Psychosom Med*, **41**, 501–514.

Huang, S. W., Plaut, S. M., Taylor, G., and Wareheim, L. E. (1981). Effect of stressful stimulation on the incidence of streptozotocin-induced diabetes in mice, *Psychosom. Med.*, **43**, 431–437.

Iimori, K., Tanaka, M., Kohno, Y., Ida, Y., Nakagawa, R., Hoaki, Y., Tsuda, A., and Nagasaki, N. (1982). Psychological stress enhances noradrenaline turnover in specific brain regions in rats, *Psychopharmacol. Biochem. Behav.*, **16**, 637–640.

Irwin, J., Bowers, W., Zacharko, R. M., and Anisman, H. (1982). Stress-induced alterations of norepinephrine: Cross-stressor sensitization, *Soc. Neurosci. Abstr.*, **8**, 359.

Jacobs, S., and Ostfeld, A. (1977). An epidemiological review of bereavement, *Psychosom Med.*, **39**, 344–357.

Jamasbi, R. J., and Nettesheim, P. (1977). Non-immunological enhancement of tumor transplantability in x-irradiated host animals, *Brit. J. Cancer*, **36**, 723–729.

Jankovic, B. D., and Isakovic, K. (1973). Neuro-endocrine correlates of immune response: I. Effects of brain lesions on antibody production, Arthus reactivity, and delayed hypersensitivity in the rat, *Int. Arch. Allergy Appl. Immunol.*, **45**, 360–372.

Jankovic, B. D., Jovanova, K., and Markovic, B. M., (1979). Effect of hypothalamic stimulation on the immune reaction in the rat, *Period. Biol.*, **81**, 211–212.

Jemmott, J. B., Borysenko, M., Chapman, R., Borysenko, J. Z., McClelland, D. C., and Benson, H. (1983). Academic stress, power motivation, and decrease in secretion rate of salivary secretory immunoglobin A, *Lancet*, 1400–1402.

Joasoo, A., and McKenzie, J. M. (1976). Stress and the immune response in rats. *Int. Arch. Allergy Appl. Immunol.*, **50**, 659–663.

Johnsson, D. L., Ashmore, R. C., and Gordon, M. A. (1981). Effects of B-adrenergic agents on the murine lymphocyte response to mitogen stimulation, *J. Immunopharmacol.*, **3**, 205–219.

Johnsson, T., Lavender, J. F., Hultin, E., and Rasmussen, A. F. Jr., (1963). The influence of avoidance-learning stress on resistance to Coxsackie B virus in mice, *J. Immunol.*, **91**, 569–575.

Johnson, T., and Rasmussen, A. F., Jr. (1965). Emotional stress and susceptibility to poliomyelitis virus infection in mice, *Arch, Gesamte Virusforsch.*, **18**, 393–396.

Kalisnik, M., Vraspir-Porenta, O., Logonder-Mlinsek, M., Zorc, M., and Pajntar, M. (1979). Stress and Ehrlich ascites tumor in mouse, *Neoplasma,* **26**, 483–491.

Kamo, I., and Friedman, H. (1977). Immunosuppression and the role of suppressive factors in cancer, *Adv. Cancer Res.*, **25**, 271.

Karczmar, A. G., Scudder, C. L., and Richardson, D. L. (1973). Interdisciplinary approach to the study of behavior in related mice types, in *Chemical Approaches to Brain Function* (Eds. S. Ehrenpreis and I. J. Kopin) Academic Press, New York.

Kasahara, K., Tanaka, S., Ito, T., and Hamashima, Y. (1977). Suppression of the primary immune response by chemical sympathectomy, *Res. Commun. Chem. Pathol. Pharmacol.*, **16**, 687–694.

Kasl, S. V., Evans, A. S., and Neiderman, J. C. (1979). Psychosocial risk factors in the development of infectious mononucleosis, *Psychosom. Med.*, **41**, 445–466.

Katz, D. H. (1978). The allergic phenotype: Manifestation of allergic breakthrough and imbalance in normal damping of IgE antibody production, *Immunol. Rev*, **41**, 77.

Kay, M.M.B. (1980). Aging and the decline of immune responsiveness, in *Basic and Clinical Immunology* (Eds. H. H. Fudenberg, D. P. Stites, J. L. Caldwell, and J. V. Wells), pp. 327–342, Lange, Los Altos.

Keim, K. L., and Sigg, E. B. (1976). Physiological and biochemical concomitants of restraint stress in rats, *Pharmacol. Biochem. Behav.*, **4**, 289–297.

Keller, S. E., Stein, M., Camerino, M. S., Schleifer, S. J., and Sherman, J. (1980). Suppression of lymphocyte stimulation by anterior hypothalamic lesions in the guinea pig. *Cell. Immunol.*, **52**, 334–340.

Keller, S. E., Weiss, J. M., Schleifer, S. J., Miller, N. E., and Stein, M. (1981). Suppression of immunity by stress: Effect of a graded series of stressors on lymphocyte stimulation in the rat, *Science*, **213**, 1397–1400.

Keller, S. E., Weiss, J. M., Schleifer, S. J., Miller, N. E., and Stein M. (1983).

Stress-induced suppression of immunity in adrenalectomized rats, *Science*, **221**, 1301–1304.

Kennett, G. A., and Joseph, M. H. (1981). The functional importance of increased brain tryptophan in the serotonergic response to restraint stress, *Neuropharmacology*, **20**, 39–43.

Kimzey, S. L., Johnson, P. C., Ritzman, S. E., and Mengel, C. E. (1976). Hematology and immunology studies: The second manned Skylab mission, *Aviation Space Env. Med.*, April, 383–390.

Kissen, D. M. (1967). Psychological factors, personal and lung cancer in men aged 55–64, *Geriatrics*, **24**, 129–137.

Klosterhalfen, W., and Klosterhalfen, S. (1983). Pavlovian conditioning of immunosuppression modifies adjuvant arthritis in rats, *Behav. Neurosci.*, **97**, 663–666.

Kobayashi, R. M., Palkovits, M., Kizer, J.S., Jacobowitz, D. M., and Kopin, I. J. (1976). Selective alterations of catecholamines and tyrosine hydroxylase activity in the hypothalamus following acute and chronic stress, in *Catecholamines and Stress*, (Eds. E. Usdin, R. Kvetnansky and I. J. Kopin), Pergamon Press, Oxford.

Kohler, P. F., and Vaughan, J. (1982). The autoimmune diseases, *J. Amer. Med. Assoc.*, **248**, 2646–57.

Korneva, E. A. (1976). Neurohumoral regulation of immunological homeostasis, *Fiziol. Chel.*, **3**, 469–481.

Korneva, E. A., and Khai, L. M. (1964). Effect of destruction of hypothalamic ares on immunogenesis, *Fed. Proc. Am. Soc. Exp. Biol.*, **23**, 88–92.

Kort, W. J., and Weijma, J. M. (1982). Effect of chronic light – dark shift stress on the immune response of the rat, *Physiol. Behav.*, **29**, 1083–1087.

Kosch, S. G. (1981). Life style variables associated with fibrocytic disease and breast cancer. Paper presented at the annual meeting of the American Psychological Association, Los Angeles, 1981.

Kusnecov, A. W., Sivyer, M., King, M. G., Husband, A. J., Cripps, A. W., and Clancy, R. L. (1983). Behaviorally conditioned suppression of the immune response by antilymphocyte serum, *J. Imunol.*, **130**, 2117–2120.

Kvetnansky (1981). Recent progress in catecholamines under stress, in *Catecholamines and Stress: Recent Advances* (Eds. E. Usdin, R. Kvetnansky and I. J. Kopin), pp. 7–20, Elsevier North-Holland, New York.

Kvetnansky, R., Mitro, A., Palkovits, M., Brownstein, M., Torda, T., Vigas, M. and Mikulaj, L. (1976). Catecholamines in individual hypothalamic nuclei in stressed rats, in *Catecholamines and Stress*, (Eds. E. Usdin, R. Kvetnansky and I. J. Kopin) Pergamon Press, Oxford.

LaBarba, R. C. (1970). Experiential and environmental factors in cancer, *Psychosom. Med.*, **32** 259–276.

Lacassagne, A., and Duplan, J. F. (1959). Le mecanisme de la cancerisation de la mamelle chez les souris, considere d'apres les resultats d'experience au moyen de la reserpine, *Compte. Rend. Hebd. Seanc. Acad. Sci. Paris.*, **249**, 810–812.

Lapin, V. (1978). Effects of reserpine on the incidence of 9,10 dimethyl–1,2,-benzanthracene-induced tumors in pinealectomised and thymectomised rats, *Oncology*, **35**, 132–135.

Laudenenslager, M. L., Reite, M., and Harbeck, R. J. (1982). Suppressed immune response in infant monkeys associated with maternal separation, *Behav. Neurol. Biol.*, **36**, 40–48.

Laudenslager, M. L., Ryan, S. M., Drugan, R. C., Hyson, R. L., and Maier, S. F. (1983). Coping and immunosuppression: Inescapable but not escapable shock suppresses lymphocyte proliferation, *Science*, **221**, 568–570.

Leherer, S. (1980). Life change and gastric cancer, *Psychosom. Med.*, **42**, 499–502.

Lewis, J. W., Shavit, Y., Terman, G. W., Gale, R. P., and Liebeskind, J. C. (1983a in press). Apparent involvement of opioid peptides in stress-induced enhancement of tumor growth.

Lewis, J. W., Shavit, Y., Terman, G. N., Gale, R. P., and Liebeskind, J. C. (1983b in press). Stress and morphine affect the growth of a mammary ascites tumor (MAT 13762B) in rats.

Lewis, J. W., Shavit, Y., Terman, G. W., Nelson, L. R., Gale R. P., and Liebeskind, J. C. (1983). Apparent involvement of opioid peptides in stress-induced enhancement of tumor growth, *Peptides*, **4**, 635–638.

Lewis, J. W., Sherman, J. E., and Liebeskind, J. C. (1981). Opioid and non-opioid stress analgesia: Assessment of tolerance and cross-tolerance with morphine, *J. Neurosci.*, **1**, 358–363.

Linn, B. S., and Jensen, J. (1983). Age and immune response to a surgical stress, *Arch. Surg.*, **118**, 405–409.

Linn, M. W., Linn, B. S., and Jensen, J. (1983). Stress and immune function in diabetes mellitus, *Clin. Immunal. Immunopathol.*, **27**, 223–233.

Locke, S. E. (1982). Stress, adaptation and immunity: Studies in humans, *Gen. Hosp. Psychiat.*, **4**, 49–58.

Locke, S. E., and Heisel, S. J. (1977). The influence of stress and emotions on the human immune response (Abstract), *Biofeed, Self-Regul.*, **2**, 320.

Locke, S. E., Hurst, M. W., Heisel, J. S., Krause, L. and Williams, M. (1979). The influence of stress and other psychological factors on human immunity. Paper presented at the 36th Annual Meeting of the Psychosomatic Society, Dallas, 1979.

Luborsky, L., Mintz, J., Brightman, V. J., and Katcher, A. H. (1976). Herpes simplex virus and moods: A longitudinal study, *J. Psychosom. Res.*, **20**, 543–548.

Lundy, J., Lovett, E. J., Wolinsky, S. M., and Conran, P. (1979). Immune impairment and metastatic tumor growth, *Cancer*, **43**, 945–951.

Luparello, T. J., Stein, M., and Park, C. D. (1964). Effect of hypothalamic lesions on rat anaphylaxis. *Am. J. Physiol.*, **207**, 911–914.

Macris, N. T., Schiavi, R. C., Camerino, M. S., and Stein, M. (1970). Effects of hypothalamic lesions on immune processes in the guinea pig, *Am. J. Phsyiol.*, **219**, 1205–1209.

Marsh, J. T., and Rasmussen, A. F., Jr. (1960). Response of adrenals, thymus, spleen and leukocytes to shuttle box and confinement stress, *Proc. Soc. Exp. Biol. Med.*, **104**, 180–183.

Martin, J. B. (1974). Regulation of the pituitary – thyroid axis, in *Endocrine Physioloy*, (Ed. S. M. McCann) Butterworth, London.

Maruyama, Y., and Johnson, E. A. (1969). Quantitative study of isologous tumor cell inactivation and effective cell fraction for the LSA mouse lymphoma, *Cancer*, **23**, 309–312.

Maslinski, W., Grabczewska, E., and Ryzewski, J. (1980). Acetylcholine receptors of rat lymphocytes, *Biochem. Biophys. Acta*, **633**, 269–273.

Mason, J. W., Maher, J. T., Hartley, L. H., Mougey, E. H., Perlow, M. J., and Jones, L. G. (1976). Selectivity of corticosteroid and catecholamine responses to various natural stimuli, in *Psychopathology of Human Adaptation* (Ed. G. Serban), Plenum Press, New York.

Mastrovito, R. C., Deguire, K. S., Clarkin, J., Thaler, T., Lewis, J. L., and Cooper, E. (1979). Personal characteistics of women with gynecological cancer, *Cancer Detect. Prevent.*, **2**, 281–287.

Mathews, K. P. (1982). Respiratory atopic disease, *J. Amer. Med. Assoc.*, **248**, 2587–2610.

McAlpine, D., and Compston, N. D., and Compston, N. D. (1952). Some aspects of the natural history of disseminated sclerosis, *Q. J. Med.*, **21**, 135–167.

McClary, A. R., Meyer, E., and Weitzman, D. J. (1955). Observations on the role of mechanism of depression in some patients with disseminated lupus erythematosus, *Psychosom Med.*, **17**, 311321.

MCClelland, D. C., Floor, W., Davidson, R. J., and Saron, C. (1980). Stressed motivation, sympathetic activation, immune function and illness, *J. Human Stress*, **6**, 11–19.

Mei-Tal, V., Meyerowitz, M. D., and Engel, G. (1970). The role of psychological process in a somatic disorder: Multiple sclerosis, *Psychosom. Med.*, **32**, 67–85.

Meyer, R. J., and Haggerty, R. J. (1962). Streptococcal infections in families, *Pediatrics*, **29** 539–549.

Minter, R. E., and Kimball, C. P. (1978). Life events and illness onset: A review, *Psychosomatics*, **19**, 334–339.

Modigh, K. (1976). Influence of social stress on brain catecholamine mechanisms, in *Catecholamines and Stress* (Eds. E. Usdin, R. Kvetnanasky and I. J. Kopin), Pergamon Press, Oxford.

Monjan, A. A. (1981). Stress and immunologic competence: Studies in animals, in *Psychoneuroimmunology* (Ed. R. Ader), pp. 185–228, Academic Press New York.

Monjan, A. A. and Collector, I. I. (1977). Stress-induced modulation of the immune response, *Science*, **196**, 307–308.

Monroe, S. M. (1982). Assessment of life events, *Arch. Gen. Psychiat.*, **39**, 606–610.

Morgan, W. W., Rudeen, P. K., and Pfeil, K. A. (1975). Effect of immobilization stress on serotonin content and turnover in regions of the rat brain, *Life Sci.*, **17**, 143–150.

Morris, T., Greer, S., Pettingale, K. W., and Watson, M. (1981). Patterns of expression of anger and their psychological correlates in women with breast cancer, *J. Psychosom Res.*, **25**, 111–117.

Muller, E. E., Nistico, G., and Scapagnini, U. (1978). Neurotransmitters and anterior pituitary function, in *The Endocrine Hypothalamus*, (Eds. S. L. Jeffcoate and J. M. S. Hutchinson), Academic Press, London.

Muslin, H. L., Gyarfas, K., and Pieper, W. J. (1966). Separation experience and cancer of the breast, *Ann. N. Y. Acad. Sci.*, **125**, 802–806.

Newberry, B. H., and Sengbush, L. (1979). Inhibitory effects of stress on experimental mammary tumors, *Cancer Detect. Preven.*, **2**, 307–366.

Nieburgs, H. E., Weiss, J., Navarrete, M., Strax, P., Teirstein, A., Grillione, C., and Siedlecki, B. (1979). The role of stress in human and experimental oncogenesis, *Cancer Detect. Preven.*, **2**, 307–336.

Otto, R., and Mackay, I. (1967). Psychological and emotional disturbance in lupus erythematosus, *Med. J. Aust.*, **2**, 488493.

Palkovits, M., Brownstein, M., Kizer, J. S., Saavedra, J. M., and Kipin, I. J. (1976). Effects of stress on serotonin and tryptophan hydroxylase activity of brain nuclei, in *Catecholamines and Stress* (Eds. E. Usdin, R. Kvetnansky and I. J. Kopin), Pergamon Press, Oxford.

Palmblad, J. (1981). Stress and immunologic competence: Studies in man, in *Psychoneuroimmunology* (Ed. R. Ader), Academic Press, New York.

Palmblad, J., Cantell, K., Strander, H., Troberg, J., Karlsson, C. G., Levi, L., Granstrom, M., and Unger, P. (1976). Stressor exposure and immunological response in man: Interferon-producing capacity and phagocytosis, *J. Psychosom. Res.*, **20**, 193–199.

Palmblad, J., Karlsson, C. G., Levi, L., and Lidberg, (1979a). The erythrocyte sedimentation rate and stress, *Acta. Med. Scand.*, **205**, 517–520.

Palmblad, J., Petrini, B., Wasserman, J., and Akerstedt, T. (1979b). Lymphocyte and granulocyte reactions during sleep deprivation, *Psychosom.* Med., **41**, 273–278.

Parkes, C. M., and Brown, R. J. (1972). Health after bereavement: A controlled study of young Boston widows and widowers, *Psychosom. Med.*, **34**, 449–461.

Paunovic, V. R., Petrovic, S., and Jankovic, B. D. (1976). Influence of early hypothalamic lesions on immune response of adult rats, *Period, Biol.*, **78**, 50.

Pavlidis, N., and Chirigos, M. (1980). Stress induced impairment of macrophage tumoricidal function, *Psychsom. Med.*, **42**, 47–54.

Paykel, E., Myers, J. K., Dienelt, M. W., Klerman, G. L., Lindenthal, J. J., and Pepper, M. P. 1969). Life events and depression, *Arch. Gen. Psychiat.*, **21**, 753–60.

Penn, I. (1981). Depressed immunity and the development of cancer, *Clin. Exp. Immunol.*, **46**, 459–474.

Peters, L. J. (1975). Enhancement of syngeneic murine tumor transplantation by whole body irradiation – A nonimmunological phenomenon, *Brit. J. Cancer*, **31**, 293–300.

Peters, L. J., and Kelly, H. (1977). The influence of stress and stress hormones on the transplantability of a non-immunogenic syngeneic murine tumor, *Cancer*, **39**, 1482–1488.

Pettingale, K. W., Greer, S., and Tee, D. E. H. (1977). Serum IgA and emotional expression in breast cancer patients, *J. Psychosom. Rds.*, **21**, 395–399.

Petty, F, and Sherman, A. D. (1982). A neurochemical differentiation between exposure to stress and the development of learned helplessness, *Drug Development Research*, **2**, 43–45.

Pierpaoli, W., Baroni, C. and Fabris, N., and Sorkin, E. (1969). Hormones and immunologic capacity. II. Reconstitution of antibody production in hormonally deficient mice by somatotrophic hormone, thyrotropic hormone and thyroxin, *Immunology*, **16**, 217–230.

Plaut, S. M., Ader, R., Friedman, S. B., and Ritterson, A. L. (1969). Social factors and resistance to malaria in the mouse: group vs. individual housing and resistance to *Plasmodium berghei*, *Psychosom. Med.*, **31**, 536–552.

Plaut, S. M., and Friedman, S. B. (1981). Psychosocial factors in infectious disease, in *Psychoneuroimmunology* (Ed. R. Ader), Academic Press, New York.

Plaut, S. M., and Friedman, S. B. (1982). Stress, coping behavior and resistance to disease. *Psychother. Psychosom.*, **38**, 274–283.

Pradhan, S. N., and Ray, P. (1974). Effects of stress on growth of transplanted and 7, 12-dimethylbenz(a)anthracene-induced tumors and their modification by psychotropic drugs, *J. Natl. Cancer Inst.*, **53**, 1241–1245.

Prehn, R. T. (1974). Immunologic surveillance: Pro and con, in *Clinical Immunology*, Vol. 2 (Eds. F. H. Bach and R. A. Good), Academic Press, New York.

Przewlocki, R., Hollt, V., Voigt, K. H., and Nerz, A. (1979). Modulation of *in vitro* release of B-endorphin from the separate lobes of the pituitary, *Life Sci.*, **24**, 1601–1608.

Purcell, K., Turnbull, J. W., and Berstein, L. I. (1962). Distinctions between subgroups of asthmatic children, psychological tests and behavioral rating comparisons, *J. Psychosom. Res.*, **6**, 283.

Quadri, S. K., Kledzik, G. S., and Meites, J. (1973). Effects of L-dopa and methyldopa on growth of mammary tumors in rats, *Proc. Soc. Exp. Biol. Med.*, **124**, 22–26.

Rabkin, J. G., and Streuning, E. L. (1976). Life events, stress and illness, *Science*, **194**, 1013–1020.

Rasmussen, A. F. Jr. (1969). Emotions and immunity, *Ann. N. Y. Acad. Sci.*, **164**, 458–462.

Rasmussen, A. F. Jr., Marsh, J. T., and Brill, N. Q. (1957). Increased susceptibility to herpes simplex in mice subjected to avoidance-learning stress or restraint, *Proc. Soc. Exp. Biol. Med.*, **100**, 878–879.

Rasmussen, A. F. Jr., Spencer, E. S., and Marsh, J. T. (1957). Increased susceptibility to herpes simplex in mice subjected to avoidance-learning stress or restraint, *Proc. Soc. Ex. Biol. Med.*, **96**, 183–184.

Reichlin, S., Martin, J. B., and Jackson, I. M. D. (1978). Regulation of TSH secretion, in *The Endocrine Hypothalamus* (Eds. S. L. Jeffcoate and J. M. S. Hutchinson), Academic Press, London.

Richman, D. P., and Arnason, B. G. (1979). Nicotinic acetylcholine receptor: Evidence for a functionally distinct receptor on human lymphocytes, *Proc. Nat. Acad. Sci. U.S.A.*., **76**, 4632–4635.

Richter, M. A. (1982). *Clinical Immunology – A Physician's Guide*, 2nd Edn., Williams and Wilkins, Baltimore.

Riley, V. (1981). Psychoneuroendocrine influences on immunocompetence and neoplasia, *Science*, **212**, 100–1109.

Riley, V., Fitzmaurice, M. A., and Spackman, D. H. (1981). Psychoneuroimmunologic factors in neoplasia: Studies in animals, in *Psychoneuroimmunology* (Ed. R. Ader), pp. 31–102., Academic Press, New York.

Riley, V., and Spackman, D. (1977). Cage crowding stress: Absence of effect on melanoma within protective facilities, *Proc. Am. Assoc. Cancer Res.*, **18**, 173.

Riley, V., Spackman, D., McClanahan, H., and Santisteban, G. A. (1979). The role of stress in malignancy, *Cancer Detect. Preven.*, **2**, 235–255.

Rimon, R., Belmaker, R. H., and Ebstein, R. (1977). Psychosomatic aspects of juvenile rheumatoid arthritis, *Scand. J. Rheumatol.*, **6**, 1–10.

Rimon, R., Viukari, M., and Halonen, P. (1979). Relationship between life stress factors and viral antibody levels in patients with juvenile rheumatoid arthritis, *Scand. J. Rheumatol.*, **8**, 62–64.

Roark, G. E. (1971). Psychosomatic factors in the epidemiology of infectious mononucleosis, *Psychosomatics*, **12**, 402–412.

Roessler, R., Cato, T. R., Lester, J. W., and Couch, R. B. (1979). Ego strength, life events and antibody titer. Paper presented at the Annual Meeting of the American Psychosomatic Society, Dallas, 1979.

Rogentine, G. N., van Kammen, D. P., Fox, B. H., Doherty, J. P., Rosenblatt, J. E. Boyd, S. C., and Bunney, W. E. (1979). Psychological factors in the prognosis of malignant melanoma: A prospective study, *Psychosom. Med.*, **41**, 647–655.

Rogers, M. P., Dubey, D., and Reich, P. (1979). The influence of the psyche and the brain on immunity and disease susceptibility: A critical review, *Psychosom. Med.*, **41**, 147–164.

Rogers, M. P., Trentham, D. E., McCune, W. J., Ginsberg, B. I., Reich, P., and David, J. R. (1979). Abrogation of type II collagen-induced arthritis in rats by psychological stress, *Trans. Assoc. Am. Physicians.*, **92**, 218–228.

Rose, N. R. (1981). Autoimmune diseases, *Scientific American*, **244**, 80–103.

Roth, K. A., Mefford, I. M., and Barchas, J. D. (1982). Epinephrine, norepine-

phrine, dopamine and serotonin: Differential effects of acute and chronic stress on regional brain amines, *Brain Res.*, **239**, 417–424.
Saavedra, J. M. (1982). Changes in dopamine, noradrenaline and adrenaline in specific septal and preoptic nuclei after acute immobilization stress, *Neuroendocrinology*, **35**, 396–401.
Saba, T. M., and Antikatzides, T. G. (1976). Decreased resistance to intravenous tumor challenge during reticuloendothelial depression following surgery, *Brit. J. Cancer*, **34**, 381–389.
Sachar, E. J., Asnis, G., Halbreich, U., Nathan, R. S., and Halpern, F. (1980). Recent studies in the neuroendocrinology of major depressive disorders, *Psychiat. Clin. Nor. Amer.* **3**, 313-326.
Sarkar, D. K., Gottschall, P. E., and Meites, J. (1982). Damage to hypothalamic dopaminergic neurons is associated with development of prolactin-secreting pituitary tumors, *Science*, **218**, 684–686.
Schlewinski, E. (1976). Studies on the influence of psychological factors on the immune system: Changes in susceptibility to infection after infantile stimulation as a function of age, *Z. Psychosom. Med. Psychoanal.*, **22**, 370–377.
Schleifer, S. J., Keller, S. E., Camerino, M., Thornton, J. C., and Stein, M. (1983). Suppression of lymphocyte stimulation following bereavement, *J.A.M.A..*, **250**, 374–377.
Schmale, A. H. and Iker, H. (1966). The effect of hopelessness on the development of cancer, *Psychosom. Med.*, **28**, 714–721.
Schmidt, D. E., Cooper, D. O. and Barrett, R. J. (1980). Strain specific alterations in hippocampal cholinergic function following acute footshock, *Pharmacol. Biochem. Behav.*, **12**, 277–280.
Shavit, Y., Lewis, J. W., Terman, G,. W., Gale, R. P., and Liebeskind, J. C. (1983). The effects of stress and morphine on immune function in rats, *Soc. Neurosci. Abstr.*, **9**, 117.
Shavit, Y., Lewis, J. W., Terman, G. W., Gale, R. P., and Liebeskind, (1982). Opioid peptides may mediate the immunosuppressive effects of stress, *Soc. Neurosci. Abstr.*, **8**, 71.
Shavit, Y., Ryan, S. M., Lewis, J. W., Laudenslager, M. L., Terman, G. W., Maier, S. F., Gale, R. P., and Liebeskind, J. C. (1983). Inescapable but not escapable stress alters immune function, *Physiologist*, **26**, A–64.
Shekelle, R. B., Raynor, W. J., Ostfeld, A. M., Garron, D. C., Bieliauskas, L., Liu, S. C., Maliza, C. and Paul, O. (1981). Psychological depression and 17 year risk of death from cancer, *Psychosom. Med.*, **43** 117–125.
Sklar, L. S., and Anisman, H. (1979). Stress and coping factors influence tumor growth, *Science*, **205**, 513–515.
Sklar, L. S., and Anisman, H. (1980). Social stress influences tumor growth. *Psychosom. Med.*, **42**, 347-365.
Sklar, L. S., and Anisman, H. (1981). Stress and cancer, *Psychological Bulletin*, **89**, 369–406.
Smith, G. R., and McDaniel, S. M. (1983). Psychologically mediated effect on the delayed hypersensitivity reaction to tuberculin in humans, *Psychosom. Med.*, **45**, 65–70.
Solomon, G. F. (1969). Stress and antibody response in rats, *Int. Arch. Allergy Appl. Immunol*, **35**, 97–104.
Solomon, G. F. (1981). Emotional and personality factors in rheumatoid arthritis and other autoimmune disease, in *Psychoneuroimmunology* (Ed. R. Ader), pp. 259–278., Academic Press, New York.

Solomon, G. F., and Amkraut, A. A. (1981). Psychoneuroendocrinological effects on the immune response, *Annu. Rev. Microbiol.*, **35**, 155–184.

Solomon, G. F., Amkraut, A. A., and Kasper, P. (1974). Immunity, emotions and stress, *Psychother. Psychosom.*, 23, 209–217.

Solomon, G. F., Levine, S., and Kraft, J. K. (1968). Early experience and immunity, *Nature*, **220**, 821–822.

Spector, N. H., Cannon, L. T., Diggs, C. L., Morrison, J. E., and Koob, G. F. (1975). Hypothalamic lesions: Effects on immunological responses (Abstract). *Physiologist*, **18**, 401.

Spector, N. N., and Korneva, E. A. (1981). Neurophysiology, immunophysiology, and neuroimmunomodulation, in *Psychoneuroimmunology* (Ed. R. Ader), pp. 449–473, Academic Press, New York.

Spergel, P., Ehrlich, G. E., and Glass, D. (1978). The rheumatoid arthritis personality: A psychodiagnostic myth, *Psychosomatics*, **19**, 79–86.

Stavrakay, K. M. (1968). Psychological factors in the outcome of human cancer, *J. Psychosom. Res.*, **12**, 251–259.

Stein, M. (1981). A biopsychosocial approach to immune function and medical disorders, *Psychiat. Clinics Nor. Amer.*, **4**, 203–221.

Stein, M., Schleifer, S. J., and Keller, S. E. (1981). Hypothalamic influences on immune responses, in *Psychoneuroimmunology* (Ed. R. Ader), pp. 429–447, Academic Press, New York,

Stone, E. A. (1975). Stress and catecholamines, in *Catecholamines and Behavior* (Ed. A. J. Friedhoff), pp. 31–72, Plenum Press, New York.

Streng, C. B., and Nathan, P. (1973). The immune response in steroid deficient mice, *Immunology*, **24**, 559–565.

Stutman, O. (1975). Humoral thymic factors influencing post thymic cells, *Ann. N.Y. Acad. Sci.*, **249**, 89–105.

Swenson, R. M., and Vogel, W. H. (1983). Plasma catecholamine and corticosterone as well as brain catecholamine changes during coping in rats to exposed to stressful footshock, *Pharmacol. Biochem. Behav.*, **18**, 689–693.

Szentivanya A., and Filipp, C. (1958), Anaphylaxis and the nervous system. Part III, *Ann. Allergy*, **16**, 143–151.

Tang, L. C., and Cotzias, G. C. (1977). Quantitative correlation of dopamine dependent adenylate cyclase with responses to levodopa in various mice, *Proc. Nat. Acad. Sci. U.S.A.*, **74**, 1242–1244.

Tang, L. C., Cotzias, G. C., and Dunn, M. (1974). Changing the action of neuroactive drugs by changing brain protein synthesis. *Proc. Nat. Acad. Sci. U.S.A.*, **71**, 3350–3354.

Terry, L. C., and Martin, J. B. (1978). Hypothalamic hormones: Subcellular distribution and mechanisms of release, *Annu. Rev. Parmacol. Toxicol.*, **18**, 111–123.

Teshima, H., Kubo, C., Kihara, H., Imada, Y., Nagata, S., Ago, Y., and Ikemi, I. (1982). Psychosomatic aspects of skin diseases from the standpoint of immunology, *Psychoterapeut. Psychosom.*, **37**, 165–175.

Thierry, A. M. (1973), Effects of stress on the metabolism of serotonin and norepinephrine in the central nervous system of the rat, in *Hormones, Metabolism and Stress: Recent Progress and Perspectives (Ed. S. Nemeth), Slovak Academy of Sciences, Bratislava.*

Thomas, C. B., Duszynski, K. R., and Shaffer, J. W. (1979). Family attitudes reported in youth as potential predictors of cancer, Psychosom. Med., **41**, 287–302.

Toge, T., Hirai, T., Takiyama, W., and Hattori, T. (1981). Effects of surgical stress on natural killer cell activity, proliferative response of spleen cells, and cytostatic activity of lung machrophages in rats, *Gann*, **72**, 790–794.

Tomasi, T. B., Trudeau, F. B., Czerwinski, D., and Erredge, S. (1982). Immune parameters in athletes before and after strenuous exercise, *J. Clin. Immunol.*, **2**, 173–178.

Tyrey, I., and Nalbandov, A. V. (1972). Influence of anterior hypothalamic lesions on circulating antibody titers in the rat, *Amer. J. Physiol.*, **222**, 179–185.

Van Den Brenk, H. A. S. Stone, M. G., Kelly, H., and Sharpington, C. (1976). Lowering of innate resistance of the lungs to the growth of blood-borne cancer cells in states of topical and systemic stress, *Brit. J. Cancer*, **33**, 60–78.

Van Dijk, H., Testerink, J., and Novrdegraff, E. (1976). Stimulation of the immune response against SRBC by reduction of corticosterone plasma levels: Mediation by mononuclear phagocytes, *Cell. Immunol.*, **25**, 8–14.

Van Loon, G. R. (1976). Brain dopamine beta hydroxylase activity: Response to stress, tyrosine hydroxylase inhibition, hypophysectomy and ACTH administration, in *Catecholamines and Stress* (Eds. E. Usdin, R. Kvetnansky and I. J. Kopin), Pergamon Press, Oxford.

Vernikos, J., Dallman, M. F., Bonner, C., Katzen, A., and Shinsako, J. (1982). Pituitary – adrenal function in rats chronically exposed to cold, *Endocrinology*, **110**, 413–420.

Vessey, S. H. (1964). Effect of grouping on levels of circulating antibodies in mice, *Proc. Soc. Exp. Biol. Med.*, **115**, 252.

Vijayan, E., and McCann, S. M. (1978). The effect of systemic administration of dopamine and apomorphine on plasma LH and prolactin concentrations in conscious rats, *Neuroendocrinology*, **25**, 221–235.

Visintainer, M. A., Volpicelli, J. R., and Seligman, M. E. P. (1982). Tumor rejection in rats after inescapable or escapable shock, *Science*, **216**, 437–439.

Voth, H. M. (1976). Cancer and personality, *Percept. Mot. Skills*, **42**, 1131–1137.

Vuolteenaho, O., Leppaluoto, J., and Mannisto, P. (1982). Effect of stress and dexamethasone on immunoreactive B-endorphine levels in rat hypothalamus and pineal, *Acta Physiol. Scand.*, **114**, 537–541.

Warejcka, D. J., and Levy, N. L. (1980). Central nervous system control of the immune response: Effect of hypothalamic lesions on PHA responsiveness in rats (Abstr), *Fed. Proc. Am. Soc. Exp. Biol.*, **39**, 914.

Warren, S., Greenhill, S., and Warren, K. G. (1982). Emotional stress and the development of multiple sclerosis: Case control evidence of a relationship, *J. Chron. Dis*, **35**, 821–831.

Weiner, H. (1977). *Psychobiology and Human Disease*, Elsevier-North Holland, New York.

Weisman, A. D., and Worden, J. W. (1975), Psychosocial analysis of cancer deaths, *Omega*, **6**, 61–75.

Weiss, J. M. (1970). Somatic effects of predictable and unpredictable shock, *Psychosom Med.*, **32**, 397–408.

Weiss, J. M. (1971). Effects of coping behavior with and without a feedback signal on stress pathology in rats, *J. Comp. Physiol. Psych.*, **77**, 22–30.

Weiss, J. M., Bailey, W. H., Pohorecky, L. A., Korzeniowski D., and Grillione, G. (1980). Stress-induced depression of motor activity correlates with regional changes in brain norepinephrine but not in dopamine, *Neurochem. Res.*, **5**, 9–22.

Weiss, J. M., Glazer, H. I., and Pohorecky, L. A. (1976). Coping behavior and neurochemical changes: An altenative explanation for the original 'Learned

Helplessness' experiments, in *Animal Models in Human Psychobiology* (Eds. G. Serbar and A. Kling), Plenum Press, New York.

Weiss, J. M., Glazer, H. I., Pohorecky, L. A., Bailey, W. H., and Schneider, L. H. (1979). Coping behavior and stress induced behavioral depression: Studies on the role of brain catecholamines, in *The Psychobiology of Depressive Disorders* (Ed. R. A. Depue), Academic Press, New York.

Weiss, J. M., Glazer, H. I., Pohorecky, L. A., Brick, J., and Miller, N. A. (1975). Effects of chronic exposure to stressors on avoidance-escape behavior and on brain norepinephrine. *Psychosom. Med.*, **37**, 522–534.

Weiss, J. M., Goodman, P. A., Losito, B. G., Corrigan, S., Charry, J. M. and Bailey, W. H. (1981). Behavioral depression produced by an uncontrollable stressor: relationship to norepinephrine, dopamine and serotonin levels in various regions of rat brain, *Brain Res. Rev.*, **3**, 167–205.

Weksler, M. E. (1981). The senescence of the immune system, *Hosp. Prac.*, **16**, 53–64.

Welsch, C. W., and Meites, J. (1970). Effects of reserpine on development of 7,12-dimethylbenzanthracene-induced mammary tumors in female rats, *Experientia*, **26**, 1133–1134.

Wick, M. M. (1977). L-dopa methyl ester as a new anti-tumor agent, *Nature*, **269**, 512–513.

Wick, M. M. (1978). L-dopa methyl ester: Prolongation of survival of neuroblastoma-bearing mice, *Science*, **199**, 775–776.

Wick, M. M. (1979), Levodopa and dopamine analogs: Melanin precursors as anti-tumor agents in experimental human and murine leukemia, *Cancer Treat. Rep.*, **63**, 991–997.

Wilder, R. M., Hubble, J., and Kennedy, C. E. (1971). Life change and infectious mononucleosis, *J. Amer. Coll. Health Assoc.*, **20**, 115–119.

Williams, R. C. (1980). *Immune Complexes in Clinical and Experimental Medicine*, Harvard University Press, Cambridge, Mass.

Williams, J. M., and Felten, D. L. (1981). Sympathetic innervation of murine thymus and spleen: A comparative histofluorescence study, *Anatomical Record*, **199**, 531–542.

Williams, J. M., Peterson, R. G., Shea, P. A., Schmedtje, J. F., Bauer, D. C., and Felten, D. (1981) Sympathetic innervation of murine thymus and spleen: Evidence for a functional link between nervous and immune systems, *Brain Res. Bull.*, **6**, 83–94.

Williams, J. M., Snyderman, R., and Lefkowitz, R. J. (1976). Identification of beta-adrenergic receptors in human lymphocytes by (-) (3H) aprenolol binding, *J. Clin. Invest.*, **57**, 149–155.

Wright, W. C., Ank, B. J., Herbert, J., and Stiehm, E. R. (1975). Decreased bactericidal activity of leukocytes of stressed newborn infants, *J. Pediatr.*, **56**, 579–584.

Wybran, J., Appelboom, T., Famacy, J-P., and Govaerts, A. (1979). Suggestive evidence for receptors for morphine and methionine-enkephalin on normal human blood T-lymphocytes, *J. Immunol.*, **123**, 1068–1070.

Yager, J., Grant, I., Sweetwood, H. L., and Gerst, M. (1981). Life events reports by psychiatric patients, nonpatients and their partners, *Arch. Gen. Psychiat.*, **38**, 343–350.

Zagon, I. S., and McLaughlin, P. J. (1981). Heroin prolongs survival time and retards tumor growth in mice with neuroblastoma, *Brain Res. Bull.*, **1**, 25–32.

Zagon, I. S., and McLaughlin, P. J. (1983). Naltrexone modulates tumor response in mice with neuroblastoma, *Science*, **221**, 671–672.
Zajaczkowska, M. N. (1975). Acetylcholine content in the central and peripheral nervous syustem and its synthesis in the rat brain during stress and post-stress exhaustion, *Acta. Physiol. Pol.*, **26**, 493–497.

Footnote

Supported by Grants MT-6486 from the Medical Research Council of Canada and A9845 from the Natural Sciences and Engineering Research Council of Canada.

Psychosocial Stress and Cancer
Edited by C. L. Cooper

Chapter 7
Stress: a Psychophysiological Approach to Cancer

Tom Cox
Senior Lecturer, Department of Psychology, University of Nottingham, Nottingham, UK

INTRODUCTION

In 1980, Currie wrote that 'cancer(s) can be described but as yet defy scientific definitions'. However, from a clinical viewpoint, their most important features are obvious. They are: the growth of cells in a disorganised fashion, the tendency for tumour cells to invade and disseminate and the apparent failure of normal growth control mechanisms. At one time the concept was of the inexorable growth of a totally autonomous and delinquent tissue mass. However, this view has now changed in the light of evidence that the interactions between host and tumour can influence the clinical progress of the malignant neoplasm, and can themselves be influenced. It is possible that the hormonal environment plays a part in these interactions, and it is also possible that the endocrine response to 'stress' (Cox and Cox, 1983; Cox *et al.*, 1983) makes a significant contribution to that environment.

However, in 1981, the well-respected cancer epidemiologists Doll and Peto wrote:

'It is possible that psychological factors could have some effect (in the production of cancer), e.g. by modulating hormonal secretions, but we know of no good evidence that they do nor that they affect the incidence of cancer in any other way, except insofar as they lead people to smoke, drink, overeat, or enjoy some other harmful habit.'

They went on to say:

'. . . it might perhaps be that some form of immunological surveillance normally controls the development of certain types of cancer so that failure of such control would affect the onset rate of such cancers and that environmental factors affect the likelihood of such failure, but for the present this is all to speculative to quantify.'

These two statements provide an effective and provocative outline of the theme of this chapter: it is concerned with the role of psychosocial factors associated with stress in the aetiology and development of cancers. It largely considers the effects of stress-sensitive hormones on immune surveillance as a possible mechanism by which that role might be expressed. It does, however, give some consideration to the part that the behavioural correlates of stress might play. This chapter develops ideas first presented by Wayner, Cox and Mackay (1979) and later by Cox and Mackay (1982).

ON THE NATURE OF THE EVIDENCE

It is recognised that it will always be difficult to provide direct evidence to support the hypothesis that stress, and its behavioural and endocrine correlates, contribute to the initiation or promotion of tumour growth. Progress is complicated because there is no single criterial state against which these various factors can be validated. Cancer is not a single disease entity: there is no one kind of cancer (Nature, 1981). The most common cancers are those of the lungs, stomach, intestines, pharynx and larynx, and of the breast, cervis and uterus in women, and leukaemia. Some of these cancers show hormone dependence.

The very nature of the hypothesis, combined with type of processes involved, may make it unlikely that *epidemiological* studies will be able to provide the critical evidence relating to endocrine effects. However, with regard to the behavioural correlates of stress there are epidemiological data of relevance. Doll and Peto (1981) have pointed to relationships between smoking, drinking, type of diet, and life-style, on one hand, and certain types of cancer, on the other. For example, smoking, they estimate, causes about 30% of U.S. deaths from all cancers. Furthermore, while the carcinogenic effects of drinking (alcohol) may be slight in non-smokers, they appear to increase the incidence of cancers of the mouth and pharynx in smokers some two- or three-fold (Rothman and Keller, 1972). In the same vein, it is probable that diet is a major factor in determining the occurrence of a high proportion of all cancers of the stomach and large bowel, as well as of the uterus, gall bladder, and, under some conditions, of the liver. The pattern of reproductive and sexual behaviour may have some relationship to the likelihood of particular cancers occurring in women. Other aspects of both general life-style and occupation may also play some significant part in the production of cancers.

The literature on the strategies that people adopt in coping with stressful experiences and situations is very much concerned with behaviours such as smoking and drinking, with the nature of diet and any exercise taken, and with general life-style and behaviour at work (see for example, Cox, 1978: Lazarus, 1976: Hamilton and Warburton, 1979). Thus to this extent, there is some indirect epidemiological evidence in favour of a link between stress and cancer (figure 1). Indeed, many of the preventive measures urged by cancer epidemiologists (see Doll and Peto, 1981) are essentially psychological (behavioural), for example, reducing smoking and drinking, and changing diet, and all may be easier to achieve if any underlying stress-related problems were dealt with.

STRESS - - → COPING BEHAVIOUR - - → EXPOSURE TO CARCINOGENS
PRODUCTION OF CANCERS ← - - - - -

Figure 7.1: Stress, Coping Behaviour and Cancer.

Much of the necessary evidence is coming from *experimental* and *clinical* studies; the former will for ethical reasons largely concern animal research. The overall situation is one in which the individual pieces of a jigsaw are being identified and fitted together, hopefully until there is sufficient to make it obvious whether or not the overall hypothesis is correct. Likely pieces will be:

(*a*) the relationship between stressful experiences and behavioural and endocrine changes;
(*b*) the role of behavioural factors in determining exposure to potential carcinogens;
(*c*) the reaction to diagnosis of cancer, and survival;
(*d*) the effects of stress-related hormones on immune system activity;
(*e*) the role of the immune system in the production of cancers; and
(*f*) the relationship between clinical state and immune system and endocine activity.

It is assumed that there is sufficient evidence available to answer the first wo questions. The last four questions are addressed in various forms in the emainder of this chapter.

The outcome of experimental (animal) studies depend to some extent on he host – tumour system chosen, on the nature, intensity and duration of he stress manipulation, on the timing of this manipulation with regard xposure to the carcinogen or tumour transplantation, and on the outcome neasures used (tumour incidence, growth rate or animal survival). All such autions need to built into our evaluation of the evidence, and an understanding of the processes involved will probably explain some of the apparently ontradictory evidence which exists (Riley, 1979).

Clinical research on hormone levels in relation to cancer is complicated ecause certain tumours such as oat cell lung carcinoma, are themselves apable of secreting tropic substances, such as CRF, LPH, and ACTH Jeffcoate and Rees, 1978). This may make it difficult to establish the initial ature of any relationship between hormonal environment and the development of these tumours. Furthermore, it is possible that in such cases positive feedback loops are established and the competence of the immune system is further impaired, increasing the individual's vulnerability to other agents or latent processes (Riley, 1981).

Some encouragement to pursue this overall approach comes from the apparent success of similar approaches to coronary heart disease. It now seems possible to describe the contribution of stress-related factors to its multifactorial aetiology, and of behavioural strategies in the rehabilitation of coronary patients (for example, Patel, 1975; Patel and North, 1975; Patel *et al.*, 1979). There is also some understanding of the mechanisms underpinning these contributions (Surwit *et al.*, 1982).

PERCEPTIONS OF AND REACTIONS TO CANCERS

The first line of the present argument concerns people's perceptions of cancer as a disease, and their psychological reactions to it. This may be one of several links between stress and cancer.

For most people cancers are among the most feared of diseases; they have been reported as the diseases which are '*most serious*' or '*most worrying*' by a substantial number of survey respondents (for example: Richardson and Woolcott, 1967; Wyler, 1968; Knopf, 1976). Their incidence is generally overestimated, and survival rates are markedly underestimated.

Cancers are associated with fears of severe and unavoidable pain, with disfigurement and disability, and with social rejection and even moral censure (Jenkins, 1968, 1976). Not surprisingly, those that suspect that they have cancer have great difficulty in handling that particularly threatening situation and of making full use of the available medical facilities. The problems of caring for cancer patients have been recently discussed by Fielding (1983).

Part of the problem is the lack of early diagnosis, and the delay in reporting symptons (Hacket *et al.*, 1973; Worden and Weisman, 1975). Many fail to take actions which would reduce early mortality.

In studies on cervial cytology, negative predictors of action have been identified as 'fear of cancer' (Kegeles, 1967; Wakefield, 1971; Paterson and Aitken-Swan, 1954), 'belief that cancer is incurable' (Wakefield, 1971 Paterson and Aitken-Swan, 1954), 'belief that professional diagnosis is n better than self-diagnosis' (Kegeles, 1967; Kegeles *et al.*, 1965), 'lack of belie in the value of early diagnosis' (Kegeles, 1967; Kegeles *et al.*, 1965; McKinlay 1972), and 'absence of felt susceptibility to cervical cancer' (Kegeles, 1967 The same attitudes and beliefs are often stated as reasons for delay in brea cancer examinations, and probably also hold true for the lack of early actio on most cancers.

While diagnosis may not be a 'biologically significant event', it may b critical psychologically. Numerous studies have reported the severe psychos cial problems experienced by cancer patients (Freidenbergs *et al.*, 1982). From the point of suspicion forward to the actual diagnosis the person, being aware of the consequences of a positive diagnosis, will undoubtedly be subject to much anxiety. Indeed, intense anxiety and suicidal pre-occupations have been described by Laxenaire and his colleagues (1971) as a common response to a positive cancer diagnosis. Craig and Abeloff (1974) also reported elevated levels of anxiety in their patients (about a third), as well as depression (about a half). The persons response to learning that they have cancer may partly determine their subsequent survival time, and the quality of that survival.

An early study by Blumberg and his colleagues (1954) compared cancer patients who died within 2 years of diagnosis with a matched group who survived for longer than 6 years. All patients were studied immediately after diagnosis during a phase of temporary well-being. The study used the MMPI, and suggested that those that died within 2 years had higher depression scores, lower neurotic outlet scores, and very low acting out scores. A later study by Stavrakay (1968) was of similar design and was based on 204 cancer patients psychologically assessed at the time of the person's first contact with the cancer clinic. Their scores on various psychological tests were related to subsequent survival times, taking into account the site and stage of development of the cancers at time of presentation. Stravrakay (1968) found general abnormalities in patients' MMPI scores. Those with the most favourable prognosis were significantly characterised on projective tests as displaying strong hostile drives without loss of emotional control under severe stress. Schonfield (1972) reported a significant correlation between patients' ability to return to work and high scores on the MMPI well-being scale: successfully treated cancer patients, in his study, had lower scores on the morale loss scale. The results of these, and other studies, tend to suggest that patients who are not severely depressed by a positive cancer diagnosis, who feel angry or hostile without losing emotional control, and who can engender some sense of well-being survive longer, and undoubtedly better, than those who do not. To what extent such reactions are inborn or can be encouraged remains to be determined, with obvious implications for the management of cancer patients.

An interesting Soviet study by Genzdilov and his colleagues (1977) suggests a link between the reaction to the stress of diagnosis and surgery, post-operative complications, and the person's endocrine response. Their data showed that the highest frequency of post-operative complications occurred in patients who showed severe psychiatric reactions when admitted to the cancer clinic. Post-operative complications were also possibly associated with high urinary catecholmaine and plasma corticosteroid levels before surgery, and with a marked decrease in catecholamine excretion on the sixth day after surgery. This latter observation may be important.

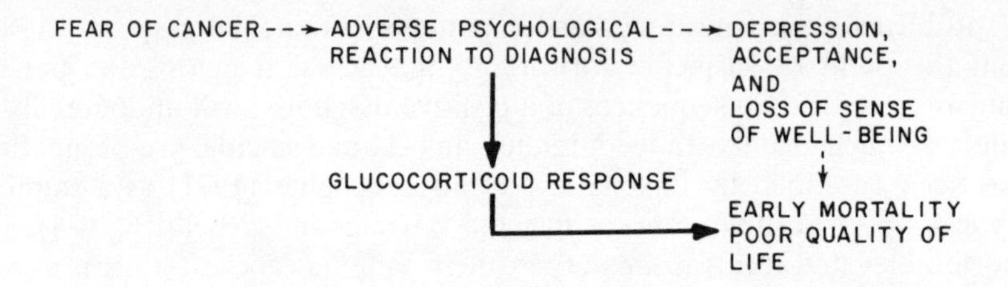

Figure 7.2: Diagnosis, Stress and Cancer Survival.

Studies such as these open up the possibility that the psychological and endocrine responses to stress may be linked to cancer survival. If so it is possible that they are involved in the development of cancers, if not their aetiology. At least part of these effects may be expressed through the immune system.

STRESS, THE IMMUNE SYSTEM AND CANCER

The person is entirely dependent on maintaining a satisfactory relationship with his total environment. The very fact of life depends on one's ability to maintain an optimum body temperature, on the intake of food, of fluids and of air, on the elimination of waste products, and on achieving a balance between activity and rest. Given the ability to fulfil these critical requirements, the person will *survive*. Beyond this, the *quality of life* is dependent on the ability both to resist disease, and to cope with the physical and psychological demands of the environment. There is thus a natural appeal in associating the response to stress and immune system activity: both share functions of adaptation and defence in this *transaction* between the person and his environment (Cox *et al.*, 1983).

There is evidence derived from *animal studies* that exposure to stress can in various ways alter immune system activity (e.g. Amkraut and Solomon, 1975; Solomon and Amkraut, 1979), and tumour incidence and growth (e.g. LaBarba, 1970). This evidence is not unequivocal. Generally, enhanced tumour growth has been reported after exposure to stress. However, it has been shown that in certain situations particular stressors can inhibit tumourigenesis. Furthermore some studies (e.g. Peters and Kelly, 1977) have failed to show any effect of stress on tumourigenesis, or of increased glucocorticoid levels or ACTH administration. These differences in the outcome of experiments may be partly attributable to differences in experimental procedures and manipulations, and the host – tumour systems chosen for study (see earlier; Riley, 1979). It is obvious that a better understanding of why these different outcomes were obtained may represent an important advance in our knowledge. Whatever the direction of effect, the evidence *does* suggest that immune system function and the production of cancers in animals can be influenced by stress manipulations.

There is *clinical evidence* to suggest that many patients with cancer show evidence of decreased immunity (Hellstrom *et al.*, 1971; Smith *et al.*, 1971), and may be immunosupressed (Britton *et al.*, 1975). Britton *et al.* (1975) suggested that immunosuppression was associated with over-production of glucocorticoids. It is possible, of course, that such effects may reflect tumour development rather than be responsible for it.

It has been severally suggested that stress effects on immune system activity and tumour production may be associated with *adrenal cortical* reactivity, and with elevated glucocorticoid levels. There is, however, some debate over whether this is so (Solomon and Amkraut, 1979). The following sections of this chapter examine the possible role of the immune system and of the adrenal cortical and other hormones in some detail.

THE IMMUNE SYSTEM

The immune system operates to protect the person against invasion by foreign cells or substances, and several different mechanisms are involved, both humoral and cell-mediated. The concept of competence may be discussed in terms of the capacity to identify and reject material foreign to the individual, and to recognise and accept material furnished with markers of self (Palmblad, 1981). The competence of the immune system may be related to susceptibility to cancers (Baldwin, 1973, 1977; Levy and Wheelock, 1974; Stutman, 1975).

A. PHAGOCYTES
Neutrophils (inc. engulfment and bactericidal action)
Monocytes-macrophages (phagocytosis, antigen presentation to lymphocytes, and cytotoxic action)

B. LYMPHOCYTES
T-cells (cytotoxic action)
B-cells (antibody production)
Others, including:
NK cells

C. HUMORAL IMMUNITY
Antibodies (IgG, IgM and IgA)

D. OTHER FACTORS
Serum complement factors
Interferon

Figure 7.3: Components of the Host's Defence Against Micororganisms (adapted from Palmblad, 1981).

Cells possibly active against tumours are known as *effector* cells. Until the early-to-mid 1970's, cell-mediated defence against tumours was thought to involve T-lymphocytes, killer (K) cells, and specifically activated macrophages. It is now known that other cells may be as, or even more important, for example, natural killer (NK) cells, and polymorphonuclear leucocytes (PMNs). Other anti-tumour substances may also contribute to such defence, for example interferon. Interferon activates NK cells, but also is a viral antagonist in its own right (Bloom, 1980).

B- and T-Lymphocytes

There are two main types of lymphocyte that can recognise and react against a wide range of antigens; these are the T-cells and B-cells.

B-cells

B-cells are derived from bone marrow, and are responsible for antibody production. Their characteristics and functions have been extensively discussed (Golub, 1980). It has been argued that alterations in B-cell function might result in the production of blocking antibodies and thus enable tumours to be protected from the host's defences (Stein *et al*., 1979). They do not, however, appear to function as direct effector cells for reactivity against tumours or microbial agents (Herberman and Ortaldo, 1981).

T-cells

T-cells are a major subpopulation of small but typical lymphocytes that are dependent on the thymus for their maturation and the acquisition of their functional activity: the thymus releases humoral factors which effect the maturation of these cells (Luckey, 1973). T-cells are a very heterogenous collection of cells, and have virtually no detectable spontaneous cytotoxic activity. Rather they have to be activated, usually by being exposed to specific antigens on accessory cells such as macrophages. Thus there may be a considerable delay before T-cells develop their primary reactivity. This often then subsides to low or undetectable levels, but on re-exposure to the antigen, T-cells show an accelerated response and high levels of reactivity are then reached relatively quickly (2—5 days). The activity of T-cells is regulated by a variety of cells and substances, including interferon.

It was thought that T-cells were involved in immune surveillance against tumours, and thus decreased T-cell activity might have allowed the proliferation of neoplastic cells and thus promote tumour growth. Exposure to stress and glucocorticoid administration have been shown to suppress antibody synthesis and various T-cell mediated immune processes (e.g. Santisteban and Riley, 1973; Monjan and Collector, 1977). Effects on T-cell function may be partly brought about through action at the level of the thymus.

Somewhat in the same vein, Bartrop *et al*. 1977) have shown that T-cell function can be depressed after the stress of bereavement in the absence of a change in T-cell numbers. Twenty-six bereaved spouses were studied 1 week and 6 weeks after bereavement. Significant changes in *responsiveness* were observed at 6 weeks. These changes were not associated with any changes in thyroxine, cortisol, prolactin or growth hormone, or in B-cell numbers or function. Following the course of this argument, there are some data to suggest there is an excess appearance of disease after bereavement, at least within the first 6 to 12 months, but possibly little excess thereafter (Jacobs and Ostfeld, 1977). Fox (1981) suggests that the time course of these effects is difficult to reconcile with that for the production of cancer (to a detectable size). It is thus unlikely, he argues, that bereavement could trigger the induction of either a precursor to cancer or cancer itself. Of course, it is still possible that it might accelerate the growth of an already developing cancer.

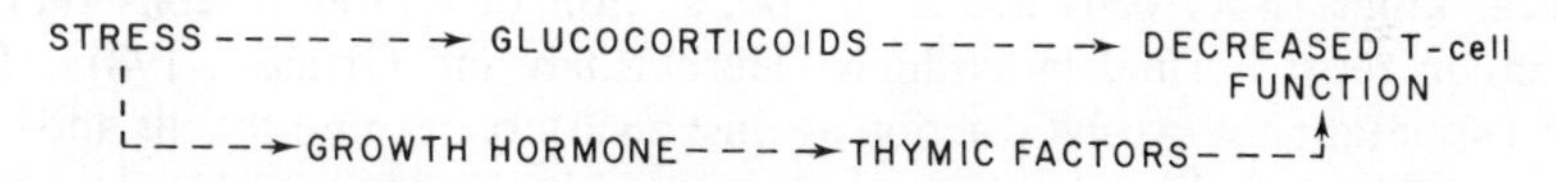

Figure 7.4: Stress, and T-cell Function.

The evidence suggests that thymic humoural factors confer immune competence upon lymphoid cells. Solomon and Amkraut (1979) have speculated that growth hormone (GH) and various steroid hormones may interact with these thymic factors in determining immune competence. If so this might define a different pathway by which the endocrine response to stress might alter immune function.

Immune Surveillance

Until relatively recently, attention has been focused on the central role of T-cells within the classical model of immune surveillance (Burnet, 1970), However, evidence now suggests that T-cell mediated immunity alone cannot account for resistance against tumours, and that T-cells may play little part in the recognition and elimination of transformed cells (Stutman, 1975). For example, neonatally thymectomised rats, with little T-cell activity, do not have particularly high incidences of spontaneous tumours, or carcinogen induced tumours, and are reasonably resistant to growth of some microbial agents (see Herberman and Ortaldo, 1981). Furthermore, the conventional cytotoxic T-cell model requires that tumours are antigenic, and provoke a classical T-cell response. Although most viral and chemically induced animal tumours possess rejection antigens, spontaneous tumours by-and-large do not. Although weak T-cell mediated immune responses against some tumour factors can be demonstrated they are not capable of dealing with the *in situ* tumour. These sort of data have led some to doubt that there is any type of immunological protection against cancers (Prehn, 1974), but it is more sensible to first consider the possible involvement of other effector cells in immune surveillance before completely rejecting the hypothesis. What has now been suggested (see Heberman and Ortaldo, 1981) is a *two phase* model of immune surveillance. Herberman and Ortaldo (1981) suggest that a primary broad-range defence system responds almost immediately to foreign cells or substances, and partially controls them until a more potent and specific immune system begins to respond adequately. They also suggest that natural killer cells, macrophages and polymorphonuclear leucocytes (PMNs) may play an important role in the primary response.

Natural Killer Cells

Natural killer (NK) cells are a sub-population of lymphoid cells that are present in most normal individuals (Herberman and Ortaldo, 1981). They have a spontaneous cytolytic action against a variety of tumour cells and some normal cells, and their reactivity can be rapidly augmented by interferon.

NK cells were first discovered during the early-to-mid 1970's through studies of natural cell-mediated cytotoxicity. It was shown in these studies that lymphoid cells of entirely normal individuals could react against some tumour cells or cells derived from tumours (Herberman and Holden, 1979; Takasurgi *et al.*, 1973). NK cells have different characteristics from the other types of lymphoid cell and are closely associated with large granular lymphocytes, which comprise about 5 per cent of blood or splenic leucoctyes. They have been postulated as an alternative to T-cells as an immune mechanism for surveillance against tumours (Herberman and Holden, 1978), and may thus mediate natural resistance to tumours.

The effects of stress on natural resistance to tumours has yet to be thoroughly researched, and there is little evidence concerning the effects of stress-related hormones on NK activity. That which does exist suggests that NK activity against *in vitro* lymphoid targets is depressed by glucocorticoids (Hochman and Cudkowicz, 1979). There is also indirect evidence to suggest that stress may effect natural immunity to *in situ* tumours. Administration of interferon or poly I:C and other interferon inducing agents significantly boost rat NK activity against lymphoid targets (Herberman and Holden, 1978), and augment NK cell activity in mice (Djeu *et al.*, 1979): interferon production may be suppressed by stress (Jensen, 1968; Chang and Rasmussen, 1976). Seemingly contradictory results have been obtained by Solomon and Amkraut (1979). They report that the stress administered during interferon production following virus innoculation in mice had little effect. The stress was caused by repeated random electric shocks preceded by a warning stimulus (buzzer). However, such stress administered for 5 hours prior to virus innoculation significantly *enhanced* interferon production.

Fox (1981) has suggested that these results can be explained in terms of the effects of prior stress on resident and passive viruses. Stress may activate such viruses, and when active they would have primed the interferon system. The interferon response to subsequent innoculation with other viruses may thus have appeared enhanced. In the studies reported by Solomon and Amkraut (1979) the administration of ACTH did not alter the interferon response, nor did corticosterone administration. However, in other studies, adrenocortical hormones have been shown to reduce both interferon (Rytel and Kilbourne, 1966), and NK cell activity (Herberman and Holden, 1978).

Other Effector Cells

Macrophages, monocytes and polymorphonuclear leucocytes (PMNs) are the other main types of effector cells. These cells have many characteristics in common, and in most regards are quite different from T-cells. Macrophages and monocytes represent different stages in the differentiation of the same cell type, and share a common origin with PMNs. Macrophages and PMNs show natural and spontaneous cytotoxic activity against tumour cells (Palmblad, 1981), and can be rapidly activated. Macrophages, at least, may be sensitive to changes in glucocorticoid levels.

ADRENAL CORTEX

It is obvious from what has been written above that much of the literature concerned with the impact of psychosocial events upon the immune system has been related to the neuroendocrine response to stress. Considerable attention has been paid to an examination of the role of the adrenal secretions, in particular the glucocorticoids, in determining immune system competence. It must be born in mind, however, that other hormones are undoubtedly involved in the mediation of any stress effects.

There is evidence to suggest that the glucocorticoids have a depressing effect on several different cellular elements of the immune system, including T-cells, B-cells and macrophages (e.g. Gisler and Schenkel-Hullinger, 1971; Monjan and Collector, 1977; Santisteban, 1978; Santisteban and Riley, 1973). However, some workers have argued that these effects on cell-mediated processes are small (Gabrielson and Good, 1967; van den Broek, 1971; Ahlqvist, 1976).

Any effects on T-cell function may be mediated by changes in thymic structure or function. The acute involution of the rodent thymus after stress is generally ascribed to the glucocorticoids (Dougherty, 1952), and data from several experiments suggest that thymus size is inversely correlated with plasma levels of (free) corticosterone (Westphal, 1971), the main glucocorticoid in rodents.

Adrenalectomy tends to enhance antibody formation (Ahlqvist, 1976; Petranyi *et al.*, 1971), and glucocorticoid administration will suppress this process if it occurs before antigen challenge (van den Broek, 1971; Ahlqvist, 1976). However, in man usual doses of glucocorticoids do not have such an effect (Frick, 1976).

Overall, the effects of glucocorticoids on the immune system are complex and, despite much research, still require further elaboration. A number of factors are important in respect to such effects: for example, time of administration and *dose*. Pharmacological doses reliably suppress immune system function both *in vitro* and *in vivo*, while the effects of physiological doses may vary (Fauci, 1975; Denckla, 1978). Pharmacological doses suppress primary and secondary antibody formation (Petranyi *et al.*, 1971), while physiological doses have been reported to enhance T-cell formation (Ritter, 1975), but cause their redistribution from the circulating pool to bone marrow (Claman, 1974; Fauci, 1975).

AN EXPERIMENTAL SYNTHESIS

Not many experimental programmes have considered the effects of different sources of stress on hormone levels, markers of immune system function, and tumour growth. One such set of studies provides an interesting synthesis of various of the pieces in the jigsaw puzzle. Research on mice at the Pacific Northwest Research Foundation by Riley (1979, 1981) has provided important data in support of the present hypothesis.

Riley (1981) has demonstrated that exposure to non-traumatic stressors, such as rotation and handling, can significantly increase plasma corticosterone levels in mice. The relationship between speed of rotation and hormonal response was shown to be linear, as was the relationship between duration of handling stress and hormonal response. The latter data also indicated the rapidity of the corticosterone response.

Two markers of immune competence were investigated. It was shown that intermittent rotation stress significantly depressed leucocyte numbers compared with unstressed controls. A 50 per cent reduction occurred within 2 hours. Animals subjected to such stress also showed a marked reduction in thymus weight, which reached a low the day after exposure. Evidence suggested that the thymocytes are destroyed by the increased concentration of plasma corticosterone that accompanies this stress.

Riley (1981) also considered the direct effects of rotation stress on the growth of implanted tumours. Lymphosarcomas in a particular substrain of mice provided a suitable model for testing the effects of stress. These mice were exposed to intermittent rotation on days 4 to 6 after implantation. Tumour volume in the stressed mice increased significantly compared to their controls. A strong effect of corticosterone implants on tumour growth was also demonstrated.

The timing of exposure to corticosterone, and possibly stress, appeared important. Most interestingly, when a synthetic corticoid was injected into the mice 7 days before tumour implantation, an enhancement of immunological competence was observed. However, when administration occurred 7 days after implantation tumour growth was accelerated, suggesting immunosuppressiion.

Riley's (1981) data also suggest that young mice are more capable of resisting tumour growth than older ones.

These studies bring together the findings of many other studies. Rasmussen (1969) has, for example, demonstrated that daily exposure to avoidance situations significantly increases susceptibility to several different viruses; herpes simplex virus, poliomyelitis virus, Coxsackie B virus, and polyma virus. This immunosuppressive response appeared related to elevated levels of glucocorticoids. Several different experiments have shown how handling, housing regimes and mild aversive stimulation may variously modify the rate of tumour growth in mice (Ader and Friedman, 1965; Levine and Cohen, 1959; Marchant, 1967; Ebbesen and Rask-Nielsen, 1967).

OTHER HORMONES

The adrenal cortical hormones are not the only ones sensitive to stressful events, and similarly others may also be important in mediating the effects of stress on the immune system. Growth hormone (GH), for example, is known to be sensitive to various stressors in man (Charters *et al.*, 1969; Yalow *et al.*, 1969; Noel *et al.*, 1972), and in other primates (Brown and Reichlin, 1972). Furthermore, the GH response is often dissociated from that of the glucocorticoids (Yalow *et al.*, 1969), and appears more related than the latter to individual differences in personality or behavioural style. GH responders have been reported to score higher than non-responders on measures of social engagement (Greene, 1970; Kurokawa *et al.*, 1977), field dependence (Brown and Heninger, 1976), and type A behaviour (Friedman and Rosenman, 1971). The GH response also appears related to neuroticism (Miyabo *et al.*, 1976). These relationships are of particular interest because there is some evidence that GH may enhance the immune response (Gisler, 1974; Denckla, 1978). Indeed, Gisler (1974) found that GH could reverse the immunosuppressive effects of glucocorticoids.

Thyroid hormones are involved in the modulation of immune responses (Denckla, 1978), and have been found to be sensitive to various stressors (Mason, 1975). Testosterone levels in males have been reported to decrease in response to a number of different stressful conditions (Mason, 1975; Repcekova and Mikula, 1977), while levels may increase in others (Mason,

1975). Testosterone appears to have a suppressive effect on immune function (Wyle and Kent, 1977; Mendelson *et al.*, 1977).

The catecholamines, adrenaline and noradrenaline, well-known for their sensitivity to both physical and psychological demand (Mason *et al.*, 1961; Frankenhaeuser, 1971; Cox *et al.*, 1983), may also alter aspects of immune function. Both have been found to decrease various immune responses, including anaphylaxis (Schmutzler and Freundt, 1975) and delayed cutaneous hypersensitivity (Kram *et al.*, 1975). They can also cause a contraction and emptying of the spleen. Part of any effects on lymphocyte activity may be related to their ability to influence intracellular cyclic nucleotide levels. Numerous studies have shown that increased cAMP levels can inhibit immune function, while decreased levels enhance immune activity (Bourne *et al.*, 1974; Watson, Epstein and Cohn, 1973). Horovitz *et al.*, (1972) have observed changes in cAMP levels in anxiety states.

It would seem that several different hormones are capable of modulating immune system function, but that their effects depend on a number of important factors. It has been repeatedly pointed out (Riley, 1979; above) that the outcome of any experiment depends on when the stress was experienced, or when hormones were administered in relation to the challenge to the immune system. The effects of hormone administration are obviously dose-dependent. Given these differences, both enhancements and impairments of immune responses have been reported with the various hormones reviewed here. Furthermore, a number of different aspects of the system have been shown to be sensitive to changes in the hormone environment.

If it is accepted that the hormonal environment is a determinant of immune system effectiveness then it remains possible that effects of stress on that environment may be of some significance. However, even accepting this, two important questions remain. First, how biologically significant are these immunological effects in animals for cancer production? Second, how far can these effects be generalised to man? These questions remain largely unanswered, although as final comment from this chapter they are addressed by Fox (1981).

The final section *assumes* that stress-sensitive hormones do effect immune system competence and cancer production, and explores what is feasible by way of an explanatory model. This model put forward was first described by Wayner, Cox and Mackay, (1979).

A MODEL FOR STRESS AND CANCER

The following model for 'stress and cancer' is proposed. There are several different ways in which the *stress process* could effect the production of cancer.

First, exposure to stress may effect the *initiation* of the cancer process and thus play an aetiological role. The way in which the person copes may effect exposure to carcinogenic stimuli. Some examples have already been suggested: increased smoking as a coping strategy, and increased drinking (alcohol) in interaction with existing patterns of smoking. Furthermore, the person's physiological response may enhance the effects of an existing carcinogen. This may involve changes in the general nature of the cellular and hormonal environments, resulting in them becoming more conducive to malignant transformation and the triggering of any latent processes.

Second, stress may effect the *promotion* of malignant transformation through the suppression of immune surveillance, and play some role in the development of cancers. These effects are most probably mediated by stress-sensitive hormones, in particular the glucocorticoids, and possibly growth hormone and the catecholamines. Stress associated blockade of immune effector cells may increase the probability of early transformed cells slipping through the host's defences. However, it could be that stress effects on anti-tumour immunity occur later in the process: spontaneous tumours may not be sufficiently different from self to be recognised by immune effector cells. This possibility would require some reappraisal of the significance of stress-sensitive hormones as malignant promoters.

Again the behavioural responses to stress (coping) may modify the endocrine environment to increase the malignant potential of any associated endocrine changes. Such behavioural (and possibly physiological) reactions may be partly conditioned by covert personality traits or differences in behavioural style: for example, the use of denial or repression as cognitive coping strategies.

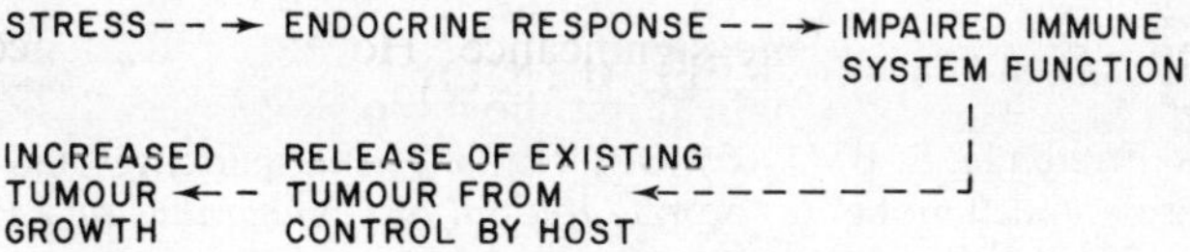

STRESS - - → ENDOCRINE RESPONSE - - → IMPAIRED IMMUNE SYSTEM FUNCTION

INCREASED TUMOUR GROWTH ← - - RELEASE OF EXISTING TUMOUR FROM CONTROL BY HOST ← - - - - - - - -

Figure 7.5: Stress-sensitive Hormones, Immune Competence and Cancer.

Putting aside any aetiological role of stress, there are several implications that can be drawn from its involvement in the development of cancer. These have been briefly discussed by Riley (1981). First, stress-associated pathologies will not be observed, despite the presence of stress, if there is no disease process already in existence. Second, even if there is an existing latent pathology, the effects of stress will not be observed unless the disease is under the control of the immune system. Third, the effects of stress will only be observed if there is some functional balance between the host's defences and the developing cancer. Where one or other is obviously dominant, any additional effects of stress may be impossible to detect. It may also be that the effects of stress will not be detectable until some way into the development of any particular cancer.

FINAL COMMENTARY

By way of conclusion, the author has adapted [] some of Fox's recent comments (1981):

'. . . there is good reason to think that PF [psychosocial factors] . . . affect the probability of a person [developing] cancer, but they do so both damagingly and protectively.'

He went on to say however that:

'. . . compared to other . . . biological events, PF may contribute a smaller amount in humans than in animals, assuming there is a contribution.'

The available data do not argue for the rejection of the hypothesis set out in the introduction. Indeed, there is support for the further study of the effects of stress-sensitive hormones on immune system competence, and its role in the development of cancers. However, the data do argue that the effects of such processes may be small compared to the others involved. Despite this, it may still prove possible to exploit our growing understanding of the stress factor in cancer production to the benefit of cancer patients. This practical spin-off may be the strongest argument for continuing research in this area.

REFERENCES

Ader, R., and Friedman, S. B. (1965). Differential early experiences and susceptibilities to transplanted tumours in the rat. *Journal of Comparative and Physiological Psychology*, **59**, 361–364

Ahlqvist, J. (1976). Endocrine influences on lymphatic organs, immune responses, inflammation and autoimmunity, *Acta Endocrinologica*, (Copenhagen), Suppl. 206.

Amkraut, A., and Solomon, G. F. (1975). From the symbolic stimulus to the pathophysiological response: immune mechanisms, *International Journal of Psychiatry in Medicine*, **5**, 541–563.

Baroni, C., Fabris, N., and Bertoli, G. (1970). Hormonal control of lymphocytic tissue development in Snell–Bagg dwarf mice, in *Progress in Immunological Standardisation*. (Ed. R. H. Reganey) Karger, Basle.

Baldwin, R. W. (1973). Immunological aspects of chemical carcinogenesis, *Advances in Cancer Research*, **18**, 1–75.

Baldwin, R. W. (1977). Immune surveillance revisited, *Nature (London)*, **270**, 557.

Bartrop, R. W., Luckhurst, E., Lazarus, L., Kiloh, L. G., and Penny, R. (1979). Depressed lymphocyte function after bereavement, *Lancet*, **i**, 834–836.

Bloom, B. (1980). Interferon and the immune system, *Nature (London)*, **284**, 593–595.

Blumberg, E. M. West, P. M., and Ellios, F. W. (1954). A possible relationship between psychological factors and human cancer, *Psychosomatic Medicine*, **16**, 277–286.

Bourne, H. R., Lichenstein, L. M., Melmon, K. L., Henney, C. S., Weinstein, Y. S., and Shearer, G. M. (1974). Modulation of inflammation and immunity by cyclic AMP, *Science*, **184**, 19–28.

Britton, S., Thorer, M., and Sjoberg, H. E. (1975). The immunological hazard of Cushing's syndrome, *British Medical Journal*, **4**, 678–680.

Van den Broek, A. A. (1971). Immune suppression and histophysiology of the immune response, unpublished Ph.D. thesis, University of Groningen.

Brown, G. M., and Reichlin, S. (1972). Psychologic and neural regulation of growth hormone secretion, *Psychosomatic Medicine*, **34**, 45–61.

Brown, G. M., and Heninger, G. (1976). Stress-induced growth hormone release: psychologic and physiologic correlates, *Psychosomatic Medicine*, **38**, 145–147.

Burnet, F. M. (1970). Immunological Surveillance, Pergamon Press, Oxford.

Chang, S. S., and Rasmussen, A. F. (1965). Stress-induced suppression of interferon production in virus-infected mice, *Nature (London)*, **205**, 623–624.

Charters, C. A., Odell, W. D., and Thompson, C. (1969). Anterior pituitary function during surgical stress and convalescence. Radioimmunoassay measurement of blood TSH, LH, FSH and growth hormone, *Journal of Clinical Endocrinology and Metabolism*, **29**, 63–71.

Claman, H. N. (1974). How corticosteroids work, *Journal of Allergy and Clinical Immunology*, **55**, 145–151.

Cox, T. (1978). Stress, Macmillans, London.

Cox, T., and Cox, S. (1983). The role of the adrenals in the psychophysiology of stress, in *Current Issues in Clinical Psychology*, (Ed. E. Karas) Plenum Press, London.

Cox, T., and Mackay, C. J. (1982). Psychosocial factors and psychophysiological mechanisms in the aetiology and development of cancers, *Social Science and Medicine*, **16**, 381–396.

Cox, T., Cox, S., and Thirlaway, M. (1983). The psychological and physiological response to stress, in *Physiological Correlates of Human Behaviour*, (Eds. A. Gale and J. A. Edwards) Academic Press, London.

Craig, T. J., and Abeloff, M. D. (1974). Psychiatric symptomatology among hospitalized cancer patients, *American Journal of Psychiatry*, **131**, 1323–1327.

Currie, G. (1980). *Cancer and the Immune Response*, Edward Arnold, London.

Denckla, W. D. (1978). Interactions between age and neuroendocrine and immune systems, *Federation Proceedings*, **37**, 1263–1266.

Djeu, J. Y., Heinbaugh, J. A. Holden, H. T., and Herberman, R. B. (1979). Augmentation of mouse natural killer cell activity by interferon and interferon inducers, *Journal of Immunology*, **122**, 175–181.

Doll, R., and Peto, R. (1981). *The Causes of Cancer*, Oxford University Press, Oxford.

Dougherty, T. F. (1952). Effect of hormones on lymphatic tissue, *Physiological Review*, **32**, 379–401.

Ebbesen, P., and Rask-Nielsen, R. (1967). Influence of sex-segregated groupings and of inoculation with subcellular leukemic material no development of non-leukemic lesions in DBA/2, BALB/C, and CBA mice. *Journal of National Cancer Institute*, **39**, 917–932.

Fauci, A. S. (1975). Corticosteroids and circulating lymphocytes, *Transplantation Proceedings*, **7**, 37–48.

Fielding, G. (1983). Professional problems of caring for the cancer patient, in *The Application of Psychology to Serious Illness*. (Eds. J. Weinman and C. Ray) Sage, London.

Fox, B. H. (1978). Premorbid psychological factors as related to cancer incidence, *Journal of Behavioural Medicine*, **1**, 45–133.

Fox, B. H. (1981). Psychosocial factors and immune system in human cancer, in *Psychoneuroimmunology*, (Ed. R. Ader) Academic Press, New York.

Frankenhaeuser, M. (1971). Experimental approaches to the study of human behaviour as related to neuroendocrine functions, in *Society, Stress and Disease*, (Ed. L. Levi) Oxford University Press, Oxford.

Freidenbergs, I., Gordon, W., Hibbard, M., Levine, L., Wolf, C., and Diller, L. (1982). Psychosocial aspects of living with cancer: a review of the literature, *International Journal of Psychiatry in Medicine*, **11**, 303–329.

Frick, O. L. (1976). Immediate Hypersensitivity, in *Basic and Clinical Immunology*, (Ed. H. H. Fudenberg) Lange Medical Publications, Los Altos, California.

Friedman, M., and Rosenman, R. (1971). Type A behaviour pattern: its association with coronary heart disease,*Annals of Clinical Research*, **3**, 300–312.

Gabrielson, A. F., and Good, R. A. (1967). Chemical suppression of adapted immunity, *Advances in Immunology*, **6**, 90–229.

Genzdilov, A. V., Alexandrin, G. P., Simonov, N. N. Evhujin, A. I., and Bobrov, U. F. (1977). The role of stress factors in the post-operative course of patients with rectal cancer, *Journal of Surgery and Oncology*, **9**, 517– 523.

Gisler, R. H. (1974). Stress and the hormonal regulation of the immune response in mice, *Psychotherapy and Psychosomatics*, **23**, 197–208.

Gisler, R. H., and Schenkel-Hullinger, L. (1971). Hormonal regulation of the immune response: II. Influence of pituitary and adrenalactivity on immune responsiveness in vitro, *Cellular Immunology*, **2**, 646–657.

Golub, E. S. (1980). *The Cellular Basis of the Immune Response: an Approach to Immunobiology*. Sinauer, Sunderland, Mass.

Greene, W. A. (1970). Psychologic correlates of growth hormone and adrenal secretory responses of patients undergoing cardiac catheterization, *Psychosomatic Medicine*, **32**, 599–614.

Hackett, T. P., Cassem, N. H. and Raker, J. W. (1973). Patient delay in cancer, *New England Journal of Medicine*, **289**, 14–20.

Hamilton, V., and Warburton, D. M. (Eds.) (1979). *Human Stress and Cognition*. John Wiley & Sons, Chichester.

Hellstrom, K. E., Hellstrom, I., Sjogren, H. O., and Werner, C. A. (1971). Cell-mediated immunity to human tumour antigens, in *Progress in Immunology*, (Ed. B. Amos) Academic Press, New York.

Herberman, R., and Holden, H. (1978). Natural cell-mediated immunity, *Advances in Cancer Research*, **27**, 305–377.

Herberman, R., and Holden, H. T. (1979). Natural killer cells as antitumour effector cells, *Journal of National Cancer Institute*, **62**, 441– 445.

Herberman, R. B., and Ortaldo, J. R. (1981). Natural killer cells: their role in defenses against disease, *Science*, **214**, 24–30.

Hochman, P. S., and Cudkowicz, G. (1979). Suppression of natural cytotoxicity by spleen cells of hydrocortisone treated mice, *Journal of Immunology*, **123**, 968–976.

Horovitz, A. P. Beer, B., and Clody, D. E. (1972). Cyclic AMP and anxiety, *Psychosomatics*, **13**, 85–92.

Jacobs, S., and Ostfeld, A. (1977). An epidemiological review of bereavement, *Psychosomatic Medicine*, **39**, 344–357.

Jeffcoate, W., and Rees, L. (1978). Adrenocorticotropin and related peptides in nonendocrine tumours, *Current Topics in Experimental Endocrinology*, **3**, 57–74.
Jenkins, C. D. (1968). Dimensions of belief and feeling concerning three diseases; poliomyelitis, cancer and mental illness: a factor analytic study, *Behavioural Science*, **13**, 372–381.
Jenkins, C. D. (1976). The semantic differential for health: a technique for measuring beliefs about diseases, *Public Health Reports*, **81**, 549– 558.
Jensen, M. M. (1968). Transitory impairment of interferon produced in stressed mice, *Journal of Infectious Diseases*, **118**, 230– 234.
Kegeles, S. S. (1967). Attitudes and behaviour of the public regarding cervical cytology: current findings and new directions for research, *Journal of Chronic Diseases*, **20**, 911–922.
Kegeles, S. S., Haefner, D. P., Kirscht, J. P., and Rosenstock, I. M. (1965). Survey of beliefs about cancer detection and taking Papanicolaou tests, *Public Health Reports*, **80**, 815–823.
Keller, R. (1978). macrophage-mediated natural cytotoxicity against various target cells in vitro. 1. Comparison of tissue macrophages from diverse anatomic sites and from different strains of rats and mice, *British Journal of Cancer*, **37**, 732–741.
Knopf, A. (1976). Changes in womens' opinions about cancer, *Social Science and Medicine*, **10**, 105–109.
Kram, J., Bourne, H., Maibach, H., and Melmon, K. (1975). Cutaneous immediate hypersensitivity in man: effects of systematically administered adrenergic drugs, *Journal of Allergy and Clinical Immunology*, **56**, 387–392.
Kurokawa, N., Suematsu, H., Tamai, H., Esakai, M., Aoki, H., and Ikemi, Y. (1977). Effect of emotional stress on human growth hormone, *Journal of Psychosomatic Research*, **21**, 231–235.
LaBarba, R. (1970). Experimental and environmental factors in cancer: a review of research with animals, *Psychosomatic Medicine*, **32**, 259–276.
Laxenaire, M., Chardot, C., and Bentz, L. (1971). Quelques aspects psychologiques du malade cancereaux, *Presse Medicine*, **79**, 2497–2500.
Lazarus, R. (1976). *Patterns of Adjustment*. McGraw-Hill, New York.
Levine, S., and Cohen, C. (1959). Differential survival to leukemia as a function of infantile stimulation in DBA/2 mice. *Proceedings of the Society for Experimental and Biological Medicine*, **104**, 180–183.
Levy, M. H., and Wheelock, E. F. (1974). The role of macrophages in defense against neoplastic disease, *Advances in Cancer Research*, **20**, 131–163.
Luckey, T. D. (1973). *Thymic Hormones*. University Park Press, Baltimore.
Marchant, J. (1967). The effects of different social conditions on breast cancer induction in three genetic types of mice by dibenz (a,h) anthracene and a comparison with breast carcinogensis by 3-methylcholanthrene. *British Journal of Cancer*, **21**, 750–754.
Marsh, J. T., and Rasmussen, A. F. (1960). Response of adrenal cortex, thymus, spleen and leukocytes to shuttle box and confinement stress, *Proceedings of the Society for Experimental Biology and Medicine*, **104**, 180–183.
Mason, J. W. (1975). Psychologic stress and endocrine, in *Topics in Psychoendocrinology*, (ed. E. J. Sachar) Grune and Stratton, New York.
Mason, J. W., Mangan, G., Brady, J. V., Conrad, D., and Rioch, D. M. (1961). Concurrent plasma epinephrine, norepinephrine, and 17-hydroxycorticosteroid levels during conditioned emotional disturbances in monkeys, *Psychosomatic Medicine*, **23**, 344–353.

McKinlay, J. B. (1972). Some approaches and problems in the study of the use of services —an overview, *Journal of Health and Social Behaviour*, **13**, 115–52.

Mendelsohn, J., Multer, M. M., and Bernheim, J. L. (1977). Inhibition of human lymphocyte stimulation by steroid hormones: cytokinetic mechanisms, *Clinical and Experimental Immunology*, **27**, 127–134.

Miyabo, S., Hisada, T., Asato, T., Mizushima, N., and Ueno, K. (1976). Growth hormone and cortisol responses to psychological stress; comparison of normal and neurotic subjects, *Journal of Clinical Endocrinology and Metabolism*, **42**, 1158–1162.

Monjan, A., and Collector, M. I. (1977). Stress-induced modulation of the immune response, *Science*, **196**, 207–208.

Nature (1981). Two views on the causes of cancers (editorial), *Nature*, **289**, 431–432.

Noel G., Suh, H. K., Stone, J. G., and Frantz, A. G. (1972). Human prolactin and growth hormone release during surgery and other conditions of stress, *Journal of Clinical Endocrinology and Metabolism*, **36**, 840–841.

Palmblad, J. (1981). Stress and immunological competence: studies in man, in *Psychoimmunology*, (Ed. R. Ader) Academic Press, New York.

Patel, C. (1975). 12-month follow up of yoga and bio-feedback in the management of hypertension, *Lancet*, **i**, 62–64.

Patel, C., and North, W. R. (1975). Randomised controlled trial of yoga and bio-feedback in the management of hypertension, *Lancet*, **ii**, 93–95.

Patel, C., Marmot, M. G., and Terry, D. M. (1979). Control trial of bio-feedback aided behavioural method in reducing mild hypertension, *British Medical Journal*, **282**, 2005–1008.

Prehn, R. T. (1974). Immunological surveillance: pro and con, *Clinical Immunology*, **2**, 191–203.

Peters, L., and Kelly, H. (1977). The influence of stress and stress hormones on the transplantability of a non-immunogenic murine tumour, *Cancer*, **39**, 1482–1488.

Paterson, R., and Aitken-Swan, J. (1954). Public opinion on cancer–a survey among women in the Manchester area, *Lancet*, **ii**, 857–861.

Petranyi, G., Gengzur, M., and Alfoldy, P. (1971). The effect of single large dose hydrocortisone treatment on IgM and IgG antibody production, morphological distribution of antibody producing cells and immunological memory, *Immunology*, **21**, 151–158.

Rasmussen, A. F. (1969). Emotions and immunity, *Annals of the New York Academy of Science*, **164**, 458–461.

Repcekova, D., and Mikulaj, L. (1977). Plasma testosterone of rats subjected to immobilization stress and/or HCG administration, *Hormone Metabolism Research*, **8**, 51–57.

Richardson, A., and Woolcott, J. F. (1967). A social survey of community attitudes to cancer, *International Journal of Health Education*, **10**, 141–144.

Riley, V. (1979). Stress – cancer contradictions: a continuing puzzlement, *Cancer Detection and Prevention*, **2**, 159–162.

Riley, V. (1981). Psychoneuroendocrine influences on immunocompetence and neoplasia, *Science*, **212**, 1100–1109.

Ritter, M. (1975). Embryonic mouse thymocyte development enhancing effect of corticosterone at physiological levels, *Immunology*, **33**, 241–246.

Rothman, K., and Keller, R. (1972). The effect of joint exposure of alcohol and tobacco on risk of cancer of the mouth and pharynx, *Journal of Chronic Diseases*, **25**, 711–716.

Rytel, M. W., and Kilbourne, E. F. (1966). The influence of cortisone on experimental viral infection, *Journal of Experimental Medicine*, **123**, 767–775.

Santisteban, G. A. (1978). Adrenal cortical and cardiovascular responses to psychosocial stress in CBA mice and albino rats, *Anatomical Records*, **190**, 530.

Santisteban, G. A., and Riley, V. (1973), Thymo-lymphatic organ response to the LDH-virus, *Proceedings of American Association of Cancer Research*, **14**, 112.

Schmutlzer, W., and Freundt, G. P. (1975). The effect of glucocorticoids and catecholamines on cyclic AMP and allergic histamine release in guinea pig lung, *International Archives of Allergy and Applied Immunology*, **49**, 209–212.

Schonfield, J. (1972). Psychological factors related to delayed return to an earlier life-style in successfully treated cancer patients, *Journal of Psychosomatic Research*, **16**, 41–46.

Smith, J. W., Steiner, A. L., and Parker, C. W. (1971), Human lymphocyte metabolism. Effects of cyclic and non-cyclic nucleotides on stimulation by phytohemaglutinin, *Journal of Clinical Investigation*, **50**, 442–448.

Solomon, G. F., and Amkraut, A. A. (1979). Neuoendocrine aspects of the immune response and their implications for stress effects on tumour immunity, *Cancer Detection and Prevention*, **2**, 197–224.

Stavrakay, K. M. (1968). Psychological factors in the outcome of human cancer, *Journal of Psychosomatic Research*, **12**, 251–259.

Stein, M., Keller, S., and Schleifer, S. (1979). Role of hypothalamus in mediating stress effects on the immune system, in *Mind and Cancer Prognosis*, (ed. B. A. Stoll) John Wiley & Sons, Chichester.

Stutman, O. (1975). Immunodepression and malignancy, *Advances in Cancer Research*, **25**, 261–422.

Surwit, R. S., Williams, R. B., and Shapiro, D. (1982). *Behavioural Approaches to Cardiovascular Disease*. Academic Press, New York.

Takasurgi, M., Michey, M., and Terasaki, P. (1973). Reactivity of lymphocytes from normal persons to cultured tumour cells, *Cancer Research*, **33**, 2898–2902.

Wakefield, J. (1971). *Seek Wisely to Prevent*, H.M.S.O., London.

Watson, J., Epstein, R., and Cohn, M. (1973). Cyclic nucleotides as intracellular mediators of the expression of antigen-sensitive cells. *Nature*, **246**, 405–409.

Wayner, L., Cox, T., and Mackay, C. J. (1979). Stress, immunity and cancer, in *Research in Psychology and Medicine*, (Eds. D. J. Oborne, M. M. Gruneberg and J. R. Eiser) Academic Press, London.

Westphal, U. (1971). *Steroid – Protein Interactions*, SpringerVerlag, Berlin.

Worden, J. W., and Weisman, A. D. (1975). Psychosocial components of lagtime in cancer diagnosis, *Journal of Psychosomatic Research*, **19**, 69–79.

Wyle, F. A., and Kent, J. R. (1977). Immunosuppression by sex steroid hormones, *Clinical and Experimental Immunology*, **27**, 407–415.

Wyler, A. R. (1968). Seriousness of illness rating-scale, *Journal of Psychosomatic Research*, **11**, 363–374.

Yalow, R. S., Varsano-Aharon, N., Echmendia, E., and Berson, S. (1969). HGH and ACTH secretory responses to stress, *Hormone Metabolism Research*, **1**, 3–8.

Section Four
Managing Psychosocial Factors in Cancer Patients

Psychosocial Stress and Cancer
Edited by C. L. Cooper

Chapter 8
Wellness and Work

Frances Lomas Feldman
University of Southern California, USA

'Work is life.' Sad and contemplative as he waited for the bush pilot who would fly him to the tiny distant hospital where the Inuit's leg probably would be amputated, he added: 'Better I not come back.' How would he hunt, fish, perform the other work essential for his family's survival through each winter? In his village, one of a handful dotting desolate tundra stretching 100,000 square miles without telephone or radio communication or medical resources, there was no alternative to a state of wellness sufficient for the performance of myriad tasks requisite for family survival. Even the age-related government subsidies that increasingly led older villagers to be viewed as assets rather than economic liabilities had not entirely changed work expectations in a subsistence economy. Villagers had responded with a mixture of eagerness and skepticism to the research team's experimental strategies to enable the Inuits to improve the quality of the economic and social life in these villages—as long as work plans were prominently included. Would a 'sick hunter' be fitted into these plans?

A decade later, an urban respondent in a cancer and work study expressed similar sentiments. 'I received a death sentence twice, once when the doctor told me I have cancer, then when my boss asked me to quit because the cancer would upset my fellow-workers.' And a letter to the Editor appearing in a major metropolitan newspaper at this writing echoed the despairing Inuit's words: 'Jobs are life.' The letter writer was protesting a reported recommendation by a highly-placed government official to place before the townspeople the decision to close or keep open a polluting factory thought by environmentalists to be a source of cancer danger to the employees and to the town. He saw need to balance environmental concerns with economic realities of the worker and of the town, and supported leaving the choice in 'jobs versus cancer' to those most intimately affected, the employees. 'Without jobs, there is no hope, and without hope, there is nothing.'

These items, spanning fewer than 15 years, reflect diverse geographic and economic settings life-styles and traditions. Yet they contain common elements: the strong pull to work; the sense of powerlessness and the not infrequent pervasive depression that accompanies job loss for reasons beyond the individual's control; and threatened self-esteem and other psychological responses to seeming failure to meet societal expectations that the individual manifest adequate social functioning (and, hence, *morality*) by work, self-support, and self-management. That such responses are not isolated in the general population is apparent in the mounting research evidence that associates job loss with higher rates of suicide, family violence, homicide, alcoholism, depression leading to admissions to hospitals for the mentally ll, and other negative sequellae of stress (Brenner, 1973, 1976; Raymon and Bluestone, 1982). The growing body of literature addressing occupational stress testifies to the presence of stress in all kinds of work but suggests that distress is not a necessary consequence (Selye, 1974; Cooper and Marshall, 1976; and others). There is reason to believe, however, that for many individuals in the work force who have experienced cancer, the psychosocial stresses related to the diagnosis and treatment of this disease compound or are compounded in number and degree of severity by the stress that is inherent or that arises in the work site or on cessation of work. In either event, work-related stress may seriously affect both the patient's success in coping with the cancer treatment and accompanying psychosocial issues, and with the quality of the patient's total life.

Yet, despite the sizeable proportion of patients whose work is vital to their emotional or economic well-being, relatively scant attention is paid to anticipating the interactions of the psychosocial stress of cancer with the individual's work life and, therefore, taking measures to avert or contain the negative consequences that arc between the work and personal segments of the patient's total being.

That is the thesis of this article. It recognizes that an individual's adequacy as an adult functioning effectively in accordance with the expectations of society is measured by many socially-developed criteria, that incorporation of these criteria influences the individual's self-perceptions and coping capacity, and that a diagnosis of cancer may heighten the individual's vulnerability to psychosocial stress because at least two of these measures (work and wellness)—and, often, a third (personal money management)—may come into question and affect the course of the patient's adjustment to work, to a medical regimen, and to life itself.

The nature and confrontation of stress the cancer patient brings to or encounters in the world of work will be presented in the following pages against a backdrop of the social and emotional meanings of work in today's society, stress in the workplace, the role of wellness versus illness as a criterion of independence and personal adequacy, and the singular role of cancer in the context of the work arena. Findings and issues identified in the author's research centered on work experiences of individuals with a cancer history will be offered to illuminate psychosocial stress relevant to attitudes and efforts to be productively attached to the workforce.

Several comments, of different orders, are offered prefatorily. One is merely cautionary: namely, that in the interest of facilitating reading, pronouns are stated in masculine—generic—form except when the subject is known to be feminine. The other comments are definitional.

'Work' properly refers to any activity in which an individual engages that produces something of value for other people (O'Toole, 1974). This definition includes the housewife who performs child-caring and other tasks for which she receives no specific remuneration. It also includes the individual who regularly volunteers services that advance the operation of an organization. Certainly these are important activities—and probably, were they not provided by volunteers (voluntarily or not), would have to be recompensed. For purposes of this paper, however, 'work' refers to paid employment, whatever its nature or locus—on the employer's premises or one's own, and whatever the schedule. It may be speculated that the housewife or the volunteer will feel distress because expected responsibilities intrinsic to their work obligations interact with psychosocial aspects of cancer in ways that resemble those to which paid workers are susceptible. However, although experience of individuals in this group have received some attention in popular anecdotal literature, only rarely has research literature (as in Greenleigh Associates, 1979, for example) addresssed them; nor are they taken into account here. Neither, except incidentally, is the topic of work settings as a course of industrially-induced malignancies within the purview of this paper despite growing emphasis on it in certain research quarters.

SOCIETAL MEASURES OF ADEQUACY

The work-orientated individual whose health is temporarily impaired may accept dependency enforced by the illness more or less gracefully or patiently, but he knows that it is time-limited, that he will be restored to a former level of functioning. An illness with possible or probable consequences of a more enduring nature may arouse in the individual considerable anger or depression because of pain and/or dependency, but as long as the condition is controllable by the exercise of proper care and is not regarded as life-threatening, this patient is likely to come to terms with it, to take steps necessary to maximize the level of his health and return to the workplace—or decide to retire from work. Within limits, certain decisions are within his control: whether he will resume work before he has been fully discharged medically, whether he will linger at home until all sick benefits have been exhausted, whether he will talk freely about his medical experiences to any sympathetic or nonsympathetic listener he can 'buttonhole' or who asks him how he feels. His absence from work may have been an inconvenience to him and to his employer, but he can be on the job, ready to resume work activities with or without medically-imposed restrictions.

The patient with a cancer history faces a different set of psychological stressors that may be both internally and externally induced. The life-threatening nature of his disease in combination with extant fears and other attitudes the presence of his cancer may evoke in others, and his own sense of having little, if any, control over the inexorable progress of the cancer these and other factors arouse in him reactions that produce further stress. How will others perceive him? Will he be taken back in the workplace on former terms? Will he be able to perform? In the face of encroaching disease, how will he be able to demonstrate that he continues to be capable of managing himself, his affairs, his work—that he is an independent, adequately functioning individual worthy of the respect of others? For the likelihood is that he has grown up incorporating the societal expectations that hold economic and psychological independence to be an essential measure of adequacy in an adult, that this independence is inseparable from working and earning, and that working and earning are contingent on reasonably continuing good health. The cancer diagnosis confronts him with two sets of stressors simultaneously: those inherent in the diagnosis itself, and those he perceives as inevitably following in the work segment of his life and, consequently, his life as a whole. If he cannot retain mastery over one, can he control the other?

WORK IN EVERYDAY LIFE

In Joseph Conrad's *Heart of Darkness*, Charlie Marlow says, 'I don't like work . . . no man does—but I like what is *in* the work – the chance to find yourself. Your own reality . . . .' (Conrad, 1976).

What is in the work?

In some form and degree, work has been essential to man's survival from his earliest beginnings. It is an instrumental and alterative activity for the dual purpose of obtaining the means of subsistence needed to maintain life, and of planfully altering certain features of the human environment so that the quality of life will be more certain, more efficient, more comfortable. To the concept of work as a means for obtaining necessities for physical survival, the Protestant Ethic stemming from the influence of Luther and Calvin during the sixteenth century—but not confined to Protestant peoples or countries—added some elements that have become an integral part of our value system. The older view, that only certain holy vocations in religious service are sacred and that ordinary work is a curse put upon mankind as a punishment for sin, was replaced with the admonition that all honest work is sacred if done well and, moreover, ordinary everyday work is essential and natural and pleasing to God and we must continue it to our last days (Luther, translated by Lenkers, 1909). This teaching not only was useful in exhorting sixteenth century European peasants to return to the fields and forgo an uprising accompanied by looting, burning and property destruction. It was especially compatible with frontier labor needs in the New World (as well as on subsequent frontiers) and became ingrained in the evolution of the work ethic as a concept implying that work is an essential component of strength of character, that such strength and independence are synonymous, that an individual's independence and capacity for self-maintenance are demonstrated through work, and that independence is reflected in employment and self-support and, therefore, symbolizes social competence and morality.

That high value is placed on work in more modern society is evident in various ways. The still-common accolade that a person is 'worth his salt' attests to the prevalent regard for one who earns his way. This being worth one's salt is not related to the valuable and indispensable one per cent suspended in human plasma. Rather, it derives from ancient forms of payment for service in salt as an important equivalent of money. Further, in antiquity, salt possessed a religious symbolism closely analogous to that of the early coin metals and was believed to possess magical qualities. The original meaning of being worth one's salt has been all but forgotten, but a certain respect has persisted for work that yields payment (in more modern money forms) that today also is viewed by many as having magical qualities. Thus, deeply rooted in American society, as in other countries circling the globe, is the social value holding that, whenever possible, individuals should earn the means of subsistence for themselves and their dependents by their own labor. Indeed, one effect of Protestantism is the conviction that idleness is suspect. In times when the economic climate pushes people to seek to assure survival through financial help from public and voluntary organizations, the old skepticism that someone might be 'poor *but* honest' either deters some from obtaining the help they require lest such action stamp them as either less than honest or not desirous of work, or induces so much self-blame for their condition that their ability to function effectively is overwhelmed by powerlessness. It is further depleted by loss of the self-esteem essential for adequate social functioning. This emotional pain is no less acute if the work ceased because the individual became ill. It is exacerbated if the nature of the illness is not immediately apparent to the observer.

In Western society, work—'the job'—has been at the center of adult life: the individual's self-image and status in the community have been nurtured by how one's living has been earned. The exception is the clearly wealthy person whose means, by their visibility, generate respectability and independence. For, although Luther had difficulty finding a functional place for the very rich in his idea of the economic system, Calvin's 1559 supplement to Luther's earlier economic ethic did charge them with (in *Institutes of the Christian Religion*) stewardship, with investment of money in enterprises which make goods and services for the people (Presbyterian Board, 1936).

Work is almost an irreplaceable element in establishing one's sense of worth, which is a vital ingredient for the adequate social functioning that comprises the psychological, social, and economic tasks performed by individuals and families in fulfillment of their respective roles in society. It also is through work that we define ourselves. We ask a new acquaintance, 'What do you do?' and a retired person or old acquaintance, 'What are you doing?' and thus infer that person's status in the community and position as an independent and responsible adult.

From time to time, expectations have changed about what is to be gotten from work: material rewards, self-fulfillment, power or prestige. During the 1960s and 1970s for example, student-generated ideas and attitudes contributed somewhat to a shift in the traditional American ethos and philosophy of life away from materialism and 'nose to the grindstone' tasks of making a living, to greater preoccupation with how to live, to discovering a life-style that precisely expresses each person's uniqueness. Yet the deep recession of the latter 1970s and early 1980s re-awakened the fear of economic instability and reinforced the work ethic not just in mature adults but also in youth.

For young people in our society still generally grow up with the expectation that they will become earners, that on their shoulders will rest the responsibility for their own support and for that of those for whom they become responsible. Parents are expected to instill in their children—in American culture, in girls as well as boys—the expectation that they will make a vocational choice which in later years will enable them to carry successfully these tasks of support and self-support. The importance of education is perceived less as an opportunity for broadening intellectual, emotional, and personal horizons than as a passport into an adult world wherein remunerative employment generally symbolizes maturity, responsibility, independence, and other qualities that signify competence in the fulfillment of adult roles.

In adulthood, having a career or holding a job is a daily reminder of independence, of retaining mastery over one's own affairs, meeting needs and obligations. Through 'earning' the respect of others, self-respect is strengthened. Work, then, plays a crucial part in most adult lives, and the adolescent's search for autonomy, visible in the development crises that punctuate the movement from childhood to adulthood, embraces the making of tentative or final vocational plans and directing much of the learning that takes place toward the career or vocational choice.

The adolescent's movement toward successfully establishing autonomy is contingent upon the resolution of two tasks. The emotionally healthy adolescent simultaneously feels a compelling push towards growth and independence and fears the loss of dependence on parents. Ordinarily, the resolution of this conflict lies in the development of emotional independence from parents and the achievement of economic independence through work. Both of these tasks are oriented to the future and involve some degree of planning from a base that has incorporated a work-related value system.

Thus, from early years our work-oriented culture equates work with adequacy and self-worth; morality with independence symbolized by self-support, good management of financial resources, and general economic self-sufficiency. Far less important to the worker is affection for, or satisfaction with the job; of overriding importance is the fact of *working* and *earning*.

What is the significance for the cancer patient reared in a work-ethic environment when the work-related value system he has incorporated does not accord him full or continuing membership? What are the implications for the young person who is diagnosed as having cancer even before he has embarked on a career or has yet begun to think about the nature and amount of schooling he should pursue? Should they resign themselves to being invalids? Regard themselves as well, despite some possible limitations on activity? Demonstrate to themselves and others that they are worth their 'salt'? are honest and, hence, to be trusted? Function adequately, as witness their identification and independence in the world of work?

WELLNESS, CANCER, AND WORK

'My life expectancy is good and I'm highly competent at my job, but the decision-makers think I'll die any minute because I have Hodgkin's disease, and they don't want to make any investment in a pariah like me!' The 24-year-old study respondent complained that his co-workers had been 'chummy enough' in the 2 years before the medical diagnosis, but now they behave 'as though I committed some great sin!' Another respondent, 20 years older, remarked that 'You learn to hide what you can hide' so that his demonstrated competence would not be challenged if anyone in the workplace learned of his cancer health history. 'I'm well, physically and psychologically; why should I feel guilty and ashamed, afraid someone might find out I'm still getting treatments, even though I go at night?'

Health must be bracketed with work as a societal measure of the level of personal functioning, although the fact that one is working generally is observable, while health (the state of being sound in body or mind) often may be more apparent than real. Yet, like the fact of working, health is sometimes overtly and sometimes subliminally perceived as a measure of morality. This is given credence by dictionary definitions of 'illness', the unabridged Oxford Universal reporting the use of the word, since the sixteenth century, as connoting 'a bad moral quality' and the unabridged

Webster-Merriam citing 'wickedness; depravity; disagreeableness'. One might wonder about the greater emphasis over the years on 'ill' as a synonym for *bad* rather than *sick*. To be sure, 'sickness' has been in common use to describe, without imputing immorality, a state of suffering from some malady. But whether sickness or illness, the condition is understood as an assault on the coping capacity of both mind and body that threatens the individual's functional ability. Health, on the other hand, implies *strength*. Just as work and effective management of one's finances imply independence, the healthy person retains mastery over personal affairs and capability for meeting needs and obligations. Health, therefore, is a virtue in which subjective judgements on worthiness and morality inhere.

In recent years, 'wellness' has been heard with increasing frequency to refer to a quality or state of physical or emotional well-being, an antonym for illness. In use for more than three centuries, the word nevertheless appears in few dictionaries—and thus lends itself to attribution of qualities that are neither negative nor otherwise judgmental. Neither cancer patient quoted in this section, for example, felt ill even though neither was cured of the cancer. Both, indeed, felt *well*—well enough to function physically and mentally at a good level. Both, however, had experienced the stress-provoking reactions induced by responses of others to the designation of their diagnosis as cancer.

Three *Work and Cancer Health Histories* studies (Feldman, 1976, 1978, 1980) disclosed the frequency with which interview subjects, whether patients or other respondents, were met in the workplace, school (and, sometimes, at home) with reactions to the word 'cancer' that seemed still tied by a thread of morality to antiquity, Sontag (1977) traces the word as a metaphor for idleness and sloth from the early Middle Ages. When this metaphor is paired with the attitudes about dependence because of failure to work, regardless of the reason, one begins to understand better how the study patients could be so filled with fear, shame and guilt fed by their own and others' perceptions of cancer as intractable, invidious, punishing perceptions surviving in literature and metaphor for centuries. One man and his wife whispered throughout the research interview, unconsciously acting out their stated apprehension that 'someone' might learn of the man's rectal cancer. They were so anxious about the prospect that the employer might learn of it that they had not even shared the information with their adult son; he might inadvertantly become the source of disseminating this shameful fact! One doctor denied the researchers permission to invite a patient to participate in the study, explaining 'I never use that word and I don't want anyone else to use it with my patients and for them to think of themselves as cancerous.' Did the patients whose cancer treatments he arranged really not suspect the nature of their diagnosis? If they did, how did they regard his avoidance of the word and his perception of their capabilities?

All three studies revealed that those patients tended to fare better in the work or school siuation who did not 'act out' the sick role and, without in any way denying the nature of the diagnosis or treatment, presented themselves as 'well and able'. There was greater likelihood that co-workers or fellow students would so view them, even if allowances had to be made for certain cancer-related conditions. The patient's posture did not necessarily alter associates' reactions to the presence of cancer; the respondent's deliberate or intuitive emphasis on wellness, however, tended to be a mitigating element.

THE WORK AND CANCER HEALTH HISTORIES STUDIES

Over a period of several years the California Division of the American Cancer Society had received letters and telephone calls from individuals who attributed to their cancer history some form of discrimination in the work arena. These incidents were accepted at face value and not verified or acted on directly, but they did suggest that a systematic examination of the nature of post-cancer diagnosis work experiences could be instructive and useful in the areas of social policy formulation, public and professional education, and development or refinement of counseling programs. The limited fiscal resources of the Division shaped decisions about the scope and criteria for sample construction in the first study: the demographic criteria were devised to avoid inclusion of individuals vulnerable to workplace problems that might be attributable to such factors as too little work experiences or ageism. Hence, because at the time of the designing of the study the employment market was favourable for white collar occupations, nursing and teaching, these were the target occupations for the study. The other criteria for inclusion in the patient sample were that the person was employed full time at time of diagnosis (pragmatic evidence of employability at that critical juncture); that age at diagnosis fell between 23 and 50 years (so that patients could point to some qualifying work experience and, under ordinary circumstances, look forward to a work life of at least 10 more years); and that the cancer site was breast, head/neck, or rectum/colon (the most common groups, with relatively favorable survival rates and sometimes overt evidence of surgical treatment). Given these characteristics of employability and likelihood of continued attachment to the work force, what work experiences would be reported and what elements would facilitate or impede successful attachment to the work force? What proportion of situations would point to discrimination, if any? And, if discrimination occurred in this random sample, what could be inferred about occupational groups with less overall favorable working qualifications or prospects?

The first study (Feldman, 1976) was followed by the similarly designed blue collar and services inquiry (Feldman, 1978). The series was rounded out with a third study that addressed the work expectations and experiences of youth whose cancer diagnoses were made when they were between 13 and 23 years old (Feldman, 1980). This study did not limit the cancer sites to those in the other two.

In all, 344 patients participated in this research. Because time and emotions so easily affect recollections and perceptions, a 20% sample of employers was interviewed in each study (some specifically about particular patient-respondents, others in employing establishments similar to those of patients but without reference to named patients). In each study, 12 patients were selected, with their permission, for pairing with actual or potential employers they identified. The purpose of these sets of dyads was to track the employment experiences and patterns of the patients and to determine the extent to which their perceptions and those of the employing establishments were congruent. Were their recollections of reasons for changes in work or its cessation the same? Were their perceptions of performance quality, work relations, events in the workplace similar? Were reports of reactions to the presence of cancer alike?

The blue collar and youth studies also included interviews with a sample of physicians. (What explanations of the diagnosis and treatment had they given the patient—or patient's family? Who answered employer or insurance carrier queries? With what kinds of information?) Samples of parents and of school personnel were interviewed with regard to the youth, again to ascertain the match or differences in perceptions. A sample of union officers and stewards was included for interview in the blue-collar study.

The process of constructing the patient samples in itself yielded insights into attitudes and other possible sources of psychosocial stress confronting patients. The protocol called for drawing from a central tumor-data repository a count, by reporting hospital, of the potential respondents who met the criteria for sample selection. The individual reporting hospital then was approached for permission to obtain the names of patients and physicians of record, so that authorization could be secured from the physician to invite the patient to participate in an interview, with such an interview to be arranged only if written permission to proceed had been procured from the patient. The written requests to the hospitals led to some outright rejections, sometimes to written or in-person solicitations to one or more hospital committees (four hospitals delegated various decisions to more than five committees) before authorization was received to proceed; other responded affirmatively without delay. Solicitations to physicians sometimes received no response at all, even after several inquiries. Others resulted in written or telephoned refusal. On occasion, limits were set about the conditions for contacting the patient ('Don't mention cancer!' 'This patient is too sick to interview; talk to his wife'); some reported the patient's death. Like the hospitals, however, most responded affirmatively.

A common attitude encountered in the hospital committees was denial by some physician-members that the patient's work life in any way was related to the patient's mode of coping with the diagnosis and or that work had any impact on him and his dependents. Some committees objected to being party to considering anything beyond just treating the cancer; several committees or their constituent doctors were unwilling to permit the patient's 'privacy violated by inquisitive researchers.' Were these reactions predictive of the data the research inquiry would yield? In point of fact, almost all of the committees voted approval of the request for the respective hospital's participation. Interestingly, the reluctant committee members tended to ignore requests sent them with regard to their own patients. Did such reluctance reflect a protective attitude on the doctor's part, or one that permitted no room—whatever the reason—for being involved with the patient in any way other than as a target for medical treatment? What could be inferred from this to sources of psychosocial stresses and their effects on the patient?

On the whole, however, hospitals as well as physicians were cooperative, some committees and individuals even constructively reviewing drafts of the interview questionnaires or supplying patients for the pre-test phase, and some physicians requesting that certain troubled patients be included in the study even though they had not fallen into the random sample. (Such patients were interviewed, but the contents were not incorporated in the findings.)

The interviews in the two adult studies were conducted from 18 to 30 months after diagnosis; in the youth study, 2 to 5 years had passed. The distortions to be found in any retrospective inquiry about past events were expected and indubitably were present. Several elements in the interview process held potential for minimizing faulty recall, however. For one thing, the interviews were conducted by highly skilled interviewers accustomed to assessing (and teaching about) behavioural affect and the consistency of pieces of information responsive to factual queries and open-ended probing. Indeed, invariably, when the completed lengthy formal questionnaire had been put aside, the patient-respondent was just 'warming up.' (This especially was the case with the youth-study respondents, some of whom apparently had no prior opportunity to unburden themselves about some of the cancer-related events that had transpired). Another was the corroboration of remembered details by others: family, fellow workers, employers, doctors, teachers, school nurses and others in the school settings.

Credence was lent by the emergence of patterns within a patient-respondent's own described feelings and experiences as well as in the aggregation of feelings and experiences. There was occasional evidence of exaggeration or understatement or other clues to the conscious or unconscious effort of the patient to persuade himself or the interviewer that he had matters in control or had been victimized by the disease or *someone*. Nevertheless, irrespective of the accuracy of the recalled details of feeling, the quality and depth of recollected and present emotions on the part of the respondent were incontrovertible and provided an index to the origin and nature of the psychosocial stress encountered by the patient, and the strategies used by the individual to cope directly or indirectly with it. A picture will be presented, first, of who among the patients were actually working and of the stressors they met and brought to the workplace. The section will conclude with inherent dilemmas, either implicit or explicit.

TO WORK OR NOT?

The nearly universal first question that occurred to the respondents, 'Why me?', was quickly followed by anxiety among some about whether or not they would be able to work and the implications of either answer. For a number, this anxiety centered on the economic aspects of their working even though they might not depend on their earnings for support. Some were apprehensive about their continued physical ability to carry out their work responsibilities—especially those whose work required physical strength or dexterity. Among the white collar respondents especially, but also in the blue collar group, it was in the workplace that their friends were; what would happen to these friendships? But a prevalent and recurring question focused on what people in the workplace would 'think' about the cancer. On occasion, this worry was paired with comments that family members or friends had turned away from them on learning the diagnosis; could associates at work be expected to behave differently?

These implicit fears not infrequently focused on *time*: what would patients do (with themselves, with their time) if probability of their return to work life were foreclosed? Like most working people, they tended to spend at least one-third of each 24-hour day at their work. Indeed, allowing for transportation to and from the job, its demands easily might consume the greater portion of their daily waking time. The male respondents described this element as particularly stressful, for not only were they not ready to be 'idle'; they speculated that their spouses, if any, would find their constant presence intolerable. (There was a similar statement from a homosexual patient whose lover threatened to leave.)

Women were less inclined to speak of how they would 'fill' their time; there were always 'plenty' of tasks for them, but they worried about boredom, missing the social give and take in the work setting, feeling unfulfilled.

While the question about the outlook for continuing in a work role was common, not all respondents found it troubling—either because they anticipated no change in the work arena, or because the idea of not working was not unwelcome. In the first group were people who took in stride the diagnosis and treatment, confident about the outcome and their ability to handle whatever would confront them. In this group were indeed a man who subsequently found attitudes in his work environment unpleasant, and a woman who was asked to resign; both established themselves in productive businesses about which they had dreamed. It had taken the sequence of life-threatening illness and work stress to give them the 'courage' to strike out for themselves, encouraged in each instance by the marital partner.

Also among those who declared they had been unconcerned were the individuals whose long-time demonstrated pattern of handling any illness that arose in the course of their work was to tell noone about it, especially the employer. Sometimes these very private persons had not utilized their health benefits in the past if to do so would mean the employer might have known about the indisposition. Sometimes vacation or other leave time had been the occasion for handling illness or surgery. They comfortably expected to deal with the cancer diagnosis no differently. Others, though, had quickly decided not to disclose the diagnosis to anyone at work. They submitted to surgical treatment during vacation periods; they obtained needed treatment during evenings, weekends, before work, or whenever it could be arranged without the employer's knowledge. These respondents generally assumed (but did not know) that negative reactions would occur on the job. As one patient put it 'I wouldn't have anything to do with people who come back from cancer. Why should I be treated differently?'

It was evident that, unlike the individuals with a life-long pattern of not sharing personal information, those who had singled out this particular illness for secrecy were anxious about being found out, depressed with the burden of silence; what if the truth were discovered?

Each study contained either three or four respondents who used the diagnosis or treatment to *not* work, for whom not working had secondary gains. Their illness supplied what could be regarded as an acceptable sympathy-promoting reason for leaving the workforce. Each commented with various degrees of vehemence about discrimination to which they were subjected, and in each instance it was the respondent's detailed description of surgical and other treatment that shaped the outcome. Thus, two individuals with colostomies emphasized with potential employers (one in building construction, the other a teacher's aide) their need to have constant access to toilet facilities and the effect of this on continuity in work routines. The former, recounting seven different rejections, including two in which the owners had sought him out because of his excellent qualifications as a construction manager, thought it was time to 'just stop looking' and devote his time to golf, his first love. The former employer of a woman with a mastectomy who regaled the coffee-shop customers with details of her experience and feelings, asked this waitress to find a job elsewhere when she failed to abide by the employer's request to talk about 'something else' with the shop's complaining customers. The patient's explanation was the employer's intolerance of cancer.

It was evident that many of the respondents, especially in the two adult studies, expected to return to work without encountering problems related to the cancer illness. Their expectations were fulfilled in some situations, but problems arose for others for which they were not necessarily prepared. Others, who expected problems, did not find their apprehensions realized. Psychosocial stress, then, developed because patients either expected it or were not prepared for its emergence. The stress was precipitated by the nature of the work or the work environment. It stemmed from the patient's own attitudes and expectations. It was a product of the attitudes of others in the work setting—employers, co-workers, gatekeepers (physicians or personnel officers, for example). Psychosocial stressors developed not only in the worksite, but also in the school setting or in the home; originating in any of these, it interacted with elements in one or more of the others locations.

At the time of the research interviews 90% of the white collar respondents were employed, nearly four-fifths of these still with the pre-cancer employer. Only 82% of the blue-collar respondents were still working, a smaller percentage with the organization that employed them before the cancer diagnosis. With few exceptions, those not working were trying to locate employment and regarded themselves as work-able. Among the respondents in the youth study, approximately half were still in school and most of the others had full or part-time employment. Many of the latter also were attending school and a remarkable half of all of the youthful respondents at time of interview were carrying a full school program in high school or college *and* working full time. This proportion of workers attending school—or the converse, students working—was higher than in the general population.

Nearly two-thirds of the respondents reported positive experiences in their work life after the cancer diagnosis. Employees and employers were helpful in a variety of ways: enabling the patient to effect a smooth adjustment to working by relieving the patient of difficult physical tasks until strength had been restored, changing work schedules to facilitate adherance to a treatment plan, modifying equipment to make it easier for the returning employee to carry out responsibilities (for example, changing the telephone equipment to accommodate the 'new' voice of an employee following throat cancer surgery). An executive secretary, hired for the job only 6 months before the unexpected surgery removed the lower part of her jaw, described her despondency when she discovered how she had been 'mutilated'. She could not look at herself; how could anyone else? How would she earn a living? How would she *live*? She found it hard to take in the admonition of her employer in a post-surgical visit to the hospital, to 'stop lolling around and get back to work!' She did and, though much of her work required meeting the public, her responsibilities and salary had steadily increased subsequently; her employer's chauffeur delivered her to and from her treatments, and 'I came back from the dead'.

But not all reported experiences were positive. Even respondents who described helpful employers or fellow workers—or, even, customers—frequently spoke of work-connected problems they associated with the cancer history: more than half of the white-collar subjects, more than four-fifths of the blue collar respondents, and in excess of half the youth-study respondents, whether as students or as members of the labor force. In fact, nearly 70% of all the employed group wanted to change jobs or occupation and, at interview, many were still searching sporadically or had abandoned the search, discouraged by rejections or prospective loss or reduction in health benefits, or because there would be no visible advantage to making a change. The wish to effect a change, whether or not translated into active effort, is of special interest in considering psychosocial stress in the workplace for, by and large, the adult workers had been with the pre-cancer employer for a considerable period of time: about 20% for less than 2 years before the cancer diagnosis and double this proportion for 10 or more years before diagnosis. For a substantial number, the pre-cancer position was the only one they ever had known. This, then, generally was a fairly stable employee group.

Perhaps because of their youth, the working respondents in the youth study had held either one or two jobs since the cancer diagnosis, tended to have been with the present employer from 1 to 12 months and, in about half the situations, to have informed the present employer of the cancer history. And as they moved from job to job (information was collected on as many as four), there was less and less tendency to let the employer know about the cancer.

SOURCES OF PSYCHOSOCIAL STRESS

The number and kinds of stressful circumstances and incidents reported by respondents contained some differences associated with the patient's cancer site and age. For example, those over 45 years of age enumerated a greater variety of examples of stress-related work problems they connected with the cancer than were described by younger respondents in any of the three studies. The very secretiveness of those with rectal/colon cancer about this site created a degree of stress that head/neck patients did not experience, for the latter's conditions rarely permitted secrecy; instead they had to deal with stressors concomitant with obvious voice or facial impairments. While the school setting was clearly different from the work setting of the youthful respondents, similar psychosocial stressors and dynamics were discernible in the work environment of the young and the older adults.

The patients' descriptions and perceptions of stress in the workplace suggested several points of origin. The patients brought some to the worksite with them in their own previously held attitude about persons with cancer and their anticipation of reactions modelled on their personal long-held ideas. Those most fearful of rejection had 'known how they (co-workers) would act', for they could judge by their own past behaviour. If the response to their return proved to be different, they were disbelieving, untrusting, and consumed with guilt because they themselves 'had not acted right'. If the response was as had been anticipated, they felt vindicated—and angry, because they did not know what they had 'done to deserve this punishment' (the cancer itself, rather than fellow workers' reaction to it). Much as the patients wished or needed to return to work, they were apprehensive: 'I didn't want to go back even though I knew I would have to. Who would want to work with me? *I* know how *they* feel about people with cancer.' Some dealt with their apprehension by isolating themselves from other employees, at work as well as socially. Some immersed themselves more deeply in their work, thus simultaneously rechanneling into it their depression and the time they otherwise would have had to socialize with 'former' friends. Some carefully denied the nature of their illness. A number projected their unhappiness and fear on others in the workplace, displaying irritability, hostility, and other defensive behaviours. And it was not uncommon to attempt to demonstrate capability and adequacy by avoidance of any time off lest it confirm what the patient was sure colleagues believed; namely, that the patient was too ill to work and could 'fall over dead' at any moment. Although for the most part these respondents did not describe themselves as victims of workplace discrimination, they sometimes saw as 'discrimination' these relationship problems stemming from their own attitudes.

A more common and serious work problem arose from the overt attitudes and behaviours of others encountered in the workplace: dismissal ('because you can't do the work anymore,' 'it's too depressing for others to be with you,' 'you no longer have the respect of your subordinates'); transfer to other, less desirable, shifts or locations where either fewer persons were located or the change might lead the employee to quit; no salary increases when automatic upward adjustments were granted to the other employees (union membership sometimes served to protect the patient's pay raise); termination of group health and/or life insurance on the generally specious grounds that the patient-employee would cause the employer's insurance rates to increase; demotion; and others.

Sometimes interacting with these gross discriminatory acts, and sometimes totally unrelated to them, were hostile actions and statements of others in the work environment. Thus, a woman in the company rest room reportedly asked an employee with a recent mastectomy, 'How does it feel to be less than a woman?' Other frequent instances were reported where fellow workers asked to have their desks or workplace moved to avoid the 'contamination' or danger of 'catching' the cancer. A teacher deliberately moved a 14-year-old with Hodgkin's Disease to one side of the room, away from the other students, to lessen the 'danger' to the other students. (The interviewed school nurse attributed this boy's subsequent unsuccesful suicide effort to this experience.) Hostility—from fellow workers, school personnel, family members—loomed large in the three studies. To illustrate: three blue collar workers, foremen in different kinds of plants, had undergone surgery that altered their voices. In each instance their artificial speaking efforts were continually mimicked by their subordinates; and supervisors of two also imitated them. One patient, mentioned above, was demoted; only the strong support from a former subordinate who now had his own business and hired the patient made it possible for him to function 'at all'. Another tried to take his life by inhaling carbon monoxide in his garage. Still with this company, he is searching for another job. The third, a skilled technician, found a night janitorial job, working alone. Yet a fourth man with impaired speech returned to his work with the announcement that he was in delayed adolescence, undergoing youthful voice changes. He laughed and the resulting laughter of his subordinates acknowledged his mastery of the situation; his planned aggressive action had cleared the air of hostility and embarrassment.

Still another kind of situation in the work environment was reported as stressful by a number of respondents in each study. They reacted with impatience and anxiety to the high degree of solicitude exhibited by many fellow workers. They could acknowledge that people simply do not know how to deal with the life-threatening illness of others, that a number of factors—including fear and embarrassment as well as compassion—motivate the over-solicitous behaviour. But to some of the patients, this was constant reminder that their independence and adequacy were in question, as well as their mortality. They reacted with anger, impatience, irritability and, sometimes, unrestrained tears. The result was heightened concern on the part of the co-worker, and compounded anger and depression in the patient. 'Why can't they treat me like anyone else? I'm well enough to do what needs to be done! I don't need all that pity!'

Of course, the nature of the work itself might be a source of stress for some patients. A cocktail waitress in a 'topless' bar delayed for 3 years before consulting a physician about what she was sure would be breast cancer. Then, when her prediction proved accurate, she was afraid to return to work because she was certain she would either be fired because she could not wear a topless garment, or she would be unable to handle the heavy trays in her upraised hands. But the employer provided her with a special costume, and busboys carried her trays until she was physically able to do so herself. Handling of machinery (especially conveyor belts), meeting the public, performing various requisite tasks were frequent stress stimuli until the patient either learned to accommodate to the given task or a cooperative employer was able to effect a reassignment to a function more compatible with the employee's physical abilities.

Another source of stress was associated with the respondent's attempts to find a different job—or, in the instance of the young respondents, a first job. When a history of cancer was acknowledged to the potential employer—either because the question was asked or the information volunteered—the job-seeker was sometimes rejected outright, regardles of whether the work required a certain health status. Various reasons were given the job-seeker, or inferred by him: possible contagion, survival beyond a training period appeared improbable, physical weakness, immorality for which the patient was being 'punished' by the cancer, and others. Surprisingly common was rejection on medical recommendation by the company physician or other 'gatekeeper' who noted the applicant had not been sympton-free for 5 years or thought the inclusion of the applicant in the retirement system could not be 'justified' because the job-seeker would not live long enough to benefit from it. For some of the respondents, such rejections were almost devastating; they remained attached to jobs in which they were unhappy but afraid to leave.

A second source of psychosocial stress was the generally inadvertant or thoughtfully 'thoughtless' response of physicians to a query by a potential employer or insurance carrier. Asked about the present health status of the respondent, the physician might answer 'Well.' Asked about the potential for reactivation or recurrence of the cancer, some physicians answered, 'I don't know; I can't give you any assurance that it won't come back,' thereby permitting the inquirer to infer that this is likely, and soon. As a consequence, the patient appeared to be a poor employment risk and was rejected.

Physician relationships with respondents contributed on occasion to patient distress for reasons other than those noted. Many of the work-oriented patients were eager to return to work. They perceived such return to symbolize their wellness, or as a rehabilitative aid to recovery and a step toward mental as well as physical health. Such return might ease an economic need. But ranking high among the reasons was that work was 'proof' of their mastery over their own affairs, despite the cancer's presence. While self-described depression was a fairly common and recurring phenomenon among the respondents, some attributed this state to the fact that they were not working even though they felt well enough to do so. They could not understand why their doctors advised against it. At time of initial diagnosis and treatment, their doctors had been asked specifically about 'When can I return to work?' One had replied, for example, 'Don't work!' The research interview with him disclosed that he had meant 'temporarily' but had not been explicit. The patient, hesitating to ask questions about her health, had feared the worst and the abbreviated statement had served to confirm her fears; she was waiting to die.

Especially significant was the anger and distrust the youthful patients ascribed to the fact that some doctors delegated to parents the task of letting the young patients know the diagnosis and prognosis. Why did doctors who, after all, were the experts, leave this responsibility to parents who often not only were unsophisticated about what was involved, but emotionally unequal to the delegated task?

Common also was the tendency among some adult patients to regard the doctor with adulation, to want the doctor to admire and respect the patient's handling of the disturbing diagnosis and treatment. There was, therefore, some hesitancy to ask questions or to share fears with the doctor. As a consequence, these patients sometimes were ill-prepared to cope with various problems, primarily in the realm of work or the relationship with the marital partner. One interviewed doctor, for example, spoke with admiration about the 'well-adjusted stoical' patient who took 'everything in his stride.' This was the foreman who attempted suicide.

In summary, the studies revealed a spectrum of psychosocial stressors that, interacting with the initial stress provoked on learning the diagnosis, were induced or exacerbated by real or perceived work-related stress. Some of the work and non-work stress was rooted in the respondent's acceptance of societal attitudes and expectations about the work ethic, independence, and personal adequacy. Some stemmed from compliance with or rejection of images and attitudes originating in antiquity about the source, nature and moral significance of cancer. Some emerged from the quality or absence of communication between the patient and physician or knowledgeable others that might have aided in dispelling feelings and attitudes that existed in the respondent's work setting and personal environment and that were inimical to the individual's well being. Some of the stress was based in reality factors; some was not—but was no less painful or frightening.

COPING STRATEGIES

Evidence was supplied in all three studies that although coping strategies varied considerably among the respondents, some common patterns bore on the successful coping—or the failure to cope with the identified psychosocial stress. Selye's view that one person's work is another's play and that stress is associated with every kind of work, but distress is not, (Selye, 1974) received support in this trilogy of studies.

It was clear that a large proportion of the respondents in all three studies turned to their work to 'prove' themselves, to channel their anxiety and depression into 'something productive,' something they 'could *do*.' A school crossing guard remarked: 'Going back to work speeded my recovery. You can't be gloomy around children.' And a lithograph worker reported: 'I returned to work full time, and overtime as well, a month before the doctor told me I could. At home I was climbing the walls; at work I didn't have time to think about anything except doing a decent job!' In contrast was the nurse's aide who did not want to go back to work 'even though I knew I would have to. They'll hire anyone for a convalescent home—overwork and underpay. They didn't question my facial disfigurement as other workplaces did and I have no special skills to offer anywhere.' But even she found that doing a job she disliked gave her 'confidence that I can keep going as long as I have to.'

'Proving' themselves was demonstrated in various ways, including intensive efforts to improve quality and productivity of performance (and getting 'high ratings') and avoidance of absence. Prior to the initiation of the *Work and Cancer Health Histories* series, the extremely limited extant literature centered on work and cancer contained two landmark reports in which two employers, Metropolitan Life Insurance Company (Wheatley *et al.*, 1972) and Bell Telephone (Stone, 1975) compared the absenteeism rates and work performance of employees who had cancer histories with fellow workers who had histories of other health conditions. Neither company found noticeable differences. The *Work and Cancer Health Histories* studies disclosed less absenteeism among the respondents. Patients and employers acknowledged that the respondents stayed on the job even when they were suffering from influenza or other conditions that would have led others to remain away from work. Treatments in process often were during non-working hours. The median of all absences that occurred among the patient-respondents—for diagnostic tests and surgery as well as subsequent therapy—was under 6 weeks. And many patients reported that they avoided utilizing group health care programs because they were unwilling to have people in their employing establishments made conscious of their health needs and associated costs even when these were unrelated to the cancer experience. Some of the respondents also worried that health insurance coverage would be discontinued.

Some patients endeavoured to handle unpleasant or hostile behaviour at the work site, or tasks physically difficult for them to perform, by looking for other work. Some were successful but, as was noted earlier, a substantial proportion abandoned frustrating efforts to relocate and tried to 'make the best' of the work situation they had. Many of these patients also were subject to recurring depression. Some had been surprised, though certainly not all, that they so quickly exceeded their physical limits, that the return to performing at their former full-capacity level took longer than they had expected. They reported symptoms of greater fatigue with strenuous work, weight gain, arm pains, nervousness, and the aforementioned depression. If the support of the individual or of the family depended on the employment, working far beyond physical capacity and coping with pain and fatigue were not uncommon experiences. This group in particular was apprehensive about recurrence or spread of the cancer. They felt a constant shadow about not passing a physical examination and worried about whether they could or should conceal the cancer history.

The respondents' ability to actively employ the work environment and their work tasks to cope with the sometimes almost overwhelming psychosocial stress—or merely to accommodate to 'managing' to remain on the job—depended on a constellation of factors. Among these were intellectual endowment, personality elements, characteristic or habitual ways of coping with stress before the onset of the cancer, strength of basic impulses (that combination of energy and need driving the individual to want and to strive), ego strength, and family and formal and informal social supports. Some carefully assessed the work situation to which they would return, planfully preparing themselves for the coping tasks. The man who used direct humor about his 'adolescent voice changes' was an example, but there were others: countering the oversolicitude of fellow workers with flat statements (repeatedly, in some instances) about being well and expecting to be treated as though the cancer had never occurred; announcing that certain physical temporary or permanent constraints did not reduce the respondents' mental capacity or ability for self-management and job performance; acknowledging the concern of others, assuring the solicitous individuals they would be called on if needed, or advised if the patient died, but meanwhile 'let's not burden ourselves with unnecessary pity.' The emphasis was on *wellness*, whether with or without some limits. Often this attitude was bolstered with the use of humor: if the patient could laugh, why not the co-worker? Some of the women with mastectomies were strengthened in their resolve to have symptoms diagnosed and undergo necessary treatment because of the models provided by Mrs. Gerald Ford and Mrs. Nelson Rockefeller. To overly-sympathetic individuals in the work setting, such patients would refer to these two prominent women whose cancer course had been detailed in the public press and add: 'If they could manage, so can I!'

The hostility, the shunning, the fear of contamination—these and other behaviours in the workplace were more difficult for the respondent to handle. Sometimes the patient openly confronted the attacker (occasionally clearing the air, but more often simultaneously deepening the other's anger and the respondent's depression), but most often tried to avoid the individual. This was not always possible in some work settings and arrangements. Withdrawal also was used by the adolescent respondents, particularly those in the developmental stage where they were acutely sensitive to body loss. Thus, one described his refusal to respond to the physical therapist's efforts by turning away from her and maintaining total silence, declining to permit her to minister to him. When the doctor confronted this 16-year-old with the possible consequences of his behaviour, the patient blurted out that no-one who talked to him about a 'stump' (a leg had been amputated) could make him into a 'whole person.'

The strong push of those effecting moderate to good adjustments was to be treated as 'normal.' This was not easy for companions, adults or young people, family members or friends or casual acquaintances; it was difficult for them to know how to approach or respond to someone 'they know is going to die.' The sensitive awareness of relatives, friends, co-workers and employers to the psychological needs of the respondent was instrumental in giving many the strength to face the stressors that were inherent in the illness, the patient's work, or precipitated by behaviour of others. Not all family members could cope with the situation and some families broke down or apart: there were divorces—of the patient, of the youthful patient's parents; sibling, adult children, friends avoided the patient. In some of these situations the patient's description suggested that the illness had merely been the 'final straw,' but in some cases the disruption in the family or the avoidance by others came as a surprise to everyone. Some patients reacted by investing themselves more fully in performing in the workplace; others were hurt, and they anticipated—and sometimes precipitated—rejecting reactions in the work setting, where they remained isolated and lonely.

The attitudes and supportive behaviour of parents played an especially important role among the youth study respondents and, also, younger respondents in the two adult studies. A notable instance among the former was the determination of a mother, herself a teacher, that her 15-year-old daughter whose leg had been amputated was to be treated in the school setting like her peers. To the school personnel's protest that the girl's prosthesis prevented her full participation in the gym-class activities, this mother replied: 'If she falls, she will pick herself up; this is what she will have to do throughout her life!' The mother's demand was met. At this writing, a note from this girl, now 19, triumphantly reported her selection as a finalist in competition for the Olympic ski team. 'If my mother had not fought for me, my life would be *terrible*.'

Among the participants in the studies were some whose coping was primarily in the form of active self-pity, exploiting the sympathy of those in their home and/or work environment. It was in this group that more dissatisfaction with work was reported, although it also was speculated by the research interviewers that for some the self-pity was a defense against obvious hostility, deflecting this by making the attacker feel guilty.

More common than the self-pity, however, was denial. This was manifest in two ways: some individuals took a variety of measures to avoid disclosure of the cancer history to others in work settings—or even to relatives or friends. As will be discussed later, others flatly denied having cancer, sometimes offering other explanations for their medical treatment, sometimes just saying 'It isn't true.' The latter occurred even in some situations where the respondent had arranged a research interview, knowing the cancer-focus of the study. (Their doctors were consulted to ascertain that there was indeed a cancer diagnosis that had been discussed with the patient.)

From among the many psychosocial stressors discernible in the *Work and Cancer Health Histories* series, depression bears special attention. It appeared as a stressor, as a response to stress, and as a coping device—albeit not one highly successful in modifying the consequences of the stress. Depression has been offered since early times as a factor in causing cancer. Galen, in 200 A.D. (Fobair and Cordoba, 1982) proposed that 'melancholic' women, as opposed to sanguine women, had a tendency toward breast cancer. Explanations have been offered (Fox, 1978; Selye, 1979) for physiological or bodily reactions and processes of stress that can be instrumental in rendering an individual vulnerable to cancer. Others (LeShan, 1966; Haney, 1977; Kissen *et al.*, 1969) suggest that adverse life events and the loss of a love object lead to 'despair, depression and hopelessness' and offer these traits as precursors of a cancer diagnosis. The *Work and Cancer Health Histories* studies neither speculated nor drew inferences about personality factors and stress as a factor in carcinogenesis. Nor were relationships drawn between carcinogenesis in persons who had lost loved ones and tended to feelings of hopelessness, depression, and low self-esteem. But respondents were queried about the occurrence of cancer among close friends or relatives and how the patient had reacted to their having cancer or to their death from cancer.

No conclusions could be drawn from these data, although certainly there were clues both to consequent depression and to the effect of the incidence of cancer in relatives or friends on how quickly the respondent had sought medical attention for his own symptoms or how prepared the respondent was to cope with his own diagnosis. Nor was it possible to learn from retrospection clouded by passage of time whether respondents to whom their work or job had tremendous meaning might have responded to work problems or work loss as they would have to the loss of a human love object. What was evident, however, was the prevalence of hopelessness, depression, and lowered self-esteem among those who perceived themselves as having work problems, regardless of their origin or their basis in reality.

How did these people cope with the depression? Many simply did nothing: the depression engulfed them, sometimes their families as well, and sometimes repelled co-workers. The consequence was that the patient was shunned or management transferred or dismissed the respondent. Some respondents, on the other hand, sought help of a psychiatrist, psychologist, or social worker and at least two turned to clergy. In some instances, it was the oncologist or another physician who observed the presence of the depression and urged the patient or family to obtain help. In some instances, it was the patient's own decision. It seems likely that the decision to obtain psychological help was actually a function of education, for the respondents who obtained help tended to be individuals with at least some college education or, if youthful respondents, to live with college-educated parents. In this connection, it also is worth noting that the youthful respondents who developed career goals which they implemented through education or work plans, also were in families in which one or both parents had college educations and who were strongly work-oriented.

A few patients turned to self-help organizations (Reach for Recovery, Make Today Count, and others) for support in the face of fear and anxiety about present and future cancer-related prospects. A few rejected the 'subjective' help proffered them; several found in it the hope and the courage to think more clearly about how to handle themselves in their work relationships as well as family and social networks.

The most persistent and common resources on which respondents called for support, however, were family members (spouse and parents, then adult children and, last, sibling or other relatives), the social support system that included friends in and out of the workplace, and certain caring physicians.

SOME DILEMMAS

How to cope with the fact and sequellae of the cancer diagnosis and treatment posed a serious and often continuing ethical problem for a number of cancer patients and, sometimes, for their employers. Two illustrations will be cited. In one, a young Air Force officer had read a news article quoting the principal investigator with reference to workplace discrimination experiences of cancer victims. He wrote to describe how alone, guilty, and ashamed he had felt in his belief that he had been singled out for special prejudicial attention, and the strength he had gained from knowing it was not an attack he had himself provoked. Seven years before, he had a malignant brain tumour which was successfully excised, with no subsequent medical problems. He had 'a feeling of pride' in 'the completeness of my recovery.' He reported his efforts to find work after he completed college and finding that 'most employers viewed my medical history as a liability. I became expert in interview situations at observing the reaction of the interviewers when I would disclose or volunteer the facts . . . .' Even using a 'protective policy of not disclosing' the medical facts, he could not obtain meaningful employment. This habit was firmly entrenched when 'I applied for entry' into the military service and was accepted after passing a medical examination in which there was no reference to the surgery. Subsequently, in relation to a pending promotion, a doctor discovered the original medical scar. 'They then tried to medically separate or discharge me from the service because of the brain tumour.' A Physical Examination Board determined he was 'not medically impaired and was completely fit for worldwide duty. Now, authorities here on base have begun legal procedures to administratively separate or fire me. They are charging me with fraudulent enlistment . . . . It is odd that first people here tried to get rid of me because I at one time had a cancerous brain tumour. Now these same people are trying to get rid of me because I didn't tell them about it when I enlisted.'

To tell or not to tell is a common anxiety of the cancer patient who wants to enter or re-enter the work force. What will be the consequences if the information is or is not revealed?

Closely allied to the dilemma on which the lieutenant was caught is the matter of health insurance in the workplace. Despite protestations to the contrary by some insurance carriers, some interviewed employers declared that their insurance rates rise if persons with cancer histories are included in the company's group plan. Some, consequently, excluded these employees from plans already in effect and that had covered them until the cancer diagnosis was revealed. Other employers thought it advisable not to choose to hire the patient-respondent if other equally qualified applicants were available. For the employee or potential employee, fear lay in the prospect that insurance might be cancelled if the cancer history were divulged, thereby also jeopardizing health insurance protection for other ailments—or for dependents who might require health insurance protection. Indeed, several respondents spoke regretfully of the fact that the employed spouse was tied to a job less desirable than others that might be available but which would mean at least a waiting period before health protection would be available, if at all, to the family member with the cancer history.

The other situation is of a different order. In an action brought before the Workers' Compensation Appeals Board (October, 1983), the widow of a small-town former police chief pressed a death claim on the grounds that work stress affected his immune system, causing deterioration in the leukemic condition that led to his death. He had worked from 12 to 20 hours a day under severe stress which had included a reorganization leading to his demotion to a deputy chief position in which he had to draw up a reorganization plan that resulted in the elimination of his own friends from the department as well as to other problems. The widow's assertion, supported by testimony of the physician who had attended the patient, was refuted by the hemotologist called as an expert witness. The latter held that there was no evidence that immunology played any specific part in the officer's chronic myelogenous leukemia. Furthermore, the hemotologist was convinced not only that work did not shorten the officer's life but, in fact, may have been the reason he survived the blast stage for such a long period. An unspoken issue here was the possible impact on employers who might be unwilling to employ workable persons with a cancer history if work stress were to be regarded as a major element in causing the employee's death from cancer.

In this situation, the issue was resolved when the court ruled against the widow. But the threat to workers' compensation rates because of claims that work stress might contribute to the deterioration of a cancer patient's mental health was a worry mentioned by several employers in the cancer and work studies: whether their anxiety was reality-based or not, they saw it as real.

AVENUES FOR RESEARCH

The psychological, social, and economic meanings of work to individuals and families in Western society have been profound for a number of centuries. The fear that cancer engenders has hardly lessened, if at all, during these centuries. Furthermore, the concern about the effect of cancer on the quality of life of the patient and the patient's family is magnified geometrically if work or work satisfactions or work opportunities are placed in jeopardy because cancer strikes the work-oriented individual or dependent family member. Yet, there is a paucity of research about the interaction of the patient's personal life and work life, about the therapeutic role of work in enabling the cancer patient to cope with the cancer or the indicated medical regimen, about whether work dissatisfaction or cessation may render an individual vulnerable to cancer in a way similar to that shown in research centering on loss of love objects (Cooper, 1982). Indeed, given available data about the high incidence of cancer that occurs in the later, post-retirement years, would longitudinal or other relevant studies disclose any significant relationship between involuntary or voluntary retirement from the work force of individuals who subsequently develop cancer? Recent years have witnessed a flurry of statutes enacted in various localities proscribing discrimination in the workplace against individuals with cancer who want to enter, re-enter or remain in the workplace. In what ways and to what extent are such statutes and their enforcement effective?

The avenues for constructive further enquiry into psychosocial stressors affecting cancer patients at work, and how they have responded to such stress, have hardly been explored, yet the size of the population affected stretches far beyond a visible horizon. The importance of such research can be encapsulated in two comments. One is the closing statement of a blue collar respondent: 'A comment I'd like to add is that more needs to be understood about cancer and what it means to the working person. *Everybody* is scared to death of cancer. They make remarks like, "Wow, are you still here?" They connect cancer with death; they think there is nothing *well* about you. But when you worry about whether you might lose your job, you wonder whether you *should* have died!'

One of the first to develop a theoretical model of what happens when an individual is subjected to stress was Freud (1930). In an earlier (1927) writing, however, he remarked: 'Work is the chief means of binding the individual to reality.' He might have been anticipating the respondents in the Work and Cancer Health Histories series—and, indeed, work-oriented individuals for whom work is a tool for coping with cancer-related psychosocial stress.

REFERENCES

Brenner, H. (1973). *Mental Illness and the Economy*, Harvard University Press, Cambridge, Mass.

Brenner, H. (1976). *Estimating the Social Costs of National Economic Policy: Implications for Mental and Physical Health and Criminal Violence*, Report Prepared for Joint Economic Committee of Congress, U.S. Government Printing Office, Washington, D.C.

Conrad, J. (1976). *Heart of Darkness*, Penguin, New York.

Cooper, C. L. (1982). Psychosocial Stress and Cancer, *Bulletin of the British Psychological Society*, **35**, 456–459.

Cooper, C. L., and Marshall, J. (1976). Occupational Sources of Stress, A Review of the Literature Relating to Coronary Heart Disease and Mental Ill Health, *Journal of Occupational Psychology*, **49**, 11–28.

Feldman, F. L. (1976). *Work and Cancer Health Histories: A Study of the Experiences of Recovered Patients*, American Cancer Society, California Division, San Francisco.

Feldman, F. L. (1978). *Work and Cancer Health Histories: A Study of the Experiences of Recovered Blue Collar Workers*, American Cancer Society, California Division, San Francisco.

Feldman, F. L. (1980). *Work and Cancer Health Histories: Work Expectations and Experiences of Youth (Ages 13–23) With Cancer Histories*, American Cancer Society, California Division, San Francisco.

Fobair, P., and Cordoba, C. S. (1982). Scope and magnitude of the cancer problem in psychosocial research, in *Psychosocial Aspects of Cancer* (Eds. J. Cohen, J. W. Cullen and L. R. Martin), Raven Press, New York.

Fox, B. (1978). Premorbid psychological factors as related to cancer incidence, *Journal of Behavioural Medicine*, **1**, 45–133.

Freud, S. (1927). *The Problem of Lay-Analysis*, Brentano's, New York.

Freud, S. (1930). *Civilization and Its Discontents*, Hogarth, London.

Greenleigh Associates (1979). *Report on the Social, Economic and Psychological Needs of Cancer Patients in California*, American Cancer Society, California Division, San Francisco.

Haney, C. A. (1977). Illness behaviour and psychosocial correlates of cancer, *Journal of Social Science and Medicine*, **11**(4), 223–228.

Kissen, D. M., Brown, R. I. F. and Kissen, M. A. (1969). A further report on personality and psychosocial factors in lung cancer, *Annals of the New York Academy of Sciences*, **1964**, 535.

LeShan, L. (1966). An emotional life-history pattern associated with neoplastic disease, *Annual New York Academy of Science Journal*, **125**, 780–793.

Luther, M. (1909). *Luther's Epistle Sermons*, translated by John N. Lenkers, Luther Press, Mineapolis.

O'Toole, J. (1973). *Work in America*, MIT Press, Cambridge, Mass.

Presbyterian Board of Christian Education (1936). *Institutes of the Christian Religion*, Philadelphia.

Raymon, P., and Bluestone, B. (1982). *The Private and Social Responsibility to Job*

Loss: A Metropolitan Study, Final Report of Research Sponsored by Center for Work and Mental Health, National Institute for Mental Health, Washington, D.C.

Selye, H. (1956). *The Stress of Life*, McGraw-Hill, New York.

Selye, H. (1974). *Stress Without Distress*, Lippincott, New York.

Selye, H. (1979). Correlating stress and cancer, *American Journal of Proctology, Gastroenterology, Colon and Rectal Surgery*, **30**(4), 18–28.

Sontag, S. (1977). *Illness as Metaphor*, Farrar, Straus and Giroux, New York.

State Compensation Appeals Board, State of California (October 23, 1983), Sojka vs. City of Simi Valley; State Compensation Insurance fund 81SD 65829.

Stone, R. W. (1975). Employing the Recovered Cancer Patient, in *Cancer July Supplement*, 36.

Wheatley, G. M., Cunnick, W. R. *et al.* (1972). *The employment of persons with a history of treatment for cancer*, Metropolitan Life Insurance Company, New York.

Psychosocial Stress and Cancer
Edited by C. L. Cooper

Chapter 9

Psychosocial Factors in the Management of Patients with Cancer

C. Allen Haney*
Professor of Sociology, University of Houston, Texas USA

INTRODUCTION

Probably no disease diagnosis is viewed by the average citizen of the western world with as much fear and dread as cancer. This group of diseases appears to evoke the same type of reactions as did the plague. The widespread fear response has multiple origins which are not necessarily related to either fact or logic. This fear may arise in part from an awareness that the incidence of cancer is extremely high: estimates indicate that approximately one-quarter of the U.S. population will develop some form of cancer in their lifetime, and roughly 20% of these will die of their cancer. A second of the bases for this fear may be the fact that cancers spare no age, sex, ethnic or economic group, and is therefore not confined to the devalued or marginal members of society, striking as it does the moral and the immoral, the noble and the ignoble, those who contribute to society as well as those who only consume society's resources. Perhaps at a less logical level, the fear response may be influenced by the extensive media coverage of cancer in its various forms and stages as 'news' and as an element in works of fiction. Finally, a fourth possibility relates to the perception that cancer treatment is disfiguring, painful, protracted, expensive and/or fruitless.

Whether because of the nature of the illness itself or the atmosphere of fear which is evoked by the concept, cancer poses special problems both for the individual's adaptation to both self and the systemic relations between the individual and those in his/her more or less immediate social environment. In this chapter I will consider, in turn, first some of the elements involved in

*The author would like to acknowledge the assistance of Deborah J. Marlowe and Louis Stern, who helped formulated the ideas expressed here, and Dr. Howard Kaplan, William Simon and Joseph Kotarba for repeatedly assisting with early drafts of this manuscript. This work is dedicated to the cancer patients who were so willing to discuss their illness.

the cancer patient's adaptation in terms of his/her own emotional and cognitive coming to terms with the diagnosed disorder, and second, with the adaptational problems posed for the patient and the significant others implicated in the circumstances surrounding the diagnosis and treatment process. The latter includes both the members of the patients' primary groups, and the personnel comprising the therapeutic environment. Within each category I will consider the implications for management of the patient's more or less effective attempts to adapt to self and others, and for the need for such adaptations in the clinical encounter occasioned by the cancer.

THE COGNITIVE AND AFFECTIVE ADJUSTMENT OF CANCER PATIENTS

Adaptation to Cancer: Self-Cognition and Self-Feeling

Simple crisis resolution models are unsatisfactory when applied to cancer

> (1) Since people with cancer are confronted with continuing stress or a series of severe stresses over an extended period of time, it is inaccurate to speak of cancer as though it were a single event, posing a time-limited crisis that requires only immediate adaptive response. (2) . . .[O]ne of the major problems posed by cancer is that the patient cannot be sure for many years whether or not a cure has been effected. This problem too involves not a single event or series of events well marked in time, but rather a continuing, unremitting condition of uncertainty about potentially disastrous and poorly predictable future events. (3) The treatment of cancer usually entails irreparable physical damage which may enforce changes in patterns of activity, habits of daily living, perceptions of oneself, and the like. In such circumstances, a return to an original equilibrium is simply precluded. (4) In fact, the majority of cancer patients regard their disease as the source of major discontinuity in their lives and report permanent changes in how they view themselves and their future existence. (Mages and Mendelsohn, 1979; p. 259).

It would appear that three basic assumptions underlie the study of the effects of cancer on patient's lives. First, cancer results in an ongoing process which unfolds over time and is characterized by numerous stages, each stage, producing numerous problems. Second, cancer's impact and the adaptations and coping strategies employed are in large measure a function of the individual's previous life contingencies and current stage of life. Third, the patient's psychosocial status is rooted in that patient's history and oriented toward what the patient sees as the future. As the disease and the treatment progress, not only are new adaptational needs imposed, but the patient must also face the difficulty of abandoning those now outmoded (Mages and Mendelsohn, 1979).

Hinton (1973) and later, Holland (1976), have described some of the unique demands and constraints attendant to the role of cancer patient. Four are offered here as being particularly problematic: (1) the recurrent need to modify reality, (2) the definition of time, (3) the management of uncertainty, and (4) coping with pain.

The Construction of Reality

All of us attempt to construct an enduring reality in which to function. The goal of socialization is to help the child learn how to perceive himself or herself and the world about him/her in a fashion that will ensure that (s)he will mesh with his/her social groups. When one is designated as a cancer patient, 'reality' must be restructured, not merely once, but repeatedly.

> It is not just 'having cancer' that is difficult, but also the implied meaning that the person attaches to the disease: pain, disfigurement, hospitalization, doubts, inability to care for one's family, dirtiness, loss of sexual attractiveness or function, disability and possible death . . . finding ways of coping with overwhelming but 'real' reality. (Holland, 1973; p. 992)

In one of the earliest works dealing with psychosocial factors in illness and medical practice, Stanley King (1962) offered a concise outline of the variables which merge to determine the way events are perceived and the meaning attached to them. Three categories of determinants are set forth: Physiologic, Psychologic and Sociocultural. Within the physiologic are the chemical imbalances and bodily states which routinely occur in human beings: hunger, thirst, fatigue and sexual arousal, for example. In the cancer patient, others must also be added, for not only can tumors interfere with normal bodily processes, but they can also secrete abnormal quantities of substances into the body. Chemotherapy is the deliberate attempt to alter the chemical balance of the body. Just as pellagra can produce disorientation, confusion, depression, and mania, so can cancer and its treatment alter perceptions of reality.

A second physiologic determinant of an individual's perception of reality rests upon genetic endowment. King spoke of height, weight, muscular strength, coordination, sensory acuity, and intelligence. To the extent that these influence perception of pain thresholds and other life contingencies, the perception of cancer can also be influenced. Perhaps more to the point is the reconstruction of reality which must be undertaken when cancer forces an alteration in one's genetic endowment through surgery or other therapeutic modalities.

Among the psychologic elements which determine reality, basic needs are perhaps paramount, needs both latent and manifest. Nearly 50 years ago Murray (1938) reported needs such as harm avoidance, sentience, autonomy, achievement, order and inviolacy—all of which can be blocked by cancer and its treatment, and each can determine perception and thus the construction of reality.

Other determinants in this category are the adaptive and defensive mechanisms on which the individual learns to rely when faced with conflicts between physiological, psychological and sociocultural demands. Repression, projections, reaction formation, situation avoidance and transference are among the traditional concepts usually considered at this point, and each have been observed in cancer patients and employed in the patient's quest for conflict resolution (cf. Westbrook and Viney, 1982). Finally, should be added the more enduring aspects of personality which provide continuity and allow one to order one's life—beliefs, values, and attitudes. Cancer can seriously challenge these long-held beliefs and emotionally charged feelings. These ordering mechanisms can become insurmountable barriers to cancer treatment.

The last factors which determine one's perception, and thus the construction of reality, are the *sociological*. Chief among these is the notion of culture itself. Ben Paul (1955) said that culture gives a people a means of classifying in a systematic way the events that occur about them and that this classification scheme may not be shared by those of another cultural group. In the dominant culture of the U.S.A., for example, pain may be classified in an extensive system of categories from sharp through gripping or searing to dull, etc. In the culture of the Navajo Indians, the distinctions are much more limited. Thus, for each group the concept of pain held by the other may be unfathomable. Not only does culture determine that range of normal, and the view of cause and effect, but language as well. This holds true for health, illness, and that wide range of diseases known as cancer. In a cultural group where life expectancy is short, cancer may be far less meaningful than the acute illnesses. Not so for those cultures where the chronic disease of aging populations are the leading causes of death.

Cancer can produce major alterations in perception and one's construction of a reality because of its impact upon another sociocultural determinant: one's social roles. Clearly the disease dictates that one be, to some extent, in the patient role and, due to the nature of role reciprocity, there is required the corresponding role of care providers; thus, new role relationships must be learned. Everyone occupies numerous roles and cancer can bring these roles into conflict—some abandoned, some overlapping, and some called into question when the rewards attendant to role performance are not forthcoming.

More easily measured is the altered reality when the fact of cancer is seen in terms of the reality created by one's social class and ethnic groups. If social class is defined by some combination of characteristics such as education, occupation, income, prestige, influence and place of residence, cancer is differential in its salience to reality. For those in a social class where health insurance is nearly universal, prior experience with medical specialists common, and health care routine, the demands of cancer therapy may fit well with existing reality. If, on the other hand, health care is seen as a luxury, or even mistrusted, and one already lives on the edge of poverty and is socially isolated, then successful cancer therapy will require a drastically revised view of reality.

Similar arguments can be made regarding ethnic group memberships, for not only is it generally associated with a unique, generally minority subculture, but often correlates with disadvantaged social class position. Consider, for example, the modification in one's view of authority figures which cancer requires.

Finally, the perception of reality can be influenced by time-honored customs and habits which contribute to group cohesiveness and feelings of belonging. Changed behaviour patterns stemming from a diagnosis of cancer and its treatment can necessitate a modification in one's sense of alienation, anomie, and estrangement.

Reliance on these determiners is the means by which one orients oneself towards the world and those about one. A uniquely constructed reality which lends meaning to events and relationships leads to the smooth flow of interaction, provides ready solutions to the contingencies of life and helps to fix our place in society and our image of self. With cancer, the prognosis may be unknown, treatment techniques may be experimental, the disease impacts on almost all facets of life, and is chronic in nature. Thus, one must repeatedly modify one's view of reality as the disease process progresses, new members are added to the treatment team, former roles must be abdicated, goals forgone, body image altered and coping strategies re-evaluated.

Time

Following the diagnosis of cancer is an acute grief reaction similar to that which accompanies any disaster or personal loss (cf. Lindemann (1944) for an early treatment of the subjcct and Holland (1976) for a more recent statement). Unlike the situation reported in the past, physicians more often than not tell the patient the true nature of the diagnosis, and this gives rise to two question of profound concern to the patient: 'Is it fatal (terminal)? How long have I got?' As Glaser (1966) points out, the patient's concern is for 'certainty' and 'time.' Sociologists have been concerned with this latter aspect for some years. Florence Kluckhohn (1955) spoke of time as one of the foundations of human values. For a patient with cancer, time becomes a much more elusive concept. For a patient receiving chemotherapy, the length of time between one treatment and the next may be all too brief, while the time spent in therapy may appear interminable.

Glaser (1966) gave clear evidence that time is crucial to a cancer patient. In his observations of terminally ill cancer patients and the techniques of adjustment he speaks of the patient who uses the time remaining to 'settle social and financial affairs,' the often younger patient who ops to attempt to live a 'full life,' and those whose denial of the inevitable leads them to attempt to play the polarity game—defined as controlling interaction with medical staff such that questions asked by the patient must be normalized by the staff. His example is the patient who asks 'Am I getting worse?', thus forcing the staff member to normalize and reply along the lines, 'Give yourself a chance—medicine takes time.' Some patients were observed to find comparative referents for their particular condition, i.e., finding someone with a similar diagnosis to 'out-live', while still others engaged in frank 'future talk,' diverting verbal interactions along lines that involve the next birthday, election, child's graduation, etc., even when objective criteria of progress would not support such an assumption of survivorship.

Holland (1973) has noted that as the illness progresses some patients begin to make a tacit accommodation to the notion of terminality, characterized by foreshortened goals, less planning heightened focus on day-to-day events. 'Successful treatment is no longer total recovery but survival extension in comfort . . . .' (p. 1001).

On some occasions the variable of time must be manipulated in the interest of motivation and the psychological well-being of both patient and family. This is particularly the case if a given patient is a participant in a research protocol. Patients must be taught to think in terms of the chronicity, that cancer is neither uniformly fatal nor acute. Davis (1956) was one of the first to indicate how time can be manipulated by medical staff. Writing about time and recovery in paralytic polio he points out that to elicit and maintain patient and family cooperation time must be redefined. In large measure this redefinition of time rests with the charismatic authority of the physician.

Regarding the child with polio, Davis said:

> . . . although a good deal of factual knowledge regarding the course of the disease is imparted to the parent, in polio, as in so many pathological conditions, much is unknown, and the practitioner is confronted by significant areas of therapeutic uncertainty. This uncertainty devolves for the most part on the socially crucial questions of the rate of recovery and the ultimate extent of disability with which the patient will be left. It is thus necessary for the doctor somehow to communicate to the parents that the uncertainty stems from the nature of the disease itself not from therapeutic incompetence or an unwillingness to speak the truth. (1956, p. 583).

This is not to say that patients and families do not 'shop around' for information. In a desperate desire for information and assurance, almost any source—nurses, aides, technicians and even other patients and families—may be sought out. Perhaps much of the discussion of x-ray results and laboratory results, which are treated in such detail, reflect less hypochondria and more of an attempt to fix time. Although Davis was writing about polio, much of what he says is equally true of the behaviour which transpires in a cancer center.

The cases they hear about display so much variability in onset and outcome that [they] soon come to feel that few, if any, generalizations are possible. All these frustrating encounters serve only to reinforce the doctor's initial injunction that 'much is unknown and only time will tell.' (1956, p. 584).

Clearly of importance in defining the metric of time are the structurally determined factors or therapeutic benchmarks which treatment entails. The schedules of CAT scans, hematology visits, inpatient stays for surgery or chemotherapy all impose a schedule to which patients must adjust. All of these force the patient and family into a time perspective in which the markers are at best vague and at worst non-existent. Events must occur in sequence and in order, but often the reason for enduring the hours, days, weeks, or months is never stated. patients wait with no sure knowledge of the goals or endpoints for which they wait. To adapt, patients often immerse themselves in a patient subculture where at least there are fellow sufferers.

Unlike traditional agricultural societies, which organize time around recurrent cycles, modern societies focus upon an ever-unfolding future. It is the disruption of this future which can accompany the diagnosis of cancer that requires the reconstruction of reality.

Uncertainty

In addition to the necessity of repeatedly creating a new reality as one's cancer progresses and treatments change, in addition to the problems of orienting oneself when time become the elusive concept that the preceding discussion suggests, the person with cancer must also manage uncertainty—the uncertainty created when one must face new threats.

Cohn and Lazarus (1979), after sifting through the work of others, generated the following list of threats which illness can create and to which the individual must respond (cope). Each of these threats can become a source of uncertainty.

1. Threats to life and fears of dying itself.
2. Threats to bodily intregrity and comfort (from illness, the diagnostic procedures, or the medical treatment itself)
   a. Bodily injury or disability
   b. Permanent physical changes
   c. Physical pain, discomfort, and other negative symptoms of illness or treatment
   d. Incapacitation.
3. Threats to one's self-concept and future plans
   a. Necessity to alter one's self-image or belief systems
   b. Uncertainty about the course of the illness and about one's future
   c. Endangering of life goals and values
   d. Loss of autonomy and control.
4. Threats to one's emotional equilibrium, that is, the necessity to deal with

feelings of anxiety, anger, and other emotions that come about as a result of other stresses described.

5. Threats to the fulfillment of customary social roles and activities
   a. Separation from family, friends, and other social supports
   b. Loss of important social roles
   c. Necessity to depend on others
6. Threats involving the need to adjust to a new physical or social environment
   a. Adjustment to the hospital setting
   b. Problems in understanding medical terminology and customs
   c. Necessity for decision making in stressful and unfamiliar situations (p.229)

Strauss and Glaser (1975), writing about chronic illness and the quality of life, point out that disease can cause multiple problems of daily living. These problems are of particular significant because problems demand solutions, and the quest for solutions creates uncertainty. Among the problems associated with any chronic illness, including cancer, cited by Glaser and Strauss are: (1) maintaining a life course geared to the anticipation and management of medical crisis; (2) controlling of symptoms; (3) carrying out a treatment regiment; (4) adjusting to social isolation; (5) adjusting to the trajectory of the disease; (6) attempting to normalize both one's interaction with others and one's style of life; and (7) finding the resources to pay for treatment and sustain a household.

These problems are accentuated where cancer is concerned, for as Holland (1973) points out, cancer's clinical course may range from complete cure, through remission of some duration to a clear downward trajectory to death. Each trajectory has associated with it unique unknowns and uncertainties and calls into play different psychosocial dynamics. In many ways the situation of the patient is not unlike that of the immigrant to a new and dramatically different culture.

Figure 9.1 is a modification of the model proposed by Holland (1973). As this model clearly suggests, each clinical course has associated with it unique sources of uncertainty, decisions to be made, new care providers with whom the patient must interact and new information to assimilate. The patient may even be faced with a new subculture, resulting, for example, from being shifted from a chemotherapy clinic to a radiology clinic. Regrettably, matters are further complicated by the fact that 'the complexities of therapeutic research often preclude full understanding on the part of the patient' (Holland, 1973, p. 495). Holland further contends that, where cancer is concerned, the situation is emotionally charged and the disease may be potentially life-threatening; thus 'it is dubious whether many individuals can make decisions objective.'

Uncertainty may also arise because, for cancer patients, response to treatment and improvement are difficult to define. A clinician can use x-ray evidence or the results of various laboratory procedures to objectify the

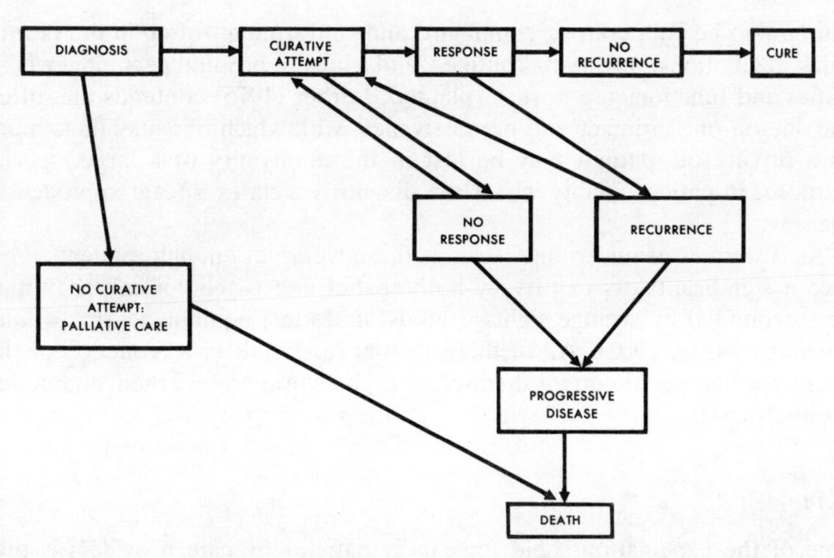

Figure 9.1: Alternative courses of cancer care (Adapted from Holland, 1973 p. 995).

progress of the disease. However, for patients and the friends and family of patients, outcomes are more problematic. Benchmarks are undefined (Roth, 1963).

Davis (1956) has demonstrated that in most circumstances we think of recovery from some ailment in terms of a spontaneous process. Clearly there may be one or more medical intervention, but 'the feeling of getting well is a subjective state which hardly requires definition' (p. 89). Often this is not the case.

> Questions can be raised as to whether the experience of recovery from any disease or ailment is ever as subjectively spontancous as we think, but, in particular, we refer to those conditions in which the precise course and extent of recovery are obscured by uncertainty factors and where, as a rule, the patients' state upon recovery [if recovery is possible] is significantly different from what it was originally. (Davis, p. 89)

Cancer—like mental disorders, some cardiac conditions, polio and other neurological conditions, such as MS—is unusual in that, without explanations and knowledge imparted by care providers, as well as the cues inherent in the treatment process, patients may be largely unaware of the progress of their disease. It may be that only when the patient receives a different institutional label that they have some marker to designate a new status.

Much of the uncertainty facing cancer patients is simply a dramatic extension of the uncertainty facing any hospitalized patient. Tagliacozzo and Mauksch (1972) argue that, to be a 'good patient,' the patient must figure out *how* to be cooperative, compliant, and conforming—often in the face of rules, regulations, unvarying routines, and a host of hospital personnel whose duties and functions are never explained. Lorber (1975) contends that often the one-on-one intimacy and permissiveness with which one may be familiar as a private out-patient may be lost in the anonymity of a large, special purpose, in-patient facility where the diagnosis dictates a team approach to therapy.

As if sources of uncertainty such as these were not enough, patients must face a significant loss of privacy both spatial and psychological; they may be surrounded by strange sights, sounds, uniforms, equipment, smells, and language (King, 1962). All of these factors can result in a reduction of the cues by which people orient themselves to the world around them and define a sense of self.

Pain

One of the expectations held for cancer patients by care providers is that pain and suffering are in some degree to be expected and accommodated. Black (1979) has pointed out that pain has a survival function, alerting individuals to injury or disease. 'In cancer, however, pain often persists far beyond its function as an initial alerting function. For the more than half the cancer patients with serious pain the pain's chronicity becomes a "debilitating and demoralizing" destructive force in the disease process' (Perrit and McDonnell, 1977). Ten years ago Melzack (1973) underscored the complex nature of pain and the crucial role played by the victim's psychosocial status in the pain process. Even earlier Leshan (1964) wrote of concomitant feelings of 'meaninglessness,' 'helplessness,' and 'hopelessness' associated with long-term chronic pain. Kotarba (1983) has offered some significant insights into the pain phenomenon which are relevant for cancer patients in general and for that 75% of terminal cancer patients who are in unremitting pain (Twycross, 1973). Kotarba points out that enduring or living with chronic pain implies coping, and coping is 'inherently a social enterprise' because (1) pain-afflicted people rarely passively accept their suffering, but rather rely on others in their attempt to give meaning to their plight, and (2) the pain may be a *constant* experience of discomfort which is carried with the patient into all social encounters. Kotarba argues:

> . . . [S]ocial meanings serve to define the pain-afflicted person's very being or self. Since the sufferer faces uncertain resolution of the dilemma, the experience of coping with chronic pain has implications for the individual's occupational and interpersonal relationships and, therefore, self-esteem and social status. In order to preserve self-esteem, the sick person attempts to present his or her condition correctly to others in interaction, according to the norms of face-to-face interaction in effect in each particular social situation. (p. 23).

As early as 1961, Davis offered the process of 'Deviance Disavowal' as the technique by which those with visible conditions attempt to normalize their conditions by removing their 'true selves' from the handicap which they define as discrediting. In an elaboration of this idea and an extension of it to the notion of chronic pain, Kotarba (1983) states:

> In situations in which pain-afflicted persons disclose their suffering to others, they feel obliged to demonstrate that they are reacting properly to their condition. Competent pain-afflicted persons, for example, demonstrate emotional control over the pain, even when in their own minds they feel that they are not coping well, and talk about their doctors as being the 'best' available practitioners even when they personally feel little confidence in the effectiveness of their doctors. Competency is also directed toward health care workers through techniques ranging from requests for help, as opposed to demands for a cure, to the display of faithful diligence to prescribed exercises whether or not these exercises are in fact undertaken. (p. 24).

Adaptation to Others

In the process of cognitively adapting to cancer, the person necessarily must re-order his relationships to others. This point is apparent when one simply lists just some of the classes of people upon whose roles cancer impacts and who in turn define the roles of the cancer patient. Twaddle (1979), writing about status definers—those who have an influence on the definition of one's level of health—has offered the following:

I. Primary Relationships
   A. Parents
   B. Spouse
   C. Children
   D. Other Relatives
   E. Friends
   F. Co-workers
   G. Neighbors

II. Secondary Relationships
   A. Religioius
   B. Commercial
   C. Medical
      Physician
      Nurses
      Technician
      Pharmacists
   D. Others.

For example, with reference to primary relationships, some patients were forced to decide how and what to discuss with family and friends, and were even faced with the burden of protecting them from the harsh realities. Even doing better than expected can create adaptive problems. Maher (1982) studied cancer patients who survived beyond the norm for their diagnosis. The recurrent themes reported indicate some of the sources of difficulty in adaptation which can emerge even under the best of circumstances. Although these findings were not presented as such, the implications are clear that patients were uncertain about such matters as the withdrawal of intense levels of social support given earlier in the disease process; the level and extent of residual disability; the need to focus on a future orientation to time after having begun to think of termination; and, finally, feelings of depression and loss when roles to which one has adapted are no longer legitimate.

Of special relevance for the management of the patient (Holland, 1976; Bean *et al.*, 1980; Cohn, 1982; Lazarus, 1982) are the mutual adaptations required of the cancer patient and helping personnel, adaptations that are to a degree required of all people who play the sick role or patient role.

The 'sick role,' discriminated from health and illness behaviours (Mechanic, 1962), may be described as those societally defined behaviours which prescribe and proscribe what are appropriate behavioural norms for a member of the group who, through no fault of his/her own, is incapable of meeting the expectations held for them. In its original formulation by Parsons (1951) the concern was more with aggregates than with individuals, and, as many critics have pointed out, it made certain assumptions about the ways in which both physicians and patients were to act. The sick person was not to be held reponsible for his or her condition, was to be excused from normal or routine role obligations, was to recognize that being sick was undesirable and was obligated to seek competent help. In fulfilling the expectations held for physicians, one was to have and apply technical competency, be affectively neutral (non-judgmental), hold a collectivity orientation (universalistic) and have functional specificity, limiting behaviour to purely medically related matters. To merge these two sets of expectations, the process was facilitated by the inherent asymmetrical nature of the relationship, with power residing with the physician.

Subsequent writing and research has modified, augmented and refuted parts of this formulation (cf. Gallagher, 1978). The dynamic nature of the relationship has been demonstrated, the middle-class bias of the formulation has been criticized and the lack of relevance for chronic conditions all have been addressed. Here the concern is that this view, while valuable for sociologists, fails to handle adequately the dynamics of a more narrow aspect of the phenomenon: the expectations held for individuals who are *patients*.

> As societal efforts to cope further with illness and injury develop, facilities and services evolve to diagnose and treat those afflicted. In the organization of these treatment settings a specific role is defined for those persons who receive their services and efforts, which is the patient role.
>
> The patient role should not be confused with the aforementioned sick role. The larger

society defines the legitimate entry into the sick role; whereas the treatment setting, as a significant component of the larger society, establishes the criteria of normative behaviour and expectations of the recipients of its attention and healing efforts, and this defines the role of 'patient' in that social organization and system. (Jaco, 1979, p. 184).

Clearly the nature of the patient role is variable, being a function of diagnosis, prognosis, therapeutic regimen, and treatment setting, All individuals in the role of patients are legitimate occupants of the sick role as well. Further, the general role of patient may carry with it a number of other more specific roles; a cancer patient may simultaneously occupy the roles of surgical patient, terminal patient, or pediatric patient, in addition to the countless other social roles, each role acquiring special adaptations to others. In short, while *disease* may be viewed as a purely biological or physical phenomenon, cancer is an *illness* and as such it is 'an event that takes place in a social context and influences and is influenced by the intimate association of the person with other people' (King, 1972, p. 129).

A major task facing the cancer patient is to learn the 'patient role,' to minimize uncertainty by learning the role expectations held for them by the care providers. Existing research would indicate that the ideal patient is expected to be dependent, but not too dependent, to deemphasize external power and prestige, to accept the fact that pain and suffering are part of treatment, etc. The work of Bean *et al.* (1980) suggests that, for cancer patients, trying to be a 'good patient' may be an attempt to deal with uncertainty. In addition to the often reported mechanisms of repression, filtering of information, 'regression, and denial a substantial number of patients appear to transfer' all decision-making power to the physician or the oncologic team—clear indications of uncertainity. Learning the patient role also reflects the adaptation to what they perceive as the expectations of more powerful treatment personnel:

[T]hese patients were concerned with the possible negative reactions of the medical staff if they learned of any critical comments. Their fears of possible retribution are symptomatic of the patients' feelings of powerlessness . . . (Bean *et al.*, 1980, p. 259)

A number of major works have been published which deal with the issue of the asymmetric relationship between the dominant care provider on the one hand, and the patient on the other. The role of cancer patient cannot be defined as apart from the reciprocal role of care provider. Talcott Parsons (1951) has in effect specified the assymmetrical basis of the physicians' superior role, high technical competence, emotional neutrality, and collectivity orientation. Fox (1957) adds that, unlike patients, physicians are trained to deal with uncertainty. Further, the physician is part of a more inclusive social network. The relative powerlessness of the patient is accented by the organization of medical practice. Historically, as Friedson (1960) has pointed out, the care provider is most usually defined as 'a colleague in the structure of institutions and organizations, the patient being an essentially minor contingency.' Such constraint as is experienced is provided by the care providers' relationship to colleagues, institutions and the state. However, the patient as consumer, *potentially* at least, exercises somo power.

> . . . [W]hile the physician may share special knowledge, identity and loyalty with colleagues rather than laymen, he is dependent upon laymen for his livelihood. Where he does not have the power to force them to use his services, he depends upon the free choice of prospective patients. But, since these prospective clients are in no position to evaluate his services as would his colleagues, and insofar as they do exercise choice, it follows that they must evaluate him by non-professional criteria and that they will interact with him on the basis of non-professional norms. (Friedson, 1959, p. 375).

This potential, however, is seldom realized. For the oncologist, as for other specialists, this potential source of client control is lessened when the patient is unable to seek care in an open-market fashion. The care provider has the option of relying less on a lay referral system and more upon the 'Community of Colleagues.' Professional values may override personal values and the practitioners' reference or audience group may be fellow physicians rather than patients.

However, the medical profession may be heir to changes that are occurring in other areas of society. The assymmetrical nature of this relationship may be changing as more patients respond to feelings of rising consumerism and equal rights for women. Pressures such as these may transform passive patients into much more active participants in the clinical encounter, more questioning or demanding—thus, eroding physician authority. The physician's social skills may take on more importance than charismatic role attributes.

Commenting on the nature of the interaction, Szasz and Hollander (1956) described the shifting nature of the interaction as dictated by the nature of the illness. Hayes-Bautista (1976b) documented the ways in which physician and patient negotiate over a treatment regimen; Stewart and Buck (1977), building on the work of others (cf. Hulka *et al.*, 1971; Hull, 1972), found that physicians are typically not very aware of the socio-emotional problems of their patients and, more importantly, even when they are, physicians are not very adept at dealing with these problems.

Engles (1977) offers six reasons why physicians must take into account the dynamic negotiation with patients over what he calls the 'biopsychosocial' aspects of the patient. First, psychosocial aspects influence diagnosis. Patients with identical physiological patterns and laboratory findings may vary in the severity of their illnesses. Second, patients' reports must be weighted on the basis of these factors to secure reliable data upon which to make an accurate diagnosis. Third, psychosocial factors, in part, determine for both the patients and patients' families the definition and meaning of illness. Fourth, psychosocial factors frequently interact with the disease to determine severity. Fifth, clinical variations in response to treatment frequently stem from psychosocial factors. And finally, the socio-emotional relationship between patient and care provider can influence the rate of recovery.

From the foregoing it is abundantly clear that the management of cancer patients rests not solely with the inherent dynamics of the patient but at least in part upon the very human constraints and dynamics which impact upon the providers of care (cf. Hayes, 1976; Davis, 1972; Krant, 1976; Greenwald and Nevitt, 1982). What is important here is the fact that the 'objective application of medical science' transpires within a sociocultural matrix, is a function of the quality of 'human interaction,' and is conditioned by the influence of the larger medical profession (Bloom, 1963).

Although stil limited, the amount of attention directed toward the physician's role in patient management has offered some important points. Studying physicians and cancer patients, Greenwald and Nevitt (1982) point out that:

> Previous inquiries in medical sociology and psychology suggest that the physician's attitude—personality, socialization, and practice surroundings, for example—can affect his or her inclination to communicate disturbing informatiion . . . . (p. 591).

Informing and educating a cancer patient about the diagnosis and prognosis is crucial if patients are to submit to needed therapies, yet some physicians are less capable, emotionally, of dealing with life-threatening conditions and to gauge, therefore, 'the form, content, and timing of commmunications as objectively as possible' (p. 591).

Over 20 years ago, Oken (1961) reported:

> Instead of logic and rational decisions based on clinical observation, what is found is opinion, belief, and conviction, heavily weighted with irrational justification. (p. 87).

More recently, Krants' observations would indicate that if there are failures in the dynamic process of interaction about cancer between doctor and patient, the difficulty lies, at least in part, in: (1) the physician's attitudinal domain, i.e., the biases and assumptions held by the physician; (2) the physician's cognitive domain, i.e., what (s)he knows or does not know about cancer management; and (3) the psychological domain—what motivates his/her behavior without conscious recognition.

Krant contends that, because of the public view of cancer, physicians are cast in the role of 'condemner of the flesh and spirit' and may reflect feelings of fatalism and pessimism. Furthermore, many physicians may have high death anxiety and feelings that any patient death represents a failure. Additionally, the emotional needs of the patient are seen as possibly creating 'a regressive need in patients for an omnipotent protecting parent physician' and the physician response may be an inappropriate sensation of power (a feeling that influences other care providers as well). To the extent that the physician finds this situation ego-gratifying, a failing patient may be blamed and avoided. The interplay of these factors and many others may result in feelings of anxiety and helplessness, and the physician may compensate by 'rushing into many experimental tasks and tests and this in turn may lead to three-way problems with patients, families, and medical staff.'

Regrettably, little in medical education is designed to prepare physicians to deal with problems such as these. Prejudices, poor attitudes and negative feelings are not systematically addressed.

To quote Krant (1976) on cancer:

> The failure to explore, even at a superficial level, some of the deep-seated feelings that physicians bring to medicine may well solidify certain attitudes behind great defensive walls. Such defended biases and perspectives, although not seen as problems by the physician, certainly produce an endless series of problems for patients and families. (p. 273)

The review by Hayes (1976) would confirm this notion.

There have been repeated calls for care providers to communicate more or better with cancer patients. Abeloff (1979) devotes an entire chapter to this subject. Speaking of primary care practitioners, Rosser and Maguire (1982) report:

> . . . [N]ot only is the practitioner's knowledge of this disease limited due to the generic nature of his work; but also, the body of knowledge which he represents, and through which he claims the trust of his patients, is full of uncertainty and controversy. Discussion of these issues with patients, therefore, presents a personal threat to practitioners themselves. Far from being ignorant of patients' and families' problems, many of the practitioners are acutely aware of the possible problems. Thus, in explaining their reluctance to investigate, they speak of opening 'Pandora's box,' a 'hornet's nest,' 'a can of worms,' or 'letting the fiend out of the bag.' (p. 321)

'Cancer specialists' are seen by Dickinson and Pearson (1979) as holding more positive attitudes toward dealing with the gravely ill. Yet there is some evidence that this generalization may not always hold. The work of McIntosh (1974) would seem to indicate that if the physician does not know the patient well enough to feel capable of predicting his/her response that the majority practice 'the ruling that patients should not be told.' Physicians too are complex human beings whose training cannot always override emotional needs and personal values.

Thomas Scheff (1963) was perhaps the first to attempt an explanation for the wide divergence between physicians based less upon patient attributes and structural characteristics and more upon the physician's value system. Although he did not specifically make the case, he did argue that a normative perspective exists, that failing to treat a 'sick' person is somehow of greater concern than needlessly treating a 'well' person. Clearly this normative perspective is one reinforced by social values, legal precedents, the self-interest of the physician, as well as the expectations of patients. The implication raised is that different physicians, for whatever reason, may differentially apply the normative perspective.

Haney (1971) elaborated on the possibility that physicians may develop a distinctive decision-making set, arguing on the bases of relevant literature, medical school curricula and the observations that at least three strategies are discernable. One strategy, put forth by Szasz and Hollander, suggested that the physician, by training or inclination, may be more adept at one mode of patient – practitioner interaction than another and thus more or less capable of dealing with specific patients' psychosocial needs. Another dimension of this decision-making set can best be described as the tendency to adopt an interventionist attitude toward diagnosis and treatment as opposed to the inclination to 'wait and see,' or a conservative orientation (similar to Scheff's discussion). Finally, is the decision-making strategy based upon the degree to which medicine is defined as art or science? If science, then the practice of medicine may tend to be disease- or organ system-specific; if art, then a more holistic view may be taken. The work of Rosser and Maguire (1982) illustrates some of these elements in regard to the general practitioner care of the cancer patient.

> . . . [T]he impact of cancer stems from its elusiveness; it challenges the claim of medicine to control disease through intervention based on scientific knowledge. Moreover, for the general practitioner, the body of knowledge upon which their expertise is based is sadly inadequate as an explanatory framework within their daily practice. It cannot account for why a particular individual should contract the disease, nor can it predict how that individual will respond to treatment. For the patient experiencing the disease and for the practitioner caring for that patient, these are crucial, unanswered questions. (p. 317)

THE INTERACTIVE NATURE OF CANCER MANAGEMENT

Clearly, the psychosocial dynamics impacting upon the cancer patient are extremely complex and subject to extreme variability. The psychological reactions and responses of the cancer patient have been extensively researched. But comparitively little has been reported on the psychosociocultural factors that influence the role of the care provider, the care recipient or the interaction among these factors. Thus, the conclusion drawn by Wortman and Dunkel-Schetter (1979) that there is no clear and consistent picture to be drawn of the cancer may still be valid.Even less is known about the interaction that transpires between patient and care provider.

That which follows is an attempt to model some of the principles and processes as they occur in the management of cancer patients. It has been argued that cancer patients face monumental psychosocial and sociocultural problems subsequent to diagnosis. It has further been suggested that those who treat cancer patients have problems of their own to contend with. This model is concerned with the outcome that results when the two are intertwined.

One of the reviews of the physician – patient relationship as a truly interactional process is that of Anderson and Helm (1979), who describe the encounter as a negotiation of reality. Based upon the assumption that 'reality is socially constructed' (Berger and Luchmann, 1967), Anderson and Helm stress the social and environmental factors influencing each participant's definition of the situation. A process of negotiation must occur for a consensus on the reality of the situation to emerge. Basic to the process of negotiation is the fact that the encounter is a social process which occurs as a given place where the exchange and evaluation of information results. Anderson and Helm concede that the relationship is asymmetrical, favoring the physician's reality; however, they maintain that the process is 'complex, conflictual, and socially defined.'

What is proposed here is a model which includes the threads of existing models of interaction, plus the salient empirical regularities observed regarding the physician – cancer patient encounter. Here, the approach to the analysis of cancer patient management is to examine the behavior of the individual participants in the system—potential recipients of treatment and 'professionals' who recommend and administer treatment—and the result of the interaction between these two. In order to understand behavior, the decision-making process of the individuals involved must be examined. It is assumed that observable behavior is preceded by decisions, either proximal or distal. Every action is not, however, necessarily the result of an immediate decision. Because individuals tend to be effort minimizers, a large proportion of behavior is habitual, i.e., reflexive or nonconscious. Garfinkel (1967) has proposed that, in the main, people respond to the world about them on the basis of decision rules, habits, and routines of daily living and do not ponder over every decision, although contextual and structural factors do modify the process. This type of behavior can be viewed as having two possible origins: either past repetitive decisions which have been made by the individual and which have resulted in a learned, often nonconscious, successful response to a given pattern of stimuli, or a successful response to a given pattern or stimulus which has been developed by a cultural group and is passed on to each generation. (The care provider may be influenced more by the former; the patient, the latter.) In either case, these habitual patterns of behavior may be re-evaluated. This may be the result of either new knowledge which provides information about previously unknown alternatives, or the failure of habitual behavior to achieve the desired results.

Cancer Patients

A first approximation to an analysis of individual decision making is shown in Figure 2. It is assumed that the purpose of individual decisions is to change the individual's state from a less preferred condition. At a given moment in time, the evaluation of an individual's state is a subjective process which is carried out in terms of his or her personal value structure. The personal value structure can be described by the willingness of the individual to choose between two sources of positive stimuli. It is based upon the complex interaction of personality, cultural background and formal education. The value structure may contain absolute, overriding positive or negative value, which frequently reflects religious beliefs.

The perceived alternatives available to an individual are derived from the adaphic, or biophysical, economic, and social environment within which the individual exists and an awareness of the conditions of the individual's own physiological state.

The raw data, i.e., stimuli received by the individual, are processed or interpreted through an interacting knowledge and perception filter. Knowledge and experience consist of the individual's understanding of the environmental system within which he or she exists and the physiological status of his or her body. This is derived primarily from the individual's cultural background and formal education. The level of sophistication of an individual's knowledge can vary along a continuum, ranging from simple prescriptions such as, 'If you speak pleasantly to others, they will be nice to you,' to complex models consiting of relationships within the environment and the interaction among relationships.

Individuals who in the past have experienced a variety of environments either by moving among cultural groups or who belong to cultural groups which exist in a rapidly changing environment will have modified their knowledge based upon these personal and group experiences. These experiences usually take the form of discovering that existing behavior prescriptions do not achieve the desired positive results, or that additional alternatives exist. A search for new behavior prescriptions is carried out and the successful ones are incorporated into the knowledge base.

The individual's perception of stimuli is a function of his or her knowledge and sensory competence. In any given situation, an individual is bombarded with stimuli. A large amount of effort would be required to process all of these data. In order to minimize this effort, the individual will classify stimuli into a relevant and an irrelevant group. The latter is either perceived and ignored or not perceived, by a subconscious process of elimination. The criteria for this classification system are derived from the individual's knowledge base, psychological needs and place in the social matrix.

In the area of health behavior the decision-making process of a potential recipient of treatment can be intially analyzed within the context of the question, 'What underlies a decision by the individual to consult a professional for advice and/or assistance, adapt to information given, and comply with advice?'

As of the time when a decision is made, two sets of influences on the individual can be identified: those which are external and those which are internal to the individual. The external influences represent the environment within which the individual exists. This can be viewed as representing the fundamental trade-offs over which the individual has no direct control. It is useful to divide the environment into two parts: first, the economic and social environment which deals with the individual's role and interaction with others in the society and is part of the subject of study of the various social sciences; second, the adaphic, or biophysical environment, differs from the economic and social environment, not only according to the classification system of traditional disciplines, but also because the individual does not always receive stimuli which can be interpreted as descriptions of the condition of this part of the environment.

The internal influences, in turn, can be divided into the physiological and psychosocial status of the person. The former is the result of the intitial genetic endowment, aging process, and past exposures to the adaphic and social environment. The latter determines the personal knowledge and perceptions through which the individual processes and interprets information about the external environment and his or her own physiological state. A complementary process is the acquisition of habitual forms of behavior. Because this type of behavior is keyed to fixed sets of stimuli, it also enters into the data interpretation process.

After being filtered through the individual's knowledge and perception, the filtered personal and environmental information represent the individual's perception of his present state and the available alternatives. The decision process consists of making a selection from the available alternatives. In order to do this, a set of personal values is required which allows the individual to identify the most desired state (or states). At a given time, these values are derived from the totality of an individual's past experiences and his personality characteristics.

Care Providers

There are two reasons for differentiating the decision process of the 'professionals' from the potential recipients of treatment. The first is that, in his or her role as a professional, the individual is making decisions within the context of a specialized knowledge base which is not completely available to other individuals in the society. The second is that professional decisions are made specifically to change the state of the recipient of the treatment. This

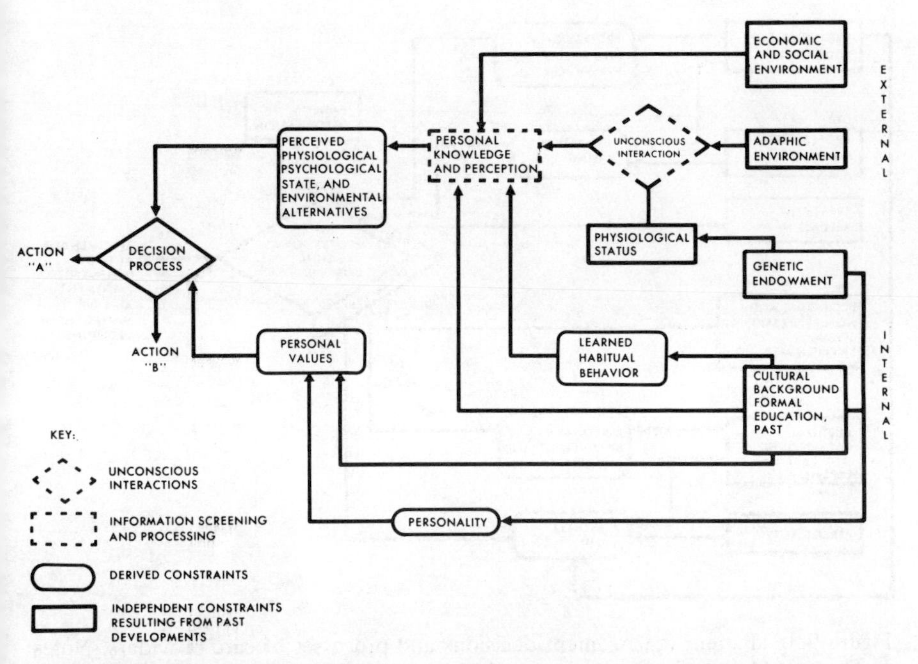

Figure 9.2: Decision Processes and adaptations of cancer patients.

requires providing information to the recipient who must, in turn, make decisions.

Figure 9.3 presents the elements of the professional decision-making process. The lower half is a summary of the personal decision-making process of any individual shown in Figure 9.2. It is included to indicate the influence of personal characteristics on the professional decision. The upper half shows the components of the professional background and environment which enter into the professional decision-making process. Separating the professional from the non-professional components of the professional decision-making process is not meant to imply that within the decision-making matrix the two sets do not interact with each other. (It should be noted that personal values are shown as being influenced by professional education. This, however, has taken place in the past and not at the time a given decision is made.)

The basic structure of the professional components of the decision-making process is the same as that of the personal components. Professional knowledge, however, is restricted to the model of the system the professional is dealing with, i.e., the 'disease model,' or 'medical models' in the case of a health professional. In this case, the model or system also provides criteria for developing an information screen.

Professional values, in contrast with personal values, represent a combination of value structures which the professional uses to make decisions of

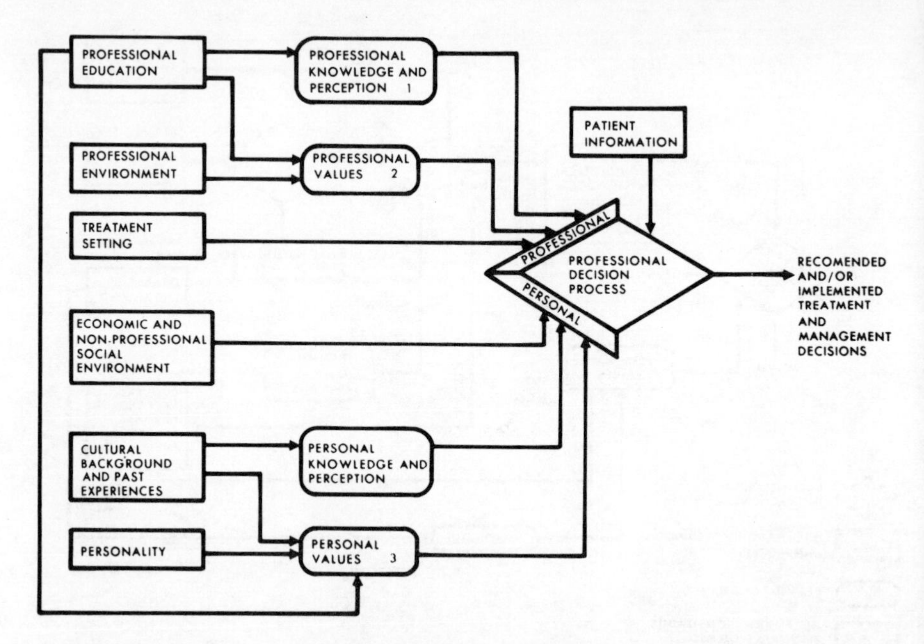

Figure 9.3: Patient management decisions and processes of care providers. Notes: 1. Disease Model. 2. Constraints and risk aversion with respect to patient cost. 3. Includes risk aversion with respect to personal cost of the professional.

the recipient of treatment, and the acceptance or non-acceptance of the professional group's constraints.

Professional decisions are based upon two sets of values with respect to risk. The first is the value placed on probable failure which will be borne by the recipient of the service. This evaluation is based upon professional values. The second is the value placed upon probable failure which will be borne by the profesional. This is based upon personal values.

Interaction Between a Provider and Recipient of Services

What can be observed is the behavior which results from the decision-making process of each participant in the transaction process (shown by the pointed boxes in Figure 9.4). This behavior is the result of initial decisions and then modified decisions based upon information received from the other member of the transaction. Information is shown going through a filter to account for language and professional vocabulary differences between the professional and the recipient of the service.

The transaction process is a feedback loop where each participant makes new decisions based upon the information received. Information flow, however, is not symmetrical for two reasons. The information filter affects

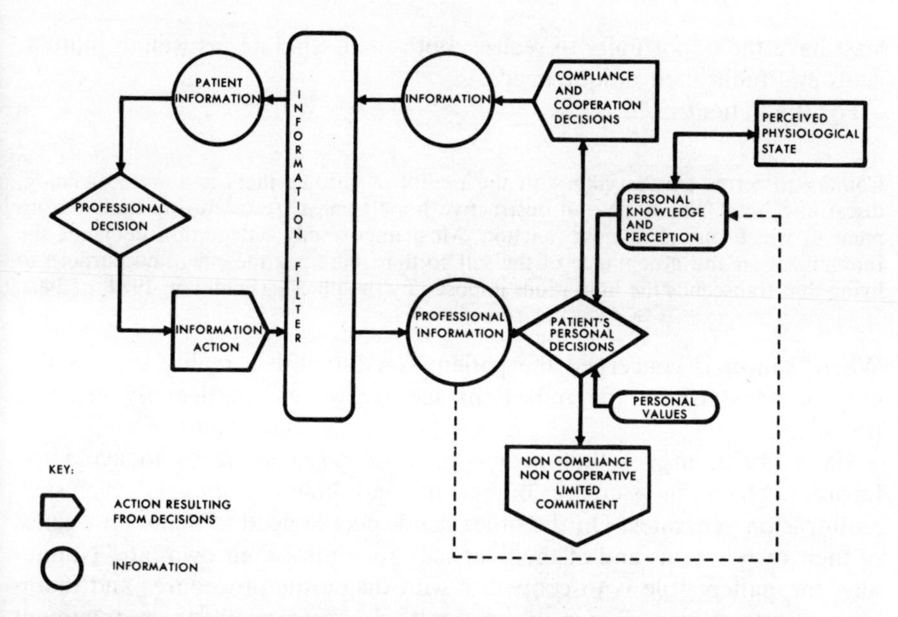

Figure 9.4: Interaction of decision of cancer patients and care providers.

the transmission of both instructions from the professional to the recipient of services and the verbal information of results from the recipient to the professional.

The sources of the information available to each party are not the same. The professional receives information either verbally from the recipient or in the form of direct machine measurements and observations of the recipient's physical state. In either case (with the exception of the problem of the information filter), the professional is in a position to process information which is independent on his or her personal situation.

The recipient receives information from two sources: the information from the professional and information about his or her personal state. The latter must be interpreted in the context of the individual's personal structure of knowledge and perceptions.

SUMMARY

Everyone in the course of life has achieved some measure of adaptation to life. When a chronic disease such as cancer disrupts this adaptation, the demands of life and the expectations of others are altered, but their intensity remains the same, or even greater than before the illness. Often, however, the capacity to respond in an effective and satisfying way is diminished (Dimond, 1983). The goal of ideal patient management is to establish a shared reality—a concordance—so that each participant can realize, or at least have the opportunity to realize, both their separate, as well as mutual, goals and fulfill their unique needs.

For the patient:

> Coming to terms existentially with the reality of chronic illess is a state of being, discarding both false hope and destructive hopelessness, restructuring the environment in which one must now function. Most importantly, adaptation demands the reorganization and acceptance of the self so that there is a meaning and purpose to living that transcends the limitations imposed by the illness. (Feldman, 1974, p. 290).

Where cancer is concerned the patient can establish a reality such as this only on the basis of the reflections seen in others, particularly the care providers.

Haan (1979) argues that people have deep-seated needs to avoid the intrusion which illness creates in their life and the powerlessness which such an intrusion generates. On the other hand, people need to maintain a sense of their own options and of their capacity to control their own fate. Nominally, the patient role is to cooperate with diagnostic procedures and therapeutic instructions. Generally, patients cooperate with their treatment regimen and try to be 'patient' while the medical staff takes the responsibility for care and cure. This is the role offered to them. In the patient role, however, there is a strong tendency for people to mute their 'natural propensities to cope' on their own behalf. They react very differently in response to patienthood than they do when faced with other, more ordinary, problems of living. This can lead to an extremely imbalanced relationship. As Parsons (1951) and Engels (1977) indicate, societal expectations are such that care providers are likely to be placed in the counter-productive, emotionally and morally untenable position of taking unilateral responsibility for the passive – receptive patient. Because this sort of one-sided relationship runs counter to human nature, both physician and patient are likely to be confused, stressed, and defensive—a negotiated reality impossible and concordance lacking.

The diagnosis of cancer stimulates the person's cognitive reconstruction of reality partly in response to the very real personal threats posed by this condition, and partly as a necessary adjustment to it. The reconstruction of reality implicates the person's interpersonal matrix, a not inconsiderable part of which is the medical management team. The course and management of the illness will depend only in part upon the technical skills of the treatment personnel. The patient's ultimate adjustment to the reality of the disorder, to the frequently unrealistic fears associated with diagnosis of the condition, and to the psychosocial stress *implicated in the treatment process itself* will also depend upon the interpersonal management skills of the professional staff. The development of these skills will follow inevitably upon their recognition of their role in the control they may exercise on the ordinarily stress-inducing treatment milieu.

REFERENCES

Abeloff, M. D. (1979). Communication with the patient, in *Complications of Cancer: Diagnosis and Management* (Ed. M. D. Abeloff), pp. 1–15, Johns Hopkins University Press, Baltimore.

Anderson, W. T., and Helm, D. (1979). The physician-patient encounter: A process of reality negotiation, in *Patients, Physicians, and Illness*, 3rd Edn (Ed. E. G. Jaco), pp. 259–271, The Free Press, New York.

Bean, G., Cooper, S., Alpert, R., and Kipnis, D. (1980). Coping mechanisms of cancer patients: A study of 33 patients receiving chemotherapy, *CA-A Journal For Clinicians*, **30**,256–259.

Berger, P., and Luchmann, T. (1967). *The Social Construction of Reality*, Anchor Books, New York.

Black, Perry (1979). Management of pain, in *Complications of Cancer Diagnosis and Management* (Ed. M. D. Abeloff), pp. 91–119, Johns Hopkins University Press, Baltimore.

Bloom, S. (1963). *The Doctor and His Patient*, Free Press, New York.

Cohn, F. and Lazarus, R. S. (1979). Coping with the stress of illness, in *Health Psychology: A Handbook* (Eds. G. C. Stone, F. Cohn, N. Adler, *et al.*), pp. 217–254, Jossey-Bass, Washington.

Cohn, M. M. (1982), Psychosocial, morbidity in cancer: A clinical perspective, in *Psychosocial Aspects of Cancer* (Eds. J. Cohn, *et al.*), pp. 117–127, Raven Press, New York.

Davis, F. (1956). Definitions of time and recovery in paralytic polio convalescence, *American Journal of Sociology*, **61**, 582–587.

Davis, F. (1961). Deviance avowal: The management of strained interaction by the visibly handicapped, *Social Problems*, **9**, 120–132.

Davis, F. (1972). *Illness, Interaction and the Self*, Wadsworth, Belmont, California.

Dickinson, G. E., and Pearson, A. A. (1976). Differences in attitudes toward terminal patients in selected medical specialties of physicians, *Medical Care*, **17**, 682–685.

Dimond, M. (1983). Social adaptation of the chronically ill, in *Handbook of Health, Health Care, and the Health Professions* (Ed. D. Mechanic), pp. 636–654, Free Press, New York.

Engels, G. L. (1977). The need for a new medical model: A challenge for bismedicine, *Science*, **196**, 129–136.

Feldman, D. (1974). Chronic disabling illness: A holistic view, *Journal of Chronic Disease*, **27**, 287–291.

Fox, R. (1957). Training for uncertainty, in *The Student Physician* (Eds. R. K. Merton, G. Reader and P. L. Kendall), pp. 207–241, Harvard University Press, Cambridge, Mass.

Fox, R. (1959). *Experiment Perilous*, The Free Press, Glencoe, Ill.

Freidson, E. (1960). Client control and medical practice, *American Journal of Sociology*, **65**, 374–382.

Gallagher, E. B. (Ed.) (1978). *The Doctor – Patient Relationship in the Changing Health Science*, U.S. Department of Health, Education, and Welfare, Washington, D.C.

Garfinkel, H. (1967). *Studies in Ethnomethodology*, Prentice-Hall, Englewood Cliffs, N.J.

Glaser, B. H. (1966). Disclosure of terminal illness, *Journal of Health and Human Behavior*, 7, 83–91.

Greenwald, H. P., and Nevitt, M. (1982). Physician attitudes toward communication with cancer patients, *Social Science and Medicine*, **16**, 591–594.

Haan, N. G. (1979). Psychosocial meanings, of unfavorable medical forcast, in *Health Psychology: A Handbook* (Eds. G. C. Stone, F. Cohn, N. Adler *et al.*), pp. 113–140, Jossey Bass, Washington, D.C.

Haney, C. A. (1971). Psychosocial Aspects in training for medical decision-making, in *Psychosocial Aspects of Medical Training* (Eds. R. H. Coombs and C. E. Vincent), pp. 404–425, C. C. Thomas, Springfield, Ill.

Hayes-Bautista, D. (1976a). Termination of the patient – practitioner relationships: Divorce, patient style, *Journal of Health and Social Behavior*, **17**, 12–22.

Hayes-Bautista, D. (1976b). Modifying the treatment: Patient compliance, patient control and medical care, *Social Science and Medicine*, **10**, 233–238.

Hayes, D. M. (1976). The impact of the health care system on physician attitudes and behaviors, in *Cancer: The Behavioral Dimensions* (Eds. J. W. Cullen, B. H. Fox and R. N. Isom), pp. 145–157, Raven Press, New York.

Hinton, J. (1973). The influence of previous personality on reactions to having terminal cancer, *Omega*, **6**, 2–10.

Holland, J. (1973). Psychologic aspect of cancer, in *Cancer Medicine* (Eds. J. F. Holland and E. Fre, III), pp. 991–1021, Lea and Febiger, Philadelphia.

Holland, J. C. B. (1976). Coping with cancer: A challenge to the behavioral sciences, in *Cancer: The Behavioral Dimension's* (Eds. J. W. Cullen, B. W. Fox and R. N. Isom), pp. 263–268, Raven Press, New York.

Hulka, B. S., Kupper, L., Cassel, J. C. and Mayo, F. (1971). A method for measuring physicians' awareness of patients' concerns, *HSMHA Health Reports*, **86**, 741–753.

Hull, F. M. (1972). How well does the general practitioner know his patients?, *Practitioner*, **108**, 688–691.

Jaco, E. G. (1979). Caring for the ill: The patient-role, in *Patients, Physicians, and Illness*, 3rd Edn (Ed. E. G. Jaco), p. 184, The Free Press, New York.

King, S. H. 81962). *Perceptions of Illness and Medical Practice*, Russell Sage Foundation, New York.

King, S. H. (1972). Social-psychological factors in illness, in *Handbook of Medical Sociology*, 2nd Edn (Eds. H. E. Freeman, S. Levine and L. G. Reeder), pp. 129–147, Prentice-Hall, Englewood Cliffs, N.J.

Kluckhohn, F. R. (1955). Dominant and Variant Value Orientations, in *Personality in Nature, Society, and Culture*, 2nd Edn (Eds. C. Kluckhohn, H. A. Murray and D. M. Schneider), pp. 342–357, Alfred A. Knopf, New York.

Kotarba, J. A. (1983). *Chronic Pain: Its Social Dimension*, Sage Publications, Beverly Hill, California.

Krant, M. J. (1976). Problems of the physician in presenting the patient with the diagnosis, in *Cancer: The Behavioral Dimensions* (Eds. J. W. Cullen, B. H. Fox and R. N. Isom), pp. 269–274, Raven Press, New York.

Lazarus, R. S. (1982). Stress and coping as factors in health and illness, in *Psychosocial Aspects of Cancer*, pp. 163–190, Raven Press, New York.

Leshan, L. (1964). The world of the patient in severe pain of long duration, *Journal of Chronic Disease*, **17**, 119–126.

Lindemann, E. (1944). Symptomatology and management of acute grief, *American Journal of Psychiatry*, **101**, 141–148.

Lorber, J. (1975). Good patients and problem patients: Conformity and deviance in a general hospital, *Journal of Health and Social Behavior*, **16**, 213–225.
Mages, N. L., and Mendelsohn, G. A. (1979). Effects of cancer on patients lives: A personological approach, in *Health Psychology: A Handbook* (Eds. G. C. Stone, F. Cohn, N. Adler *et al.*), pp. 255–284, Jossey-Bass, Washington, D.C.
Maher, E. L. (1982), Anomic aspects of recovery from cancer, *Social Science and Medicine*, **16**, 907–912.
McIntosh, J. (1974). Process of communication, information seeking and control associated with cancer: A selective review of the literature, *Social Science and Medicine*, **8**, 167–187.
Mechanic, S. (1962). the concept of illness behavior, *Journal of Chronic Disease*, **15**, 189–194.
Melzack, R. (1973). *The Puzzle of Pain*, Penguin, Harmondsworth, England.
Murray, H. A. (1938). *Explorations in Personality*, Oxford University Press, New York.
Oken. D. (1961). What to tell cancer patients, *Journal of the American Medical Association*, **86**, 86–94.
Parsons, T. (1951). *The Social System*, The Free Press, Glencoe, Ill.
Paul, B. D. (Ed.) (1955). *Health, Culture and Community*, p. 467, Russell Sage Foundation, New York.
Perritt, G., and McDonnell, D. (1977). Neurosurgical control of pain in the patient with cancer, *Current Problems in Cancer*, **1**, 1–27.
Rosser, J. E., and Maguire, P. (1982). Dilemmas in general practice: The care of the cancer patient, *Social Science and Medicine*, **16**, 315–322.
Roth, J. A. (1963). *Timetables: Structuring the Passage of Time in Hospital Treatment and Other Careers*, Bobbs-Merrill, Indianapolis.
Scheff, T. J. (1963). Decision rules, types of error, and their consequences in medical diagnosis, *Behavioral Science*, , 97–107.
Stewart, M., and Buck, C. (1977). Physicians' knowledge of and response to patients' problems, *Medical Care*, **15**, 578–585.
Strauss, A. L., and Glaser, B. G. (1975). *Chronic Illness and the Quality of Life*, C. V. Mosley, Saint Louis.
Sutherland, A. M. (1981). Psychological impact of cancer and its therapy, *CA-A Journal For Clinicians*, **31**, 159–171.
Szasz, T., and Hollander, M. (1956). A contribution to the philosophy of medicine: The basic models of the doctor-patient relationship, *Journal of the American Medical Association*, **97**, 585–588.
Tagliacozzo, D. L., and Mauksch, H. (1979). The patient's view of the patient's role, in *Patients, Physicians, and Illness* (Ed. E. G. Jaco) pp. 185–201.
Tazarus, R. S. (1982). Stress and coping as factors in health and illness, in *Psychosocial Aspects of Cancer* (Eds. J. Cohn, *et al.*), pp. 163–208, Raven Press, New York.
Twaddle, A. C. (1979). The concept of health status, in *Patients, Physicians, and Illness* (Ed. E. G. Jaco), pp. 145–161, Free Press, New York.
Twycross, R. G. (1973). Terminal care of patients with lung cancer, *Postgraduate Medical Journal*, **49**, 732–737.
Westbrook, M. T., and Viney, L. L. (1982). Psychological reactions to the onset of chronic illness, *Social Science and Medicine*, **16**, 899–905.
Wortmann, C. B., and Dunkel-Schetter, C. (1979). Interpersonal relationships and cancer: A theoretical analysis, *Journal of Social Issues*, **35**, 120–155.

Section Five
Methodolocical Overview of Studies in Psychosocial Stress and Cancer

Psychosocial Stress and Cancer
Edited by C. L. Cooper

Chapter 10
On Comparing Apples, Oranges and Fruit Salad: a Methodological Overview of Medical Outcome Studies in Psychosocial Oncology

Lydia Temoshok and **Bruce W. Heller**
Department of Psychiatry and Langley Porter Institute, University of California San Francisco, USA

Numerous authors have provided theory, clinical observations, and research data pertinent to the relationship of psychosocial factors to cancer initiation and/or progression. Further, there are several excellent reviews and critiques of the literature in this area (e.g., Bahnson, 1980, 1981; Blaney, in press; Cox and Mackay, 1982; Crisp, 1970; Fox, 1978; Levy, 1983a).

Despite these efforts, no psychosocial construct has emerged for cancer with the coordinated and systematic investigation, nor with the strength and weight of empirical evidence as has the Type A Behavior pattern (TABP) for coronary heart disease (CHD), atherosclerosis, and cardiovascular pathophysiology. One striking difference between the literatures on psychosocial factors in cancer and in CHD is the adherence of research in the latter area to the Type A construct, which has acquired increasing refinement and validity since it was first introduced by Friedman and Rosenman (e.g., 1959). This observation has led us to speculate that the more individualistic endeavors and diversified research perspectives in psychosocial oncology may obscure whatever common themes exist, or even discourage search for such a theme.

It is also possible, however, that the subject of cancer itself is more complex than the cardiovascular area. In this case, the noncongruent, nonreplicated, and sometimes contradictory findings may be accurate reflections of very different phenomena, and not merely artifacts of methodologically problematic, uncoordinated, or uncooperative research efforts.

This chapter is concerned first, with discussing methodological issues in psychosocial oncology that may contribute to the noncomparability of studies.

Then, these methodological issues will be structured so as to frame a summary and comparison of representative studies in psychosocial oncology. Finally, we will examine the resulting construction to explore common themes, determine which conclusions are warranted, and formulate recommendations for future research.

The discussion will include studies in which the focus is on the endogenous psychosocial etiology and exacerbation of human cancer. 'Endogenous' is used here in the sense posed by Fox (1981) to mean arising from internal states stemming directly from influence on or by the psyche. Thus, excluded from this discussion are: (a) studies of exogenous factors such as diet, smoking, or contamination by occupational exposure; (b) studies of the psychosocial impact or sequellae of cancer; or (c) studies of factors associated with behaviors (e.g., those affecting cancer prevention, screening, early detection, or treatment) when such behaviors are studied as dependent variables, even though these may be associated with cancer initiation or progression.

METHODOLOGICAL ISSUES

Independent Variables

Type or Site

One possible source of the lack of coherence in psychosocial oncology is that investigators have not researched the same phenomenon, yet often discuss their results as if they had. If we assume the common denominator is cancer, one set of numerators consists of type or site of cancer, e.g., breast, lung, Hodgkins, or malignant melanoma. Types, as well as sites, of cancer vary considerably with regard to etiology, incidence, risk factors, symptomatology, course, mortality, and demographics. Breast cancer, for example, is a different biological phenomenon than skin cancer. Even controlling for sex or age differences that are associated with these two types of cancer and that may influence psychosocial factors, it seems unlikely to us that the common denominator of cancer will provide sufficient universality to encompass patients with breast cancer and those with skin cancer entirely under one psychosocial rubric.

A less obvious difference between types of cancers is the degree to which they may be influenced, theoretically, by psychosocial factors, relative to clinical or epidemiological risk factors. For example, 44 persons in a 52-home subdivision near Detroit contracted various forms of cancer over a period of years (Associated Press, 1983). If much of the variance in cancer incidence may be explained by their living across the road from a toxic chemical burial site, there is little variance left to be explained by psychosocial factors. A less dramatic example is the relative contribution of smoking to lung cancer. Kissen (1964) found that, among lung cancer patients, non-inhalers had a significantly poorer outlet for emotional discharge than inhalers at all levels. He concluded that less exposure to cigarette smoke was required to induce cancer in persons with this psychosocial pattern.

Another complicating factor is that, according to Anderson (1974), most cancers have a heritable as well as a nonheritable form. A study of breast cancer that, by chance, includes a high percentage of daughters of breast cancer patients may produce quite different psychosocial results than a study of patients lacking a family history of breast cancer.

Age

Several authors (e.g., Abse *et al.*, 1974; Becker, 1979; Morris *et al.*, 1981) have reasoned that if psychosocial factors play a role in the initiation and/or course of cancer, then this role wil be most evidence in younger subjects for whom the disease process would be presumably less influenced by long-term exposure to environmental risk factors, or by age-related deterioration of the immune system (Burnet, 1961). Indeed, we (Temoshok, Heller *et al.*, 1983) found that correlations between several psychosocial variables and tumor thickness in malignant malanoma were strong and significant for subjects less than age 55, but were weak or nonexistent for subjects aged 55 and over. The general point being underlined here is related to but different from the warning posed by Fox (1978) about the confounding effects of medical risk factors and psychosocial variables. His well-taken argument is that certain epidemiological variables (e.g., socioeconomic class) might contribute to or even account wholly for any found relationships between psychosocial or stress factors and cancer. Therefore, controlling for such variables by analysis of covariance, partial correlations, or forced entry regression techniques is desirable.

Dependent Variables

Initiation or Progression

Another set of numerators over the common denominator of cancer includes points in the disease process. In her overview of behavioral – social variables contributing to cancer, Levy (1983a) differentiated cancer *initiation* from *progression* as dependent variables or criterion measures. Factors contributing to cancer initiation may vary from those contributing to cancer progression and/or death. Such heterogeneity may be more readily recognized for biological and epidemiological variables. For example, excessive exposure to solar radiation may contribute to the initiation but not to the progression of malignant melanoma. However, there may also be discrepancies between the contribution of psychosocial variables to cancer initiation or progression. Thus, it may not be valid to compare the results of studies having initiation as a dependent variable with those having progression as a dependent or criterion variable.

As an illustration of this point, we will discuss in some detail two studies which produced apparently contradictory results regarding depression. Shekelle *et al.* (1981) found that a depressive MMPI profile was associated with a two-fold increase in odds of death from cancer during 17 years of follow-up for middle-aged men. Dattore *et al.* (1980) reported that male cancer patients had significantly *lower* premorbid depression scores on the depression (D) scale of the MMPI than non-cancer patients, and that less self-reported depression was the second best discriminating variable between cancer and non-cancer groups in a discriminant analysis. Leaving aside potential problems in comparing the two studies because of different procedures used to assess depression from the MMPI (this problem will be discussed later in this chapter), a striking difference between the two studies is that the study by Shekelle *et al.* was focused on risk of *death*, whereas in the study by Dattore *et al.*, subject records were chosen to represent two groups of cancerous and non-cancerous individuals. There is no indication in the latter study that any of these patients had died, but whether they had or not, the study is more appropriately considered a study of cancer initiation rather than progression.

A point we want to underline is that while the difference between initiation and progression is crucial, it is often blurred in later discussions of the study. For example, in discussing the two studies above, Blaney (in press) referred to 'cancer outcome' groups in both studies, even though the outcome in the Shekelle study was death, and the outcome in the Dattore study was carcinogenesis. Levy (in press) interpreted the Shekelle study as examining later cancer incidence, and similarly refers to the 'cancer outcome' group in that study. In discussing an earlier version of the Shekelle report, Bahnson (1982) used the phrases 'subsequent development of cancer' and 'prediction of malignancy' to refer to the group of subjects who *died* from cancer. Of parenthetical but perhaps telling note considering the misinterpretations cited above is that the running head for the Shekelle study is 'Depression and risk of cancer,' although the full title is precise: 'Psychological depression and 17-year risk of death from cancer.'

Stage of Disease or Severity

Another medical status variable—stage of disease or severity as assessed by prognostic indicators—has been used as a dependent variable in our studies of psychosocial factors in malignant melanoma (Temoshok, DiClemente *et al.*, in press; Temoshok, Heller *et al.*, 1983), and in several studies of breast cancer (Worden and Weisman, 1975; Balachandra *et al.*, 1973; Wilkinson *et al.*, 1979). It is logical to propose that stage of disease of severity can only be used as a dependent variable for cancers in which this can be reliably and validly measured, and ideally when this measure has a strong and linear relationship with survival or mortality. This type of study is relatively rare in psychosocial oncology.

Design

Prospective

Prospective studies evaluate psychosocial and stress factors in healthy subjects who are followed until they develop cancer and/or die. This design is usually highly recommended because it circumvents the issue of the psychosocial effects of knowing one has cancer, or of the somatopsychic influence of cancer absent such conscious knowledge. Unfortunately, prospective studies are expensive and extremely time-consuming to run. Prospective studies of cancer initiation (e.g., Hagnell, 1966; Thomas, 1976) usually include multiple sites and types of cancer because of the enormous difficulty in following initially disease-free subjects until they finally develop or succumb to cancer, and the relatively small number of subjects who manifest disease compared with the intitial subject sample. This 'fruit salad' of subject variables may distort or wash out any significant findings. Often, prospective studies have not utilized state-of-the-art, appropriate, reliable, or valid measures.

Retro-prospective

One way to avoid the time and cost problems inherent in prospective designs is to utilize what we call a 'retro-prospective' design. Both Shekelle *et al.* (1981) and Dattore *et al.* (1980) utilized pre-existing MMPI records collected years before subjects developed cancer to investigate the association of depression and cancer incidence and mortality, respectively. Some weaknesses of this approach include: (a) restriction of measures to commonly administered, multi-purpose tests such as the MMPI; (b) restricted subject pools—usually veterans to whom such tests are routinely given—which limit generalizability of findings; and (c) multi-type, multi-site confounds.

Quasi-Prospective

In what we designate as the 'quasi-prospective' design, the time between psychosocial evaluation of subjects and diagnosis of cancer is collapsed into a matter of days. Subjects with suspicious lump or lesions are evaluated on psychosocial variables before a biopsy is made. These variables are then correlated with and/or used to predict diagnosis of cancer in certain individuals. Thus, while these studies are prospective in intention, they are really retrospective in that some subjects had cancer at the time of interview or testing. What is predicted, or more often postdicted, is the *diagnosis* rather than the initiation of cancer.

Because only 'at risk' subjects are evaluated, this design yields a statistically adequate number of cancer diagnoses in a short period of time. This feature allows one site/type of cancer to be studied, which is a decided advantage over the 'true' prospective design. While quasi-prospective studies are able to control for the effects of conscious knowledge that one has cancer, the potentially confounding effect of biological influences (e.g., of the tumour itself, or of physical, hormonal, viral, or chemical stimuli that contributed to carcinogenesis) on psychosocial factors (the somatopsychic critique; cf. Fox, 1978) remains an issue.

Retrospective

In controlled retrospective studies, subjects diagnosed or being treated for cancer are compared with non-cancer controls (or more precisely, non-cancer comparison or contrast groups). Such studies have been criticized (e.g., Crisp, 1970; Fox, 1978) because they imply that characteristics identified in cancer patients existed premorbidly. One argument frequently posed against this idea is that knowledge that one has cancer, and the subsequent disruption of one's life, provokes psychological upset that biases findings of certain psychosocial factors in cancer patients versus comparison subjects. Theoretically, however, personality or attitudinal *trait* factors should not be altered substantially, except perhaps to be more strongly manifested, by knowledge of cancer, whereas emotional *state* factors should be more affected. Other variables may also be affected by knowledge of cancer. Regarding assessment of recalled events (e.g., of past or recent stresses) in retrospective studies, Fox (1978) cautioned that 'any anamnestic data derived from cancer patients are suspect as to validity and must have ironclad verification' (p. 114).

Further, as in quasi-prospective studies, the somatopsychic critique may be a problem, particularly because retrospective in contrast to quasi-prospective studies include patients further advanced in the malignant process, or even more problematically, in treatment.

Control or Comparison Groups

An important but rarely noted concomitant feature of these different designs is the nature of the comparison or 'control' group. In prospective or retro-prospective studies, subjects who develop or die from cancer are compared with disease-free subjects or those with other physical or mental disorders. In quasi-prospective studies, the comparison is between subjects who are diagnosed with cancer versus those diagnosed with benign tumors. When results are reported, as they usually are, in terms of strength of group differences, it is apparent that results may differ from study to study depending on the particular comparison group(s) used.

Findings about psychosocial differences among these groups in prospective studies cannot really be compared with psychosocial differences in studies of cancer progression or severity, in which the comparison groups are other cancer patients (i.e., those who die or have disease progression versus those who survive or who are apparently disease-free at follow-up; or patients with less versus more advanced stages of disease). In these studies, there may be a restriction of range effect that further limits comparability to prospective studies.

Psychosocial Theories and Constructs

A major source of difficulty in comparing studies in psychosocial oncology is not just that they employ different psychosocial measures, but that their use is based on different underlying *constructs*, and ultimately different theoretical perspectives. It may be obvious to observe that studies in the psychodynamic tradition (e.g., Abse *et al.*, 1974; Bahnson and Bahnson, 1969; Kissen, 1966; Greer and Morris, 1975) will have few, if any points of comparison with studies taking a behavioral perspective (e.g., Casileth *et al.*, 1982; Derogatis *et al.*, 1979; Rogentine *et al.*, 1979). Psychodynamically conceived studies generally focus on personality traits or defense mechanisms as constructs, and use measures derived from clinical interviews. The constructs in behaviorally oriented studies are apt to be cognitions (attitudes, beliefs), mood, behaviors, symptoms, or stress. Measurement ranges from self-report scales to potentially 'objective' behavioral assessments (e.g., delay in seeking treatment, compliance with medical regimens). Studies using stress as a major independent variable cut across both psychodynamic studies—in which stress is apt to be conceptualized in terms of stressful family history and emotional experiences, and behavioral perspectives—in which stress is assessed on the basis of more recent life changes. In sum, it may be problematic to compare studies using measures that operationalize dissimilar constructs, which are themselves based on noncomparable (although not necessarily opposing) theories.

Forms of Measures

Almost without exception, reports in psychosocial oncology have interpreted results and drawn conclusions based on *what* was being measured, rather than *how* it was measured. We feel there are important differences between measures derived from self-report questionnaires and those derived from coding of interviews.

For example, there are apparently contradictory studies which find depression either positively or negatively associated with cancer progression. Greer *et al.* (1979) found that four out of five breast cancer patients who expressed feelings of helplessness in an interview 3 months after diagnosis had died by 5-year follow-up, in contrast to only two out of 20 women who expressed either denial or fighting spirit. On the other hand, studies by Derogatis *et al.* (1979) and Levy (1983b) found that 1-year survivors versus non-survivors of metastatic breast cancer reported significantly *lower* levels of depression and other dysphoric moods.

These discrepancies may be attributed to differences in the type of assessment used to measure dimensions of depression. The studies by Derogatis *et al.* and Levy used self-report mood measures (respectively, the Affect Balance Scale and the Profile of Mood States), while the study by Greer *et al.* used independent rating by two observers of a structured patient interview.

In order to resolve these discrepancies, a meta-prediction could be developed as follows. Patients who are judged by observers to be depressed but who do not rate themselves as depressed (either because they are not conscious of it, because they consciously want to present a happy front, or because their way of coping with these feelings is to suppress them) have the worst outcomes. Another possible explanation could be derived from Bahnson's (1981) conclusion that 'it is not loss and depression alone that usher in cancer, but the combination of depleting life events with a particular ego-defensive and coping style' (p. 213). In either case, *interactions* of variables are involved.

One way to test such interactions would be in a study that administered to subjects both self-report measures and structured interviews to be rated by observers. While this has been done in several studies, the variables so derived were considered separately rather than in interaction. Kneier and Temoshok (in press) used a combination of relatively low self-reported perturbation in response to an experimental stressor with relatively high physiological arousal to define a repressive coping reaction.

Another method, using only self-report measures, is inspired by a non-cancer study by Weinberger *et al.* (1979). These authors proposed that one source of discrepancies between reports on trait anxiety scales and actual behavioral and physiological responding could be the 'predictably inaccurate' self-perceptions of persons with a *repressive coping style*. This suggestion is germane to the present discussion in that a number of reports in the literature on psychosocial oncology converge in describing cancer patients as repressive (e.g., Bahnson and Bahnson, 1969; Dattore *et al.*, 1980; Abse *et al.*, 1974;

and Kissen *et al.*, 1969). Persons with this defensive/coping style consistently avoid disturbing cognitions and report relatively little anxiety on measures such as the Taylor Manifest Anxiety Scale (MAS). Weinberger *et al.* used the Marlow – Crowne (M – C) Social Desirability Scale (Crowne and Marlowe, 1960) in conjunction with the MAS to discriminate 'truly' low-anxious persons (low M – C and low MAS) from repressors (high M – C and low MAS).

Temoshok, Heller *et al.* (1983) were interested, as well, in the other two cells (high M – C and high MAS; low M – C and high MAS) created by contrasting high and low scorers on these two tests. We found that defensive high anxious subjects (high M – C and high MAS) had significantly thicker and more invasive melanoma lesions than patients in the other three cells. The overall picture which emerged about the individual whose primary melanoma lesion has the least favorable prognosis is someone whose defensive coping style may too rigid or otherwise unable to contain the high anxiety present. This picture is consistent with that sketched by much earlier studies (e.g., Blumberg *et al.*, 1954; Klopfer, 1954; Perrin and Pierce, 1959; West, 1954), which portrayed patients with fast versus slow growing cancers as defensive, inhibited, anxious, overly controlled persons with no ability to release tension through motor or verbal discharge. Whether this psychologically unexpressed anxiety then 'leaks out' from behind the dam of defensiveness into somatic expression that may exacerbate tumor growth is heuristic speculation.

A STRUCTURED COMPARATIVE SUMMARY OF REPRESENTATIVE STUDIES

Table 10.1 outlines representative studies over the last 20 years that have focused on the psychosocial etiology or exacerbation of human cancer. We categorized studies according to their design (prospective, retro-prospective, quasi-prospective, retrospective, longitudinal), stage of cancer focused on (e.g., pre-biopsy, post-diagnosis, in treatment, death), and site and/or type of cancer (various, breast, lung, cervix, or malignant melanoma). The theoretical constructs, the measures by which these constructs were operationalized, and the findings on each measure are indicated for each study. In order to facilitate comparisons, studies with similar designs are associated in a first level grouping; within each design, similar types or sites of cancer are grouped together. This table is intended to be illustrative rather than exhaustive of the numerous potentially relevant studies.

Table 10.1 Summary of representative studies

Author(s)	Design	Stage/Site	Constructs	Measures	Major Findings
Hagnell (1966)	Prospective. Initial $N=2550$ Follow-up 10 years later: 20 males and 22 females who developed cancer matched with healthy controls on age and sex.	Stage: post-diagnosis up to death. Site/type: various.	Personality factors: 1. intellectual ability 2. emotional control 3. abstract thinking and suggestibility 4. energy.	Sjobring's (Swedish): four personality dimensions assessed by interviewer on behavioral observation.	Compared with controls, a significantly higher incidence among women (only) who were low on factor 2; i.e., were concrete, interested in people, industrious, social, warm, hearty, effective in everyday affairs, and tended to inertia and inhibition when depressed.
Thomas (1976)	Prospective. Initial $N=1337$ med. students (87% male). Follow-up 11–26 years later (from 1st to last cohort studied). 48 males with cancer matched with healthy controls, and those who developed hypertension, coronary occlusion, mental illness cr who suicided.	Stage: post-diagnosis, including death. Site/type: various.	1. Reactions to stress 2. Emotional life history patterns 3. Personality.	1. Habits of Nervous Tension (self-report) 2. Family attitude questionnaire (self-report) 3. Rorschach (projective).	1. No significant differences between cancer and other subjects on HNT scales, including depression, anger, and anxiety. 2. Lack of closeness to parents similarly low for cancer, suicide, and mental illness groups; (2) and significantly different from the hypertension group. 3. Cancer and suicide subjects have more cancer, tumor, death responses.
Thomas *et al.* (1979)	Prospective, as above, but follow-up 14–29 years later. 913 white males: 48 with cancer; 59 with benign tumors. Cancer group divided into 20 with 'major cancer' and 28 with skin cancer (not malignant melanoma).	Stage: as above. Site: various.	Emotional life history pattern.	Family Attitudes Questionnaire.	1. More negative attitudes and fewer positive attitudes in the cancer group. 2. Total cancer and major cancer groups significantly lower than total healthy Ss on closeness-to-parents scale, especially for father–son: Benign tumor group similar to skin cancer group; major cancer group mean similar to suicide/mental illness means.
Thomas and McCabe (1980)	As above, but follow-up 15–30 years later. 1046 white males, 55 with cancer. Comparison groups: 120 healthy Ss 29 major cancer 26 skin cancer (not malignant melanoma).	Stage as above. Site: Various.	Reaction to stress.	Habits of Nervous Tension Questionnaire.	1. Major cancer group sig. different from healthy controls on *pattern* of specific HNT items: more exhilaration, more exhaustion, more depression, more loss of appetite, more urge to eat, less nausea, greater tendency to check and recheck work. Only *single* variable to sig. diff. groups: loss of appetite. 2. Skin cancer group sig. diff. from healthy controls on *pattern* of specific

					HNT items: more exhaustion, less nausea, more urge to eat, more checking and rechecking work. No single var. sig. diff. groups. 3. Total cancer group sig. diff. from controls on *pattern* of specific HNT items: more exhaustion, more urge to eat, less nausea, less concern for health, more tendency to check and recheck work. Only *single* var. sig. diff. groups: tend. check, rechk. wrk.
Dattore *et al.* (1980)	Retro-prospective. Initial *N*= 200 premorbid males. Follow-up 1–10 yrs. later 75 developed cancer, 125 non-cancer: benign neoplasms, essential hypertension, G-I ulcers, schizophrenia, no dx. (25 each).	Stage: post-diagnosis. Site: various lung, prostate, and 'multiple carcinomas.'	– 'Cancer-prone personality.' – Repressive defenses.	1. MMPI (Depression scale) 2. Byrne's Repression–Sensitization Scale.	Ca. pts. (all sites) vs. non-ca. group had scores indicating greater repression and less self-report of depression.
Greenberg and Dattore (1981)	Retro-prospective. Initial *N*= 162 premorbid males. Follow-up 1–10 yrs. later (Mean=4). 58 with cancer, 25 essential hypertension, 17 ulcer, 25 benign, 37 no disease.	Stage: post-diagnosis Site: 19 lung, 20 prostate, 19 'multiple carcinomas' (various).	Dependency needs (oral dependent traits).	MMPI: 'special scales' related to dependency, its opposite, or its denial.	1. Men who later contracted 1 of 6 illnesses vs. healthy Ss scored sig. higher on all measures related to dependency in the dependent direction. 2. No differences between cancer and other diseases.
Shekelle *et al.* (1981)	Retro-prospective Initial *N*= 2020 premorbid middle-aged white males. Follow-ups for mortality 1–5, 6–11, and 12–17 yrs. later. 82 died of cancer, 198 of ischemic heart disease, 19 from accidents, etc., 62 other.	Stage: death from cancer. Sites: various 13 bronchgenic carcinoma, 10 colon, 7 rectum, 17 other sites.	Psychological depression.	MMPI (profile: high point D).	1. Men depressed at baseline had two-fold increased odds of dying of cancer (not site specific) for all follow-up periods. 2. Psych. depression is not associated with increased risk of death from other causes. 3. Association of depression with cancer death was independent of traditional risk factors. 4. Association specific to depression, not general psychological disturbance.
Ragland *et al.* (in press)	Retro-prospective 3154 men aged 39–59 from Western Collaborative Group Study Initially interviewed 1960–1,	Stage: disease-free at initial testing; dead at follow-up. Site: various 22 lung 75	1. Behavioral pattern of coping with stress. 2. Standard clinical risk factors for	1. Type A or B Behavior Pattern assessed through structured interview.	Age unadjusted cancer death rate was 2.28 for Type A's vs. 1.56 for Type B's (relative odds = 1.46, sig. Chi^2) Adjusted for age, relative odds = 1.32 (Chi^2 not

Table 10.1 Summary of representative studies—*continued*

Author(s)	Design	Stage/Site	Constructs	Measures	Major Findings
	followed through 1977 (16–17 yrs). 1589 Type A Behavior Pattern 1565 Type B 97 cancer deaths.	other.	coronary heart disease.	2. Obesity, cholesterol, smoking habits.	sig.).
Horne and Picard (1979)	Quasi-prospective. 130 males. 44 later dx. with malignant pulmonary lesion; 66 with benign lesions (T.B., bacterial pneumonia, fungal dis.); 20 with COPD or no lung disease.	Stage: pre-diagnosis Site: lung Type: 28 squamous cell carcinoma; 13 undifferentiated carcinoma; 2 adenocarcinoma.	Combined selected psychosocial risk factors (vs. trad. risk factors).	Semi-structured interview discussing: – childhood instability, – job stability, – future plans, – recent sig. losses Scored 1–5 on each scale and combined.	– Composite scale correctly predicted diagnosis of 80% of patients with benign disease and 61% of patients with lung cancer. – Psychosocial factors were 1 to 2X as important as smoking history in predicting diagnosis of cancer.
Muslin *et al.* (1969)	Quasi-prospective. Matched pairs: 37 women later diagnosed with malignant lesions, 37 with benign lesions.	Stage: pre-biopsy Site: breast.	Significant separation experiences.	Permanent loss of 1st degree relative or significant other: 1. self-report 2. standard interview format rated by two coders from transcript.	No statistically significant differences between groups for early, recent or combined experiences using either type of measurement.
Schonfield (1975)	Quasi-prospective. 112 Israeli women: 27 later diagnosed with cancer, 85 with benign lesions.	Stage: pre-biopsy Site: breast.	Loss of significant others.	1. Interviewers read Hebrew trans. of Holmes–Rahe Recent Experiences Scale (SRE) 2. Hebrew trans. of 68 MMPI items (re: Morale loss, severe depressive tendencies, well-being, and Lie scales) 3. Hebrew trans. of IPAT scale for measuring overt and covert chronic anxiety.	1. No sig. differences between ca. and non-ca. Ss on loss of sig. others or number of stressful events in yrs. immed. prior to development of disease. 2. No sig. differences on MMPI measures of dependency & well-being – For European-American vs. Middle East-born ca. pts.: higher scores on Lie Scale. 3. In under 42 age group, ca. vs. non-ca. Ss. had sig. increased covert anxiety scores.

Greer and Morris (1975)	Quasi-prospective. 160 women: 69 later dx. with breast cancer, 91 with benign breast disease. Similar in marital state and social class, but ca. pts. older. Double-blind.	Stage: pre-biopsy Site: breast.	Abnormal release of emotions.	1. Hamilton rating scale for depression. 2. Eysenck Personality Inventory. 3. Hill-Mill Test (verbal intelligence) 4. Caine and Foulds Hostility and Direction of Hostility Quest. 5. Structured interview: – experience of emotion – social adjustment – reaction to stress.	1. No differences between ca. and non-ca. Ss. on depression. 2. No sig. differences between groups on EPI dimensions. 3. No sig. differences on verbal intelligence. 4. No sig. differences on hostility. 5. Sig. more ca. than non-ca. Ss were assessed as either 'extreme suppressors' of anger or 'extreme expressors,' while sig. more non-ca. Ss vs. ca. pts. were 'apparently normal' in release of anger. – Extreme suppression of other feelings found in higher proportion of ca. than non-ca Ss. – No association between ca. and loss or stress.
Morris *et al*. (1981)	Quasi-prospective. 50 white females aged 30–69: 17 breast ca., 33 benign breast disease. Also divided sample into: Age under 40 (benign only) (N=8) Age 40–49 (N=23) Age 50–59 (N=11) Age 60–69 (N=7).	Stage: prior to definite diagnosis. Site: Breast.	Suppression of Anger.	1. Structured interview— transcript rated by three coders in terms of expression of anger. 2. Eysenck Personality Questionnaire. 3. Spielberger State-Trait Anxiety Inventory (STAI).	1. Ca. vs. non-ca. pts. had sig. less expression of anger. This tendency more marked among younger pts. (age 40–49 vs. 50–69). 2. Mean EPQ Neuroticism score sig. lower for ca. vs. non-ca. pts. N, Lie, and Anxiety-trait scores don't show expected relations with age. 3. Elevated STAI A-State and Trait scores in all pts. except young ca. patients (could be interpreted as 'denial').
Abse *et al*. (1974)	Quasi-prospective 59 male patients: 31 later dx with lung cancer; 28 with other thoracic problems (T.B., bronchiectasis). Similar in age, SES. Double-blind; predictive. Divided into age groups: 14 young ca. pts. (≤57) 17 old ca. pts. (≥58) 15 young controls (≤56) 13 old controls (≥57).	Stage: pre-biopsy Site: lung	– Repression (measure #3; – Expression of emotional conflict (few predicted: #4,5,6) – Difficulties in self-assertion (#7,8) – Conservatism and conventionality (#9,14,15,16) – Traditional risk factors (#1,2,6).	Interview schedule scored by interviewers: 1. Daytime smoking. 2. Night-time smoking. 3. Dream recall. 4. Accident proneness. 5. Psychosomatic illnesses. 6. Use of alcohol. 7. Assertion.	1 & 2. Ca. vs. non-ca. pts. smoked 3X as many cigarettes, 3. Ca. pts., especially younger ones, remembered fewer dreams. 4. Ca. pts. with dependency and rigid self-control had more accidents. 5. Ca. pts had fewer psychosomatic illnesses. 6. No differences in amount consumed, but in drinking habits. 7. Younger ca. pts. were more rigid and overly controlled. 8 & 9. Mixed results.

Table 10.1 Summary of representative studies—*continued*

Author(s)	Design	Stage/Site	Constructs	Measures	Major Findings
				8. Occupational accomplishment. 9. Work attendance. 10. Social and spouse interaction. 11. Dependency. 12. Social activity. 13. Recreation. 14. Sexual satisfaction. 15. Frequency of orgasm. 16. Marital stability.	10 & 11. No real differences between ca. and non-ca. pts., but younger ca. pts. had more impairment in personal relationships than older ca. pts. 12 & 13. Ca. pts. reported fewer recreational activities but this was accounted for by smoking in that group. 14 & 15. Younger ca. pts. reported less satisfying sex. relns. than older ca. pts. 16. Ca. pts. had fewer separations or divorces.
Schmale and Iker (1971)	Quasi-prospective 'healthy' women predisposed to ca. of cervix. Age 20–50. 3 series: *N*=40, *N*=11, *N*=17. First 51 Ss used to select interview characteristics that sig. discriminated ca. from non-ca. pts. These were used to predict ca. (*N*=10) and non-ca. (*N*=7) Ss in Series 3.	Stage: pre-biopsy; suspicious cervical cells. Site: cervix.	1. Hopelessness; 2. Various demographic and psychological characteristics.	1. Interview diagnosis of reported evidence of high hopelessness potential, and/or reaction of hopelessness 6 mo. prior to suspicious smear. 2. Interview questions on demographic and psych. characteristics.	1. For the 3 series of patients, % correct prediction based on hopelessness criterion =73.6% (vs. 50% accuracy over ca. base — rate for group). 2. Post-hoc interview characteristics of ca. vs. non-ca. Ss. derived from Series 1 & 2 *and* sig. discriminating ca. & non-ca. Ss. in Series 3 were: past history of benign tumors, left home or school to advance self/support family, married older or inferior men, perfectionistic, religious beliefs important. 3. No sig. differences on MMPI, but a trend for ca. vs. non-ca. Ss to have increased depresssion and lower ego strength scores.
Bahnson and Bahnson (1969)	Retrospective, controlled 30 white males with ca.; 64 randomly selected well white males; 26 white males hospitalized for various serious diseases (mixed sick); 33	Stage: in treatment Sites: 4 lung 6 colon 2 bladder 2 rectum	Repressive ego defenses.	Bahnson Adjective Checklist and Bahnson Projective Checklist. (Both used to compute a Projection score for 5 dimensions of	– Ca. group vs. well controls scored sig. lower on projection, hedonic level, anxiety, guilt, & hostility. – Ca. group vs. mixed sick and coronary groups combined scored lower on each of the 5 dimensions with the exception of

	white males hospitalized following M.I. (coronary group). Similar age range (35–64).	2 neck others = 1 ea. (various).		emotion (less projection = more repression).	guilt. – Ca. group vs. coronary group scored sig. lower on hostility and social interaction (dominance).
Smith and Sebastian (1976)	Retrospective, controlled. 88 hospitalized men: aged 26–60: 44 with cancer; 44 non-ca. controls with 'physical anomalies.' Matched on age, SES, race, and education. Interviewer blind to dx.	Stage: in treatment. Site: not specified; mixed assumed.	History of emotional states.	2-hr. structured interview re: intensity and duration of emotional states. Critical Incidents (CI) = the most intense emotion-producing events. Rated by interviewer and one other rater.	Ca. pts. vs. controls had more Critical Incidents in life history (107 vs. 40).
Jacobs and Charles (1980)	Restrospective, controlled 50 children/youth aged 3 to 17: 25 with ca.; 25 seen at med. facility for physical complaints (commonly sore throats, respiratory infections). Matched on sex, age, SES.	Stage: in treatment Type: 15 leukemia, 4 lymphoma, 3 Hodgkins 3 other (various).	1. Life change experiences. 2. Personality and family characteristics.	1. Holmes–Rahe Life Schedule of Recent Events (1 yr. prior to dx.) Parent report. 2. Semi-structured interview schedule: – medical hx. of pt. and family; – personality characteristics – psychological symptoms: pt. and family – life changes 2 yrs. prior to diagnosis – pt.'s and parents' relations prior to dx.	1. Ca. pts. vs. comparison group had sig. higher mean Life Change Units. Notable: families of 72% of ca. pts. vs. 24% of comparison group had moved within 2 yrs. prior to ca. diagnosis.
Becker (1979)	Retrospective, internal comparison of age groups. 49 females aged 28–69: 25 younger pts. (28–48) 24 older pts. (50–69).	Stage: final 1/3 of post-irradiation treatment phase. Site: breast.	1. Loss of close relative 2. Family atmosphere 3. Sexual relations 4. Mother role 5. Stress prior to illness.	Semi-structured interview inquiry.	1. Sig. higher % of younger vs. older group had death of or separation from a parent. 2. Sig. higher % of younger vs. older group had non-harmonious, non-close family relations & saw family as 'loveless.' 3. Sig. higher % of 'abnormality and disturbedness' in marriage and sexual relns. in younger group.

Table 10.1 Summary of representative studies—*continued*

Author(s)	Design	Stage/Site	Constructs	Measures	Major Findings
					4. Sig. higher % of complications in attitudes towards children, childbirth, and breastfeeding in younger vs. older group. 5. Only one sig. difference between older and younger pts. on events preceding illness.
Kissen (1966)	Retrospective, controlled Investigator blind to dx. *N*= 519 males aged 25 & over: 220 lung cancer, 204 other chest unit, 95 non-ca. non-chest unit. Approx. matched for age and social class.	Stage: post hospital admission. Site: lung.	Outlet for emotional discharge.	Short Maudsley Inventory (MPI) Neuroticism score = ability to discharge emotion (Kissen). N score usually = general emotional liability, liability to break down under stress, over-responsiveness.	– Lung ca. vs. other chest unit pts. had sig. poorer outlets for emotional discharge. – Lung ca. vs. non-ca. non chest unit pts. had sig. poorer emotional outlets. – When graded in descending order of exposure to cigarette smoke, there were progressively poorer outlets for emotional discharge in the lung ca. group.
Kissen *et al.* (1969)	Retrospective, controlled Total *N*=439: 221 lung ca., 218 controls.	Stage: hospital admission for diagnosis and treatment. Site: Lung.	1. Outlet for emotional discharge 2. Adversities in adulthood and childhood 3. Denial or repression.	1. Eysenck Personality Inventory (replaced MPI above) – Neuroticism (N) – Extraversion: Lie Scale (social desirability) 2. Interview 3. Awareness of Autonomic Activity Scale.	1A. Lung ca. pts. vs. controls had lower N scores. 1B. No sig. difference for extraversion scores. 2. No sig. differences between pts. and controls for 55–64 age group. 3. Ca. pts. vs. controls sig. less aware of aut. activity (less awareness correlated with lower neuroticism).
Grissom *et al.* (1975)	Retrospective, controlled. 90 V.A. males: 30 lung ca.; 30 emphysema; 30 well controls. Controlled for smoking history; approx. same age	Stage: in treatment Site: lung.	1. Influence of environmental factors, es. stressful ones 2. Internal personality structure.	1. Recent Life Changes Questionnaire (RLCQ). 2. Tennessee Self-Concept Scale (Clinical and Research	1. No differences between groups on RLCQ. 2A. Most important variable discriminating the 3 groups was the Personal Integration Score: ca. lowest, well controls highest 2B. Ca. group had higher scores on High

	range (23–87).			Form): 29 subscales.	moral-Ethical self concept ('defensively high').
Kneier and Temoshok (in press)	Retrospective, controlled 60 Ss. in outpatient med. clinics: 20 follow-up ca. pts.; 20 follow-up cardiovascular disease pts.; 20 disease-free friends and relatives of pt. groups. Pt. groups matched on sex, approx. age, and relative severity of disease (chance of dying within 5 yrs.).	Stage: 4 mo. to 7 yrs. post dx and rx. No evidence of disease. Site: skin Type: malignant melanoma.	1. Repressive coping reactions to stressors; 2. More characteristic coping tendencies.	1. High physiological arousal (skin conductance) and low self-report of perturbation in response to anxiety-provoking statements 2A. Byrne Repression Sensitization Scale 2B. Taylor Manifest Anxiety Scale 2C. Marlowe-Crowne Social Desirability Scale 2D. Difficulty in Adjustment Scale (one item from RLCQ).	1. Melanoma pts. had. sig. more repressive coping (combination of high arousal and low self-report than either comparison group. 2A. Melanoma pts. sig. more repressed on R-S scale than C-V group. 2B. Melanoma pts. had sig. lower MAS scores. 2C. No sig. differences between groups on M-C. 2D. Melanoma pts. vs. C-V group sig. minimized adjustment difficulty of their disease and its treatment.
Stavraky *et al.* (1968)	Longitudinal: progression 204 pts. followed 40–66 months. Most and least favorable, and average outcome defined for each site-stage group: 23 most favorable outcome, 46 stage-matched controls, 30 least favorable 90 stage-matched controls of average outcome. (Age comparable across groups).	Stage: follow-up (outcome = duration of survival from date of 1st clinic admission). Sites: 83 breast, 36 cervix 28 lung 57 other (various).	1. Outward personality manifestations. 2. Basic (underlying) personality characteristics. 3. Intelligence.	1. MMPI 2. Differential Diagnostic Technique (projective) – Control Index (control of emotional drives) – Differential Index (predomination of hostility or dependency drives.	1. Minimal differences between extreme outcome groups and their controls. 2. High % of ca. pts. shows loss of emotional control &/or hostility. MF outcome vs. their average outcome group had more underlying hostility without loss of emotional control. 2 & 3. MF outcome vs. all other groups had combination of hostility and above-average IQ. 3. MF group vs. their controls had high % (not sig.) of persons with above-average IQ.
Achterberg *et al.* (1977)	Longitudinal 12 pts. who lived at least 24 months past diagnosis (Category 1); 10 patients who died within 13 months (Category II).	Stage: Stage IV, widely metastatic, or 'incurable.' Sites: various original sites with mets. to different organs.	–Control (measure #1) – Conformity: (#1) – Ego strength (#1) – Hopeless/helpless (#2) – Need for satisfying relationships (#4)	1. MMPI 2. Levenson's Locus of Control Scale 3. Bem Sex-Role Inventory 4. Schutz' FIRO-B (interpersonal)	1. Cat. I vs. II higher on 'control': psychological insight, not rigid, not over-conventional: High on psychopathic deviance (= nonconforming): Higher on Barron's Ego Strength. 2. Cat. I vs. II not different on internal control scale; Placed sig. less emphasis

Table 10.1 Summary of representative studies—*continued*

Author(s)	Design	Stage/Site	Constructs	Measures	Major Findings
			– Defensiveness (#7) – Denial (#7) – Energy level (#7)	5. Profile of Mood States 6. Human Figure Drawings. 7. Non-standardized inventory assessing medical background, social history, and 'spiritual attitudes.'	on powerful others as controlling agents. 3. Not reported. 4. Cat. I vs. II. had very low scores on Inclusion. 5 & 6. Not reported. 7. Cat. I vs. II had less denial and higher energy level.
Derogatis *et al.* (1979)	Longitudinal: survival Baseline tests correlated with length of survival: 13 short-term survivors (<1yr.) 22 long-term survivors (>1 yr.) No sig. differences in physical characteristics affecting prognosis.	Stage: in treatment for metastatic disease to 1-yr. follow-up. Site: breast.	1. Pt. 's psychological adjustment, attitudes, and expectances re: disease and treatment. 2. Psychological distress and symptoms. 3. Mood and affect.	1. 40-min. structured interview rated by interviewer on: – Global Adjustment to Illness – Patient Attitude, Information, and Expectancy Form (both also rated by treating oncologist). 2. Psychological symptoms: SCL 90-R 3. Affect Balance Scale.	1. Oncologists rated LTS vs. STS as less well adjusted and having more negative attitudes. Interviewers rated LTS vs. STS as having sig. poorer attitudes towards their physicians. 2. LTS vs. STS had sig. higher psychological distress levels, high levels of anxiety, sig. high levels of hostility & of psychoticism, more sense of alienation. 3. LTS vs. STS scored sig. higher on anxiety, depression, guilt, and hostility, as well as total negative affect and vigor. STS vs. LTS had higher scores on joy, contentment, and affection (not sig.)
Greer *et al.* (1979)	Longitudinal: progression including death. Consecutive series of 69 women under age 70 5 year follow-up.	Stage: dx clinical stage I & II. lump 5 cm.; no distant metastases. Initial testing pre-operatively and 3 mo. post-op. Site: breast.	Psychological responses to breast cancer.	Structured interview. Pre-op: 1. Standard demographic data. 2. Reactions on discovering lump. 3. Delay in seeking treatment. 4. Characteristic responses to stress. 5. Expression of anger and other feelings.	– No sig. association between 5-yr. outcome and any psych. or demographic variables assessed pre-operatively with the exception that unmarried (and non-cohabitating) pts. or those with poor marital relations at time of diagnosis had less favorable outcomes. – Sig. association between pt's initial psychological responses to cancer dx. assessed 3 mo. post-operatively and 5 yr. outcome. Favorable outcome associated with pts. who had denial or fighting spirit

				6. Depressive illness or psych. stress within 5 yrs. of lump. Rating scales: 7. Hamilton Depression Scale. 8. Caine and Foulds Hostility and Direction of Hostility Questionnaire. 9. Eysenck Pers. Inv. 10. Mill Hill Vocabulary Scale. 11. Marital, sexual, work, and interpersonal adjustment. 3 mo. post-op interview: Psych. responses to dx. of cancer: Denial, Fighting Spirit, Stoic Acceptance, Feelings of Helplessness/ Hopelessness.	(esp. strong for extreme outcome groups).
Funch and Marshall (1983)	Longitudinal: length of survival until death. 352 white women seen consecutively during 1958–1960. Follow-up 1979 (19–21 yrs. later). Age divisions: 15–45 (youngest) 46–60 (menopausal) over 60 (oldest) 20% of Ss not included in analyses because death not known.	Stage: Initially Stage I or II to death. Site: breast.	1. Life stresses 2. Social support.	Structured interview: 1A. Number of stressful events 5 yrs. preceding dx. 1B. 3 objective stressors and 3 types of stress based on pts.' perceptions. 2. Marital status number of relatives and friends, organizational involvement. 3. Health history. 4. Indirect measure of SES.	1A. 83% correct predictions of more stresses and decreased survival in youngest age group. 1B. Both subjective index and total stress index sig. related to survival time for all pts. – Occurrence of 3 objective stresses (death, illness, unemployment of household member) associated with decreased survival in oldest age category. – Perception of 3 subjective stresses (number of months pt. felt tied, upset, or felt family income inadequate) associated with decreased survival in youngest age category. 2. Esp. for youngest and oldest categories, social involvement is related to increased survival.

Table 10.1 Summary of representative studies—*continued*

Author(s)	Design	Stage/Site	Constructs	Measures	Major Findings
					3 & 4. No sig. differences.
Rogentine *et al.* (1979)	Longitudinal: progression ('prognosis') Two consecutive series of 50 male and 17 female white pts. aged 16–67: 31 in Group I 33 in Group II Follow-up 1 year after lymph node dissection.	Stage: clinical Stage I or II, all apparently disease-free. Tested 1 week after initial surgery. Site: skin Type: malignant melanoma.	1. Coping with stress of cancer. 2. Biological and other factors associated with melanoma survival. 3. SCL-90-R (psychiatric symptom checklist). 4. Locus of Control Questionnaire.	1. Recent Life Changes Questionnaire (RLCQ) 2. Number of positive lymph nodes, clinical stage, clin. enlargement of nodes, tumor histology, level of invasion, location of primary, age, sex, and delay in seeking treatment.	1. Nonrelapsers vs. relapsers in Group 1 had higher Melanoma Adjustment Score—expected more life adjustment to cope with their melanoma. – This finding was replicated in Group II (statistically sig.) 2. Number of positive lymph nodes was the only clinical factor that influenced prognosis. This was independent of Melanoma Adjustment Score. 3 & 4. Did not distinguish relapsers from non relapsers.

General Structural Impressions

In constructing the table, we were struck by how arduous it was to summarize these 29 studies according to our categorization system. Because our system is rather straightforward and not particularly idiosyncratic, we felt that other readers of the literature would be equally hard put to make comparisons among apples, oranges and fruit salad. These comparisons were made even more difficult by reports in which such critical information as sample size, hypotheses, and major findings were often enmeshed in verbiage, ambiguously stated, or even entirely missing. We originally had a category for 'hypotheses,' but so few studies stated explicit hypotheses that we felt the most editorializing warranted was to extract or highlight *constructs* (usually taken from introductions or conclusions of studies). Further, as can be seen in the table, the links between constructs and measures are often tenuous.

Another strong impression is that even with all the structural differences in design, subjects, type, site and stage of cancer, construct and measures, some common themes emerge. Thus, although retrospective studies have been criticized as methodologically problematic, their findings are generally congruent with those from prospective or longitudinal studies. We feel this is because controlled retrospective studies offer certain advantages over prospective designs; that is, one type or site of cancer can be studied economically, and more than one or two measures or forms of measures (i.e., both interview *and* self-report measures) can be administered. A prospective design in itself contains no methodological magic: a retrospective study with well-defined subject groups, specified hypotheses, well-operationalized constructs, and rationally selected measures is more scientifically respectable than a prospective study that lacks these features.

Upon surveying the table, we feel that the longitudinal design focused on cancer progression or mortality contains the best features of prospective and retrospective designs: offering, respectively, conceptually sound comparison groups for which differences have clinical meaning, and economy/efficiency. Retro-prospective studies can also be both economical and informative, combining the advantages of prospective and quasi-prospective designs if explicit hypotheses, representative subject groups, multiple psychosocial measures, and appropriate data analytic techniques are used.

Summary of Specific Findings

Prospective Studies

Empirical findings from prospective and retro-prospective studies of initially healthy subjects who later developed various types of cancer suggest that such individuals are characterized as 'nice,' pro-social, warm, hearty, effective in managing everyday affairs, who tend toward inertia and inhibition when depressed (Hagnell, 1966 – for women only), as well as industrious and conscientious (Hagnell, 1966; Thomas and McCabe, 1980). While they do not report themselves to feel dysphoric emotions, such as anxiety, sadness, and especially anger (Dattore, *et al.* 1980; Thomas, 1976; Thomas and McCabe, 1980), they appear to show vegetative signs of depression (Hagnell, 1966; Shekelle *et al.*, 1981; Thomas and McCabe, 1980). Healthy males who later contracted one of six diseases, including cancer, scored significantly higher on a measure of dependency than healthy controls, though cancer victims were not specifically distinguished from sufferers of other diseases (Greenberg and Dattore, 1981). There appears to be little difference between initially healthy subjects typed A or B on the Type A structured interview when age is controlled for (Ragland *et al.*, in press). On a projective measure, initially healthy subjects who later contracted cancer or suicided showed more cancer, tumor, and death responses than healthy controls or other disease groups (Thomas, 1976).

Findings by Dattore *et al.* (1980) of *less* depression and Shekelle *et al.* (1981) of *more* depression among individuals who later developed cancer appear to be contradictory. In fact, they are not. Both used the MMPI to measure depression, but each employed different scales. Dattore *et al.* focussed on self-reported feelings of sadness; while Shekelle *et al.* found vegetative and behavioral signs of depression to differentiate groups. To further support this point, Thomas and her colleagues found that specific patterns or clusters of specific items on their Habits of Nervous Tension Questionnaire significantly discriminated subjects who contracted cancer from healthy controls; several of these items are classed as vegetitive or behavioral signs of depression (exhaustion, increased urge to eat, and loss of appetite).

In terms of their emotional life history pattern, initially healthy subjects who later contracted cancer reported a lack of closeness to their parents (Thomas, 1976; Thomas *et al.*, 1979).

Quasi-Prospective Studies

Patients who were found to have cancer of the breast versus those who had benign tumors showed significantly less expression of anger on judges' ratings of semi-structured interviews, a finding most prominent for younger patients (Morris *et al.*, 1981), or a pattern of inappropriate affective expression including extreme suppression or extreme expression of anger and other emotions on the same sort of measure (Greer and Morris, 1975). No significant differences between groups were found on self-report measures of depression, psychoticism, extroversion, hostility, dependency, intelligence, or well-being in the above studies, although significantly lower overt anxiety and neuroticism for younger patients with cancer were found. Schonfield (1975), however, reported significantly higher covert anxiety scores and no difference on overt anxiety for younger breast cancer sufferers versus controls. Elevated scores on the MMPI lie scale (a measure of deception, rigidity, and/or pathological need to present a 'good front') were also noted for European and American-born but not Middle Eastern-born cancer patients on the basis of self-report measures.

On the basis of interview ratings, patients, especially younger patients, found to have cancer of the lung showed more repression and inhibition of emotion (Abse *et al.*, 1974). Patients found to have cancer of the cervix had high levels of hopelessness, self-sacrifice, perfectionism, and religious belief, on the basis of interview ratings, and trends toward increased depression and lower ego-strength scores on a self-report instrument (Schmale and Iker, 1971).

In terms of emotional life history pattern, breast cancer versus benign tumor post-biopsy groups showed no significant history of loss or recent stressors on a self-report measure (Schonfield, 1975), on interview ratings (Greer and Morris, 1975), or on both kinds of measures (Muslin *et al.*, 1969). Patients with diagnosed lung cancer versus controls were rated, on the basis of a semi-structured interview, to show more childhood instability, more recent losses, more marital stability, and more plans for the future (Horne and Picard, 1979). Using a similar technique, Abse *et al.* (1975) also found lung cancer versus control groups to have more stable marriages, and for younger versus older lung cancer patients to report less satisfying sexual experiences and more impairment in social relations in general. Schmale and Iker (1971) found women with cancer of the cervix versus controls to marry older or 'inferior' men more frequently, have a past history of benign tumors, and to have left home to support self/family more often, on the basis of interview ratings.

Retrospective Studies

Retrospective studies of cancer initiation for groups of patients with various types of cancer have found patients versus controls to show significantly lower projection (interpreted as higher repression) level, lower hedonic level, and lower anxiety, guilt, and hostility (Bahnson and Bahnson, 1969) on self-report and projective measures. In terms of emotional life history pattern, cancer patients were found to have more critical emotional incidents in their life history, on the basis of a semi-structured interview (Smith and Sebastian, 1976), and higher mean life change units on a self-report measure (Jacobs and Charles, 1980).

Studies of lung cancer and personality found patients with cancer versus controls to have lower neuroticism scores on a self-report instrument, a finding interpreted to reflect these patients' poorer outlets for emotional discharge (Kissen, 1966). This same finding was even more pronounced for younger patients (Kissen *et al.*, 1969), and was negatively correlated with exposure to cigarette smoke (Kissen, 1966). Cancer patients versus controls were also found to have lower personal integration scores and 'defensively' higher moral – ethnical self-concepts (Grissom *et al.*, 1975) as well as less awareness of their autonomic system functioning, suggesting greater capacity for denial (Kissen *et al.*, 1969).

Becker (1979) found that a significantly greater percentage of younger versus older breast cancer patients, on the basis of a semi-structured interview, reported experiencing death of or separation from parents, and problematic familial, marital, and sexual relations.

Kneier and Temoshok (in press) found that recovered malignant melanoma patients versus controls demonstrated significantly higher levels of repressive coping strategies on the basis of physiological and self-report measures, significantly lower self-reported anxiety, and minimized the difficulty of adjusting to their disease and its treatment on a self-report measure.

Longitudinal Studies

Longitudinal studies utilizing judges' ratings of patients who progress more slowly through the course of their disease than controls indicate these individuals are less well-adjusted, display significantly poorer attitudes toward their physicians (Derogatis *et al.*, 1979), and have either greater denial or more fighting spirit (Greer *et al.*, 1979). Utilizing self-report measures, Derogatis *et al.* (1979) and Stavraky *et al.* (1969) found long-term versus short-term survivors to manifest higher levels of psychological distress and negative effect, including higher levels of hostility, anxiety, psychoticism, alienation, depression, and vigor. Achterberg *et al.* (1977) reported that long-term versus short-term survivors showed higher levels of psychological insight, cognitive flexibility, nonconventionality, ego strength, and vigor, as well as less denial and emotional introjection, on self-report measures. No significant differences on locus of control self-report measures were found (Achterberg *et al.*, 1977; Rogentine *et al.*, 1979). Non-relapsers versus relapsers showed an expectation that more adjustment would be needed in order to cope with their disease and its treatment (an indication of less denial, it is inferred), and no significant differences regarding psychological symptomatology (Rogentine *et al.*, 1979).

In terms of emotional life history patterns, patients who were unmarried, non-cohabitating, or unhappy in their marriages had significantly less favorable outcomes (Greer *et al.*, 1979), as did patients with less social involvement in general, and with greater reported life stresses on a standard self-report measure (Funch and Marshall, 1983).

Emergent Themes

While the picture is still somewhat obscure, quite complex, and multi-determined, as well as marked by contradictory findings, some generalizations and themes emerge from the 29 studies reviewed in Table 10.1:

1. One is struck by the paucity of positive findings, given the number of variables studied and the effort invested. Many of these 'negative' findings, however, support one consistently appearing theme: that cancer patients have difficulty in expressing emotions, or even feeling them.
2. There is enough convergent evidence, from prospective, longitudinal, and retrospective studies, to discern a constellation of factors that appears to predispose some individuals to develop cancer or to progress through its stages more quickly.
3. Recent controlled studies support many earlier hypotheses derived mainly from clinical impressions.
4. Evidence from prospective and retrospective studies converges, for the most part, suggesting that there is little substance to the argument that knowing one has cancer (or has knowledge without conscious awareness) results in psychological and physiological reactions that compromise the validity of retrospective findings.
5. In addition to the emotional expression patterns noted in 1, personality traits or long-standing characteristics of persons who develop cancer or have a less favorable course include niceness, industriousness, perfectionism, sociability, conventionality, and more rigid controls of defensiveness.
6. Underlying attitudes or tendencies of helplessness/hopelessness and of giving up rather than fighting are characteristic of persons with a more unfavorable course of cancer.
7. The existence and number of past or recent life events appears to be less important than how these were cognitively, emotionally, or behaviorally dealt with.

Parenthetically, several of these themes are echoed in our 'Type C' construct (Temoshok and Heller, 1981; Temoshok, Heller *et al.*, 1983), which we have described as the opposite of the Type A Behavior Pattern associated with coronary heart disease. However, our notion of Type C as a *constellation* of emotional, cognitive, and behavioral dimensions is not strictly parallel to the Type A Pattern, which emphasizes behaviors. We have operationalized the Type C construct in several completed and ongoing studies (summarized in Temoshok and Fox, 1983) of prognostic indicators and progression of malignant melanoma. It remains to be seen from future research whether the notion of different dimensions within a wider 'Type C' constellation is a valid, useful, and/or unifying construct that reflects the themes emerging from Table 10.1.

Recommendations for Future Research

Incorporating our discussions of methodological and content themes are some recommendations for future research in the area of psychosocial oncology related to initiation and progression:

1. Researchers in this area need to define theoretically and operationally, and to distinguish among the following related terms: denial, repression, non-expression (of emotion), minimization, and avoidance. If a study focuses on one or more of these concepts, the author(s) should compare their findings with those of previous literature reports that have employed the same or related terms.

2. The same general recommendation holds for concepts in the 'depression' cluster: helplessness/hopelessness, 'given up,' depressed mood, depressive cognitions, vegetative signs of depression, and psychiatrically diagnosed depression.

3. There is a need for greater specification of:

A. the independent variables of interest—psychological, behavioral, social, stress, and other factors;

B. the independent variables to be controlled for or taken into account—biological (including age), genetic, environmental, and other non-psychosocially or stress-related factors; and

C. the dependent variable(s) to be used as criteria—cancer initiation, prognostic indicators, progression, or mortality.

4. There should be greater specification of hypotheses to be tested, theories from which these hypotheses were derived, and how hypotheses/constructs were operationalized so that they could be quantifiably evaluated.

5. Researchers should strive for more commonality of measures across studies, as well as the use of more standard, reliable, and valid measures.

6. Using *both* interview and self-report derived measures within a single study provides different, converging, and/or interacting methodological perspectives on a given construct, and may be the only way to reveal certain important differences between comparison groups.

7. More efforts should be taken to replicate previous findings, and to extend findings from one site, type, or stage of cancer to other sites, types, or stages.

Science moves forward by the disconfirmation of hypotheses. Hypotheses are derived from models or theories of the specific relations among variables relevant to the phenomenon under investigation, within a particular paradigm. Hypotheses can only bc evaluated by measures that operationalize them appropriately. In order for psychosocial oncology to progress as a field, it is essential to delineate our models, hypotheses, and the logic for the specific measures used to test them. One's model, hypotheses, or measures may not be correct or appropriate. But if they are not stated explicitly and crisply, they can not be disconfirmed, modified, or replicated.

REFERENCES

Abse, D. W., Wilkins, M. M., Van de Castel, R. L., Buxton, W. D., Demars, J. P., Brown, R. S., and Kirschner, L. G. (1974). Personality and behavioral characteristics of lung cancer patients, *J. Psychosom. Res.*, **18**, 101–113.

Achterberg, J., Matthews, S., and Simonton, O. C. (1977). Psychology of the exceptional cancer patient: A description of patients who outlive predicted life expectancies, *Psychother.: Theory, Res., Prac.*, **14**, 416–422.

Anderson, D. E. (1974). Genetic study of breast cancer: Identification of a high risk group, *Cancer*, **34**, 1090–1097.

Associated Press (1983). Cancer sweeps subdivision, *San Francisco Chronicle*, December 28, 1983.

Bahnson, C. B. (1980). Stress and cancer: The state of the art, Part 1, *Psychosom.*, **21**, 975–981.

Bahnson, C. B. (1981). Stress and cancer: The state of the art, Part 2, *Psychosom.*, **22**, 207–220.

Bahnson, C. B., and Bahnson, M. B. (1969). Ego defenses in cancer patients, *Ann. N.Y. Acad. Sci.*, **164**, 546–559.

Bahnson, C. B. (1982). Psychosomatic issues in cancer, in *The Psychosomatic Approach to Illness* (Ed. R. L. Gallon), Elsevier North Holland, New York.

Balanchandra, V. K., Schottenfeld, D., Berg, J. W., *et al.* (1973). Patterns of delay and extent of disease in radical mastectomy patients, *Clin. Bull.*, **3**, 10–13.

Becker, H. (1979). Psychodynamic aspects of breast cancer: Younger and older patients, *Psychother. Psychosom.*, **32**, 287–296.

Blaney, P. H. (in press). Psychological considerations in cancer, in *Behavioral medicine: A Multi-Systems Approach* (Ed. N. Schneiderman), Erlbaum, New York.

Blumberg, E., West, P., and Ellis, F. (1954). A possible relationship between psychological factors and human cancer, *Psychosom. Med.*, **16**, 277–286.

Burnet, F. M. (1961). Immunological recognition of self, *Science*, **133**, 207.

Cassileth, B. R., Clark, W. H., Jr., Heiberger, R. M., March, V., and Tenaglia, A. (1982). Relationship between cancer patients' early recognition of melanoma and depth of invasion, *Cancer*, **49**, 198–200.

Cox, T., and Mackay, C. (1982). Psychosocial factors and psychophysiological mechanisms in the aetiology and development of cancers, *Soc. Sci. Med.*, **16**, 381–396.

Crisp, A. H. (1970). Some psychosomatic aspects of neoplasia, *Br. J. Med. Psychol.*, **43**, 313–331.

Crowne, J. P., and Marlowe, D. (1960) A new scale of social desirability independent of psychopathology, *J. Consult. Psych.*, **24**, 349–354.

Dattore, P. J., Shantz, F. C., and Coyne, L. (1980). Premorbid personality differentiation of cancer and noncancer groups: A test of the hypothesis of cancer proneness, *J. Consult. Clin. Psychol.*, **48**, 388–394.

Derogatis, L. R., Abeloff, M. D., and Melisaratos, N. (1979). Psychological coping mechanisms and survival time in metastatic breast cancer, *J. Am. Med. Assoc.*, **242**, 1504–1508.

Fox, B. H. (1978). Premorbid psychological factors as related to cancer incidence, *J. Behav. Med.*, **1**, 45–133.

Fox, B. H. (1981). Psychosocial factors and the immune system in human cancer, in *Psychoneuroimmunology* (Ed. R. Ader), Academic Press, New York.

Friedman, M., and Rosenman, R. H. (1959). Association of a specific overt behavior pattern with blood and cardiovascular findings, *JAMA*, **169**, 1286.

Funch, D. P., and Marshall, J. (1983). The role of stress, social support, and age in survival from breast cancer, *J. Psychosom. Res.*, **27**, 77–83.

Greenberg, R. P., and Dattore, P. J. (1981). The relationship between dependency and the development of cancer, *Psychosom. Med.*, **43**, 35–43.

Greer, S., and Morris, T. (1975). Psychological attributes of women who develop breast cancer: A controlled study, *J. Psychosom. Res.*, **19**, 147–153.

Greer, S., and Morris, T. (1981). Psychological response to breast cancer and survival: Eight-year follow-up, presented at the 89th Annual Convention of the American Psychological Association, Los Angeles.

Greer, S., Morris, T., and Pettingale, K. W. (1979). Psychological response to breast cancer: Effect on outcome, *Lancet*, **2**, 785–787.

Grissom, T. T., Weiner, B. J., and Weiner, E. A. (1975). Psychological correlates of cancer, *J. Consult. Clin. Psychol.*, **43**, 113.

Hagnell, O. (1966). The premorbid personality of persons who developed cancer in a total population investigated in 1947 and 1957, *Ann. N.Y. Acad. Sci.*, **125**, 846–855.

Horne, R. L., and Picard, R. S. (1979). Psychosocial risk factors for lung cancer, *Psychosom. Med.*, **41**, 503–514.

Jacobs, R. J., and Charles, E. (1980). Life events and the occurrence of cancer in children, *Psychosom. Med.*, **42**, 11–24.

Kissen, D. M. (1966). The significance of personality in lung cancer in men, *Ann. N.Y. Acad. Sci*, **125**, 820–826.

Kissen, D. M., Brown, R. I. F., and Kissen, M. A. (1969). A further report on the personality and psychological factors in lung cancer, *Ann. N.Y. Acad. Sci.*, **164**, 535–545.

Klopfer, B. A. (1954). Results of psychological testing in cancer, in *The Psychological Variables in Human Cancer: A Symposium* (Eds. J. A. Gengerelli and F. J. Kirkner), pp. 62–65, University of California Press, Berkeley.

Kneier, A. W., and Temoshok, L. (In Press). Repressive coping reactions in patients with malignant melanoma as compared to cardiovascular patients, *J. Psychosom. Res.*, (in press).

Levy, S. M. (1983a). Host differences in neoplastic risk: Behavioral and social contributors to disease, *Health Psychol.*, **2**, 21–44.

Levy, S. M. (1983b). Emotional expression and survival in breast cancer patients: Immunological correlates, presented at the 91st Annual Convention of the American Psychological Association, Anaheim.

Levy, S. M. (in press). The expression of affect and its biological correlates: Mediating mechanisms of behavior and disease, in *Emotions in Health and Illness: Applications to Clinical Practice.* (Eds. C. Van Dyke, L. Temoshok, and L. S. Zegans). Grune and Stratton, New York.

Morris, T., and Greer, H. S. (1980). A 'Type C' for cancer? Low trait anxiety in the pathogenesis of breast cancer, *Ca. Detection Prev.* **3**, Abstract No. 102.

Morris, T., Greer, S., Pettingale, K. W., and Watson, M. (1981). Patterns of expression anger and their psychological correlates in women with breast cancer, *J. Psychosom. Res.*, **25**, 111–117.

Muslin, H. L., Gyarfas, K., and Pieper, W. J. (1969). Separation experience and cancer of the breast, *Ann. N.Y. Acad. Sci.*, **164**, 802–806.

Perrin, G. M., and Pierce, I. R. (1959).Psychosomatic aspects of cancer: A review, *Psychosom. Med.*, **21**, 397–421.

Ragland, D. R., Brand, R. J., Rosenman, R. H., Fox, B. H., and Moss, A. R. (in press). Type A behavior and cancer mortality: A preliminary report, in *Perspectives in Behavioral Medicine, Vol. III* (Ed. A. Baum), Academic Press, New York.

Riley, V. (1981). Psychoneuroendocrine influences on immunocompetence and neoplasia, *Science*, **212**, 1100–1109.

Rogentine, S., Boyd, S., Bunney, W., Doherty, J., Fox, B., Rosenblatt, J., Van Kammen, D. (1979). Psychological factors in the prognosis of malignant melanoma, *Psychosom. Med.*, **41**, 647–658.

Schmale, A. H., and Iker, H. (1971). Hopelessness as a mediator of cervical cancer, *Soc. Sci. Med.*, **5**, 95–100.

Schonfield, J. (1975). Psychological and life-experience differences between Israeli women with benign and cancerous breast lesions, *J. Psychosom. Res.*, **19**, 229–234.

Shekelle, R. B., Raynar, W. J., Ostfield, A. M., Garron, D. C., Bieliauskas, L. A., Liu, S. C., Maliza, C., and Paul, O. (1981). Psychological depression and 17-year risk of death from cancer, *Psychosom. Med.*, **43**, 117–125.

Smith, W. R., and Sebastian, H. (1976). Emotional history and pathogenesis of cancer, *J. Clin. Psychol.*, **32**, 863–866.

Stavraky, K., Buck, C., Lott, J., and Wanklin, J. (1968). Psychological factors in the outcome of human cancer, *J. Psychosom. Res.*, **12**, 251–259.

Temoshok, L., DiClemente, R. F., Sweet, D. M., Blois, M. S., Sagebiel, R. W. (in press). Factors related to patient delay in seeking medical attention for cutaneous malignant melanoma, *Cancer*, (in press).

Temoshok, L. and Fox, B. F. (1983). Coping styles and other psychosocial factors related to medical status and to prognosis in patients with cutaneous malignant melanoma, in *Impact of Psychoendocrine Systems in Cancer and Immunity* (Eds. B. H. Fox and B. H. Newberry), pp. 258–287, C. J. Hogrefe, Inc., Toronto.

Temoshok, L. and Heller, B. W. (1981). Stress and 'Type C' versus epidemiological risk factors in melanoma, Paper presented at the 89th Annual Convention of the American Psychological Association, Los Angeles, California. (August 25, 1981).

Temoshok, L., Heller, B. W., Sagebiel, R. W., Blois, M. S., Sweet, D. M., DiClemente, R. J., and Gold, M. L. (1983). The relationship of psychosocial factors to prognostic indicators in cutaneous malignant melanoma, submitted for publication.

Thomas, C. B. (1976). Precursors of premature disease and death: The predictive power of habits and family attributes, *Ann. Int. Med.*, **85**, 653–658.

Thomas, C. B., Duszynski, K. R., and Shaffer, J. W. (1979). Family attitudes reported in youth as potential predictors of cancer, *Psychosom. Med.*, **41**, 287–302.

Thomas, C. B., and McCabe, O. L. (1980). Precursors of premature disease and death: Habits of nervous tension, *Johns Hopkins Med. J.*, **147**, 137–145.

Weinberger, D. A., Schwartz, G. E., and Davidson, R. J. (1979). Low-anxious, high-anxious, and repressive coping styles: Psychometric patterns and behavioral and physiological responses to stress, *J. Abnorm. Psychol.*, **88**, 396–380.

West, P. M. (1954). Origin and development of the psychological approach to the cancer problem, in *The Psychological Variables in Human Cancer: A Symposium* (Eds. J. A. Gengerelli and F. J. Kirkner), pp. 17–26, University of California Press, Berkeley.

Wilkinson, G., Edgerton, F., Wallace, H., Reese, P., Patterson, J., and Priore, R. (1979). Delay, staging disease and survival from breast cancer, *J. Chron. Dis.*, **32**, 365–373.

Worden, J. W., and Weisman, A. D. (1975). Psychosocial components of lagtime in cancer diagnosis, *J. Psychosom. Res.*, **19**, 69–79.

Index